About the Author

William G. Crook, M.D., received his medical education and training at the University of Virginia, the Pennsylvania Hospital, Vanderbilt and Johns Hopkins. He is a fellow of the American Academy of Pediatrics, the American College of Allergy and Immunology and the American Academy of Environmental Medicine. He is a member of the American Medical Association, the American Academy of Allergy and Immunology and Alpha Omega Alpha.

As a practicing physician, medical writer and lecturer, Dr. Crook is concerned about problems which affect millions of people all over the world. These include children with repeated ear infections and with behavior and learning problems; and adults who feel "sick all over" yet have been unable to find help.

Dr. Crook is the author of 10 previous books and numerous reports in the medical and lay literature. For 15 years he wrote a nationally syndicated health column, "Child Care" (*General Features* and the *Los Angeles Times* Syndicates).

Several of his publications have been translated into Norwegian, German, French and Japanese. *Chronic Fatigue and the Yeast Connection* is his first major work since *The Yeast Connection*, a bestseller with over one million copies in print.

Dr. Crook has also appeared on numerous radio and TV programs including Oprah Winfrey, Sally Jessy Raphael, Regis Philbin, Good Morning Australia, TV Ontario and the British Broadcasting Company.

He has also addressed professional and lay groups in 35 states, 6 Canadian provinces, England, Mexico, Australia, New Zealand and Venezuela. He has served as a visiting professor at Ohio State University, and the Universities of California (San Francisco) and Saskatchewan.

Having been referred to as a preventive medicine crusader, Dr. Crook says, "The road to better health will not be found through more drugs, doctors and hospitals. Instead it will be discovered through better nutrition and changes in lifestyle."

Dr. Crook lives in Jackson, Tennessee, with his wife Betsy. They have three daughters and four grandchildren. His interests include golf, oil painting and travel.

"Though the medical establishment may balk, beleaguered patients will find much to cheer in Dr. Crook's new book.

"To start, he believes CFS 'is for real,' that the symptoms 'are caused by organic changes that affect the immune system, the nervous system, the musculoskeletal system and many other parts of the body.' He disagrees with conventional medicine wisdom that CFS is 'simply a state of mind,' just another name for depression.

"But even more valuable to patients may be his prescription for a hefty dose of common sense, as he explores the various approaches that seem to help many patients—everything from diet and nutritional supplements to newer therapies on the horizon, plus, of course, his appeal that physicians and patients consider yeast infection as a potential contributor to CFS."

Mary Hager
Newsweek

"This book is the most understandably presented and well-rounded discussion to date of the relationship of yeast infections to CFS/CFIDS.

"The illustrations are a wonderful help and the nutritional advice and diet instructions are based on common sense. Most appreciated and unusual is the time and space devoted by Dr. Crook to patient support and advocacy organizations."

Sharon Lee Moyer Horejs, R.N.
Interim Director, CFIDS Awareness
and Support Services
Laguna Niguel, California

"Chronic Fatigue Syndrome and the Yeast Connection is not only a very enjoyable read, it is packed with well organized, useful historical and holistic information for patients suffering from Chronic Fatigue Syndrome (Myalgic Encephalomyelitis, or Fibromyalgia Syndrome)."

Byron Hyde, M.D.
Chairman, Nightingale Research Foundation
Ottawa, Canada

"This is a uniquely interesting book. The accumulation of information on these important topics is written in a concise, readable style and the illustrations add so much to its enjoyment. Dr. Crook's prolific pen has again added to the depths of our understanding and enlightenment. This book will make a great contribution to the increased knowledge and the ability to make informed decisions. I highly recommend it."

Charles Kellenberger
Southern Health Organization
Cape Coral, Florida

Chronic Fatigue Syndrome

and the

Yeast Connection

A Get-Well Guide For People with This Often Misunderstood
Illness—and Those Who Care For Them.

by
William G. Crook, M.D.
Illustrated by Cynthia Crook

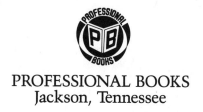

PROFESSIONAL BOOKS
Jackson, Tennessee

I've written this book to serve as a general guide for persons with CFS and those who are working to help them. For obvious reasons, I cannot assume the medical or legal responsibility for having the contents of this book considered as a prescription for anyone.

To conquer and overcome your health problems, you'll need assistance from a knowledgeable and interested physician or other licensed health care professional. Accordingly, you and those who work with you must take full responsibility for the uses made of this book.

Text © 1992, William G. Crook, M.D.
Illustrations © 1992, Cynthia P. Crook

Library of Congress Cataloging-in-Publication Data

Crook, William G. (William Grant), 1917-
    Chronic Fatigue Syndrome and the yeast connection : a get-well guide for people with this often misunderstood illness—and those who care for them / by William G. Crook : illustrated by Cynthia Crook.
        p.   cm.
    Includes bibliographical references (p. 400) and index.
    ISBN 0-933478-20-8 : $14.95
    1. Chronic fatigue syndrome—Popular works.   2. Candidiasis—Popular works.   3. Food allergy—Popular works.   I. Title.
RB150.F37C76   1992
616'.047—dc20   92-5051
                                                                                         CIP

Manufactured in the United States of America
Published by Professional Books, Inc.
Box 3246, Jackson, Tennessee 38303
901-423-8366

3 4 5 6 7 8 9 10 —97 96 95 94 93

This book is dedicated to the millions of people all over the world with CFS, CFIDS, M.E., FM and related disorders and those who are working to help them.

Contents

Foreword

Chronic Fatigue Syndrome and the Yeast Connection is Dr. William Crook's most recent undertaking to help both patients and clinicians understand one of the most perplexing problems of the 20th Century, "Chronic Fatigue Immunodysfunction Syndrome." This book does not claim that the common yeast, *Candida albicans,* is *the* cause of CFS. However, it does explain the role of multiple entities: yeast overgrowth, intestinal parasites, unchecked viral infections, food allergies and chemical sensitivities—and how these can result in the immune dysregulation we refer to as CFS.

Chronic Fatigue Syndrome is a devastating illness which has affected young and middle-aged people in increasing proportions over the past few decades. Epidemic and endemic reports of this illness and the number of affected patients seem to be rising steadily. Most clinicians working with CFS believe it is unlikely that one cause, or for example one virus, is responsible for this syndrome.

Having worked with CFS patients for almost 10 years, I believe this illness may simply represent the 10 to 15% of our species who have not yet adapted to the rapid and startling changes in the environment, and the subsequent changes in our internal intestinal environment.

Since 1950 we've seen the development and overuse of antibiotics; the use of hormones and birth control pills; the development of immunosuppressive drugs; the introduction of various chemicals and toxins into our environment; and significant changes which have occurred within our diets, leaving us foods tainted with pesticides, depleted in nutritional value and loaded with sugars and dyes.

Can we really continue to believe these incredible changes have not affected the wellbeing of some and eventually perhaps all of us?

In this book, Dr. Crook reviews information presented at medical conferences and published in medical journals which discuss the correlation of intestinal yeast overgrowth and resultant toxic and immunological effects. He makes suggestions to patients which help them clarify whether food allergies, candida or mineral deficiencies are contributing to their illness.

Many of the suggestions in this book will prove most helpful to my patients. The use of antifungal medication is becoming more common among clinicians treating CFS patients and nutritional supplements are gaining widespread support. Clinicians who are overwhelmed by patients with multiple systemic complaints may find that having their patients read this book will guide them toward a more stable course in their illness.

Ten years ago I was very frustrated working with CFS patients because of deeply ingrained skepticism about theories such as the "yeast connection." However, following further research and a trial of some of these therapeutic interventions with my patients, my work has become both intellectually rewarding and fun.

Hopefully this book will be the springboard to help many clinicians and patients understand this devastating illness.

Carol Jessop, M.D.
El Cerrito, CA
Diplomate, American Board of Internal Medicine
Assistant Clinical Professor of Medicine, University of
    California, San Francisco
American College of Physicians
American Society of Internal Medicine

Chronic Fatigue Syndrome
and the
Yeast Connection

A Special Message to the Reader:

Someone once said, "Fools step in where angels fear to tread" and some readers (especially researchers who are studying Chronic Fatigue Syndrome) may feel that this old quotation fits me. So I'd like to acknowledge up front that I'm not claiming that the common yeast *Candida albicans* is the cause of CFS. Yet, based on the experience of thousands of professionals and nonprofessionals, antiyeast therapy (as a part of a comprehensive treatment program) can help most people with CFS regain their health.

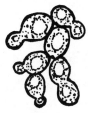

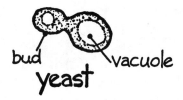

bud ····· ···· vacuole
yeast

The two essential parts of such therapy are: a special diet that must initially eliminate sugar, corn syrup and other quick-acting carbohydrates; prescription and nonprescription medications and other substances that discourage the proliferation of yeast in the digestive tract.

In Section I, *Overview*, I discuss CFS and some of its causes. I also talk about how I developed an interest in the relationship of food sensitivities to fatigue, headache, irritability, muscle aches and short attention span over 30 years ago. Then I tell how I learned about the yeast connection to disorders of the immune, endocrine and nervous systems.

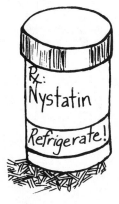

3

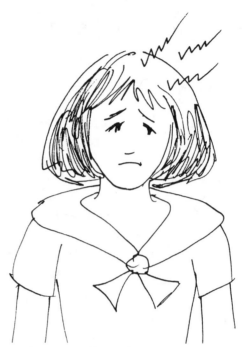

Section II, *The Yeast Connection*, begins with a questionnaire, "Are Your Health Problems Yeast Connected?" In this section you'll find a brief discussion of *Candida albicans* and how it plays a part in making you sick.

In Section III, *Support for the Yeast Connection to CFS*, you'll find brief references to scientific articles, and comments by professionals and nonprofessionals in Japan, the United States, England and New Zealand which document the relationship of *Candida albicans* to immunosuppression; the relationship of gut yeast to recurrent vaginal infections; the relationship of *Candida albicans* to PMS, food sensitivities, fatigue and depression; the response of persons with CFS to antiyeast medications and a special diet.

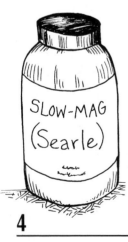

Section IV, *Regaining Your Health*, summarizes the treatment program which I've found helps many patients with CFS and related disorders.

In Section V, *More Information*, I discuss nutrition, indoor air pollutants, allergies, nutritional supplements, prescription and nonprescription medications and psychological support. This section will also include questions and answers about elimination diets.

In Section VI, *Other Therapies,* you'll find a discussion of other therapies which may help the person with CFS, including magnesium, essential fatty acids, probiotics, garlic, Coenzyme Q$_{10}$, vitamin B$_{12}$, vitamin C, viral vaccines, Prozac, Ampligen and Kutapressin™. You'll also find a summary of recommendations by four physicians who have been on the cutting edge of Chronic Fatigue Immune Deficiency Syndrome research and who have treated several thousand persons with this illness.

Section VII, *The Yeast Connection Controversy,* discusses both sides of this subject.

In Section VIII, *Other Topics of Interest,* you'll find a discussion of intestinal microbes and systemic immunity, Fibromyalgia (FM), viral studies and mercury/amalgam fillings.

Section IX, *Potpourri.* In this section you'll find an assortment of information including a summary of the article, "Chronic Fatigue Syndrome: A Working Case Definition" from the Centers for Disease Control (CDC); comments on CFS from the National Institute of Allergy and Infectious Disease (NIAID); comments by Mike Iverson, president of the CFIDS Association, Inc.; information on hormonal disorders in CFS; comments on CFS and Lyme disease; *Candida albicans* laboratory studies in CFS; tests for food sensitivities; intravenous immunoglobulin therapy; rubella virus vaccine therapy; sugar and yeast growth; more on Prozac; food sensitivities and brain dysfunction; comments about CFS by physicians; publications from New Zealand; and CACTUS—a coalition of CFIDS organizations and leaders, and a postscript.

A Special Comment About Names

While I was writing this book, I kept asking myself, "What shall I call this disorder?"

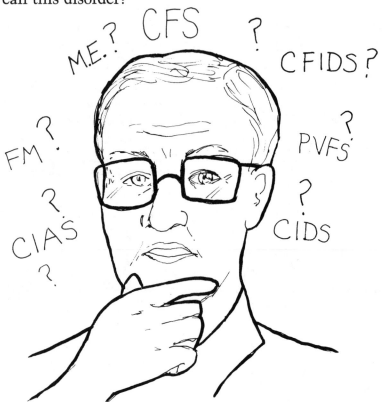

In 1986, along with most other folks interested in the subject, I called it the Chronic Epstein-Barr Virus (CEBV). Then research studies published in the medical literature showed that the Epstein-Barr Virus (EBV), although involved in making some people sick, wasn't *the* cause. Then in 1988, the Centers for Disease Control (CDC) suggested the name *Chronic Fatigue Syndrome (CFS)*.

CFS is the name I used until I attended the conference on the Chronic Fatigue and Immune Dysfunction Syndrome (CFIDS) (sponsored by the CFIDS Association, Inc.) in Charlotte, North Carolina, on November 17-18, 1990.

At this conference I heard scientific presentations that showed clearly that the immune system is adversely affected in patients with this disorder. I also read the superb newsletter, the *CFIDS Chronicle* published by the CFIDS Association Inc., P.O. Box 220398, Charlotte, NC 28222. So I said to myself, "*CFIDS* seems to be the best name."

But then, in the spring of 1991 I reviewed the lecture notes I took at the conference. And one of the speakers said, "We need a better name than *CFIDS*. We should eliminate the word 'fatigue' from the title because it trivializes this disease." And several observers suggested the name CIDS (Chronic Immune Deficiency Syndrome).

Scientific presentations showed that the immune system is adversely affected in persons with this disorder.

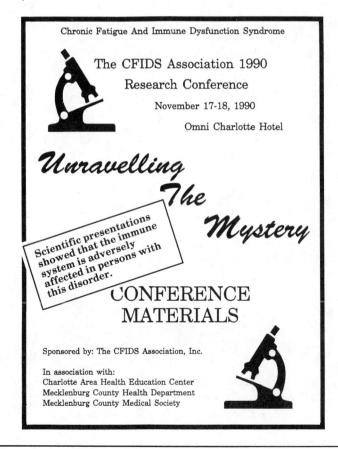

Chronic Fatigue And Immune Dysfunction Syndrome

The CFIDS Association 1990
Research Conference

November 17-18, 1990

Omni Charlotte Hotel

Unravelling The Mystery

Scientific presentations showed that the immune system is adversely affected in persons with this disorder.

CONFERENCE
MATERIALS

Sponsored by: The CFIDS Association, Inc.

In association with:
Charlotte Area Health Education Center
Mecklenburg County Health Department
Mecklenburg County Medical Society

Then I corresponded with Dr. Byron Hyde and Lydia Neilson of the Nightingale Research Foundation. They sent me many informative materials, including copies of their newsletters. They also sent me a copy of the April 9-12th, 1990, program, "The Cambridge Symposium on Myalgic Encephalomyelitis (M.E.) Chronic Fatigue Syndrome (CFS)."

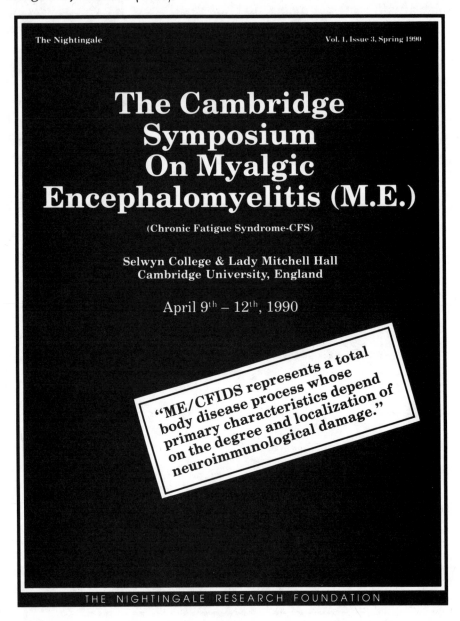

The Nightingale — Vol. 1, Issue 3, Spring 1990

The Cambridge Symposium On Myalgic Encephalomyelitis (M.E.)

(Chronic Fatigue Syndrome-CFS)

Selwyn College & Lady Mitchell Hall
Cambridge University, England

April 9th – 12th, 1990

"ME/CFIDS represents a total body disease process whose primary characteristics depend on the degree and localization of neuroimmunological damage."

THE NIGHTINGALE RESEARCH FOUNDATION

In reviewing the program brochure, I found presentations by many professionals with impeccable credentials from the United States, Canada, Great Britain, England, Ireland, Australia and New Zealand. The diversity and caliber of the presentations were impressive.*

In his introductory comments, Dr. Hyde, the conference chairman said,

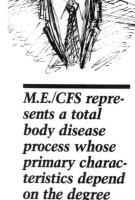

> "There have been too many names. Today, the single disease presently described as Chronic Fatigue Syndrome (CFS) in the United States and M.E. in England and much of the world, still imposes both an unnecessary complexity and a misunderstanding of what is a fairly common disease process.
>
> "M.E./CFS represents a total body disease process whose primary characteristics depend on the degree and localization of neuroimmunologic damage. The chronic and relapsing features of M.E./CFS depend on the level and ability of the patient to recover from both structural and viral-immunological damage. . . .
>
> "In this process, patients may vary as to the degree of illness, from major clinical, neurological and possibly cardiac injury to simply that of minor fatigue. These extremes are often discounted, arbitrarily considered to be not part of the M.E./CFS disease process. It is those patients in between these two extremes that are categorized as having M.E./CFS."

M.E./CFS represents a total body disease process whose primary characteristics depend on the degree and localization of neuroimmunologic damage.

I reread the 1989 book *Why M.E.?* by my good friend, the Australian/British physician Belinda Dawes and her coauthor Damien Downing. I reviewed the New Zealand publication *Meeting-Place*** and I learned that people in the United Kingdom, Australia and New Zealand favored the name M.E. Yet other people in the UK, including the Scottish researchers Peter and Wilhelmina Behan, and David Horrobin use still another name, Post-Viral Fatigue Syndrome (PVFS).

Then in the spring of 1991, I read David Bell's superb book *The*

---

*Copies of the complete papers given at the Cambridge Symposium plus papers from other conferences are available from the Nightingale Research Foundation, 383 Danforth Ave., Ottawa, Ontario, Canada K2A 03I for $35 postpaid in the U.S.
**Meeting-Place* is produced and edited by Jim Brook and Toni Jeffreys, and published by ANZMES, (NZ), P.O. Box 35-429, Browns Bay, Auckland 10, New Zealand. You'll find further information about *Meeting Place* in Section IX.

The Disease of a Thousand Names
CFIDS
Chronic Fatigue/Immune Dysfunction
Syndrome

by David S. Bell, M.D.

Also Known As

Disease of a Thousand Names and comments of J. A. Levy, M.D.[*] who said, "We also recommend renaming this disorder "Chronic Immune Activation Syndrome" (CIAS) . . . we believe that this name, . . . while it may not be perfect, at least defines laboratory data that fits all of our cases of CFIDS . . ."

I also talked to Janet Bohannon of the National Chronic Fatigue Syndrome Association[**], who told me that they liked and used the name Chronic Fatigue Syndrome (CFS) because it's easier for people to understand.

I also read and heard about Fibromyalgia (FM), a disorder which seemed to closely resemble CFS. And just before sending this book to the printer, I received more information on FM from Kristin Thorson, publisher of the Fibromyalgia Network.

So with all these different names to choose from, in November 1991, I sat down with my staff and asked, "What will we call this illness?" Almost with one voice they said, "Let's stick with the Chronic Fatigue Syndrome (*CFS*). After all, that's the name used in dozens of medical reports and hundreds of newspaper and magazine articles during the past several years."

So *Chronic Fatigue Syndrome*, or *CFS*, is the name I've used in this book.

Chronic Fatigue Syndrome is the name used in dozens of medical reports and hundreds of articles in the press.

[*]*CFIDS Chronicle*, Spring 1991, page 69.
[**]3521 Broadway, Suite 222, Kansas City, MO 64111.

Acknowledgments

If I listed all the sources which have contributed to this book, the Bibliography would be massive and the names legion.

Many colleagues will come across their ideas on these pages. When they do, they'll know how much I appreciate their sharing their ideas with me. I'm especially indebted to food allergy pioneers Albert Rowe, Theron Randolph, Frederic Speer and Bill Deamer.

I'm equally indebted to C. Orian Truss whose pioneer observations first made me aware that *Candida albicans* could be related to chronic fatigue and many other health disorders. I'm also grateful to Sidney Baker, James Brodsky, Leo Galland, Elmer Cranton, Ken Gerdes, Daniel Kinderlehrer, Keith Sehnert, George Kroker, Charles Resseger, George E. Shambaugh, Jr., Young Shin, Jack Woodard, Aubrey Worrell, Ray Wunderlich and countless other physicians who have shared their knowledge about food sensitivities, environmental allergies and their management of patients with the Candida Related Complex.

Particular thanks are due to Robert Hallowitz and Carol Jessop for sharing their observations on the use of antiyeast medications and a special diet in treating and helping hundreds of their patients with CFS. I first met Dr. Hallowitz at the Rhode Island CFS Conference in October 1988 and Dr. Jessop at the San Francisco CFIDS Conference in April 1989. I've visited with each of these physicians in person and by phone since that time.

I also appreciate and acknowledge the leadership of David Bell, Paul Cheney, Elaine DeFreitas, Jorge Flechas, Jay Goldstein, Seymour Grufferman, Walter Gunn, Byron Hyde, Nancy Klimas, Anthony Komaroff, Hilary Koprowski, Charles Lapp, Jay Levy, John Martin, Harvey Moldofsky, Daniel Peterson, Curt Sandman and many other researchers and clinicians. The clinical observations and laboratory studies of these individuals have played a critically important role in making the scientific community and the public realize that CFS is an organic disorder that affects the immune system, musculoskeletal system, the brain and many other parts of the body.

Special praise is also due to many others who have worked unselfishly to bring the plight of persons with CFS into the medical, public and government mainstream. Included are Marc M. Iverson, publisher; K. Kimberly Kenney, Managing Editor, and Caryn H. Freese, publisher and editor of the *CFIDS Chronicle*, and other members of staff of the CFIDS Association, Inc. of Charlotte, North Carolina, and Lydia M. Neilson, Communication Director, the Nightingale Research Foundation, Ottawa Canada, Gidget Faubion and others of the CFIDS Association of Portland, Oregon, Jan Montgomery and other members of the staff of the CFIDS Society of San Francisco, Janet Bohannon and other members of the staff of the National Chronic Fatigue Syndrome Association of Kansas City, Larry Sakin and the staff members of the United Federation of CFS/CFIDS/CEBV organizations, Tucson, Arizona, Belinda Dawes and Damien Downing, London, England, authors of the book *Why M.E.?*, Barry Sleight, of Washington, D.C., Jim Brook, editor and publisher of *Meeting Place*, Auckland, New Zealand, and many others.

As with my other publications, I appreciate the charming art work of my daughter Cynthia, who helps make what I write "come alive." And again I thank John Adams and the entire staff at ProtoType Graphics, Inc., Nashville, Tennessee, for their skillful production services. Special words of appreciation are due to Gregg Bender, editorial cartoonist of the *Jackson Sun* for his delightful illustrations, including the elephants and the cascades. Thanks also to Jere Perry and the staff of Tennessee Industrial Printers for their help and collaboration with many of the additional graphics. Finally I'm grateful to my Professional Books staff, Janet Gregory, Brenda Harris, Ken Keim, Tara Mitchell and Nell Sellers who helped me in various ways in putting this book together.

SECTION I

Overview

Chronic Fatigue Syndrome—
An Enigma

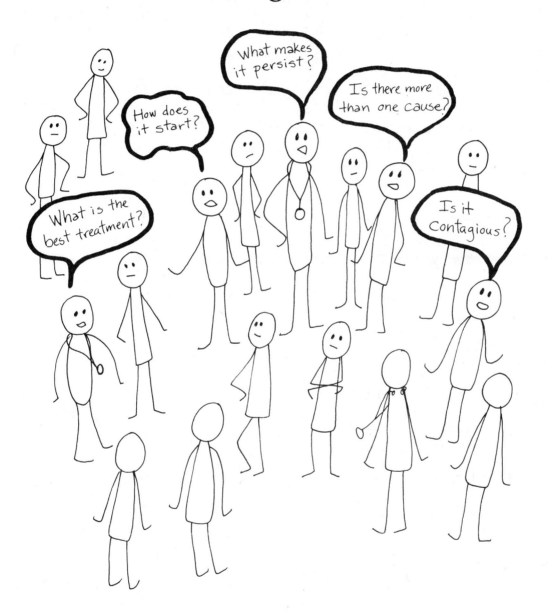

Many professionals and nonprofessionals are asking these questions . . . and searching for answers.

It appears that an illness cascade may take place in the person with CFS. Here are common sequences:

An epidemic viral infection may trigger an illness cascade.

Many people in a localized area may be affected by an infectious agent. This seemed to be the case at the Los Angeles County Hospital in 1934 when nearly 200 persons developed what appeared to be an acute viral infection. Following this infection, many individuals remained disabled for 6 to 12 months or longer.

A similar epidemic occurred in Iceland in 1948 near the town of Akureyri, where over a thousand persons became ill with a polio-like disease without paralysis. Here again, prolonged fatigue, malaise and other symptoms persisted in many of these individuals.

Still other epidemics have occurred in many parts of the world including the Royal Free Hospital in England in 1955 where 292 medical and administrative staff members fell ill.

Outbreaks of a similar type of illness were also reported in many other countries, including Greece, Scotland, Australia, South Africa and the United States. Then in 1984, some 200 people in Incline Village, Nevada on the shores of Lake Tahoe developed a lingering illness which attracted national and international attention.

Following each of these outbreaks of an acute illness, many individuals were troubled by persistent symptoms, including exhaustion, impaired thinking, anxiety, vertigo, numbness, tingling and other symptoms.

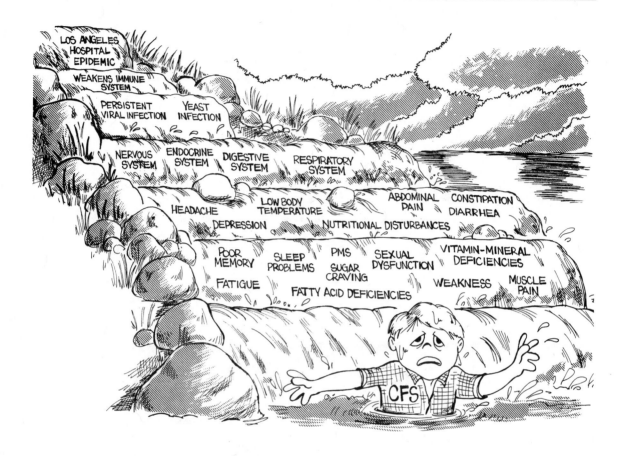

During the last 40 years, dozens and perhaps hundreds, of similar epidemics have occurred all over the world. Here are a few of them.

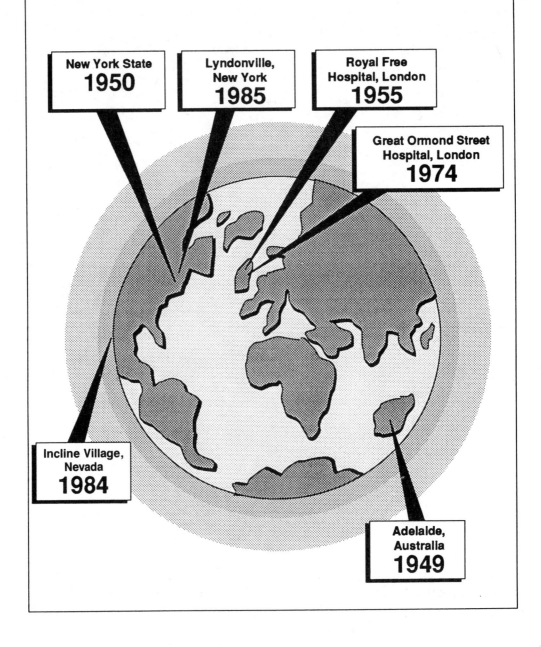

New York State
1950

Lyndonville, New York
1985

Royal Free Hospital, London
1955

Great Ormond Street Hospital, London
1974

Incline Village, Nevada
1984

Adelaide, Australia
1949

In these epidemics it seems clear that one or more infectious disease agents played an important role in causing the illness. This agent appears to have been a virus. And it seems probable that the polio virus was involved in some of these epidemics.

Symptoms that developed in people during these epidemics were caused by disturbances in many parts of the body, including the immune system and the, endocrine, nervous, musculoskeletal, digestive and respiratory systems.

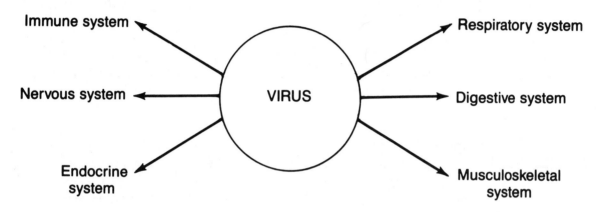

The most common symptoms in patients with acute or relapsing CFS noted by Carol Jessop, M.D.*, were: exhaustion/fatigue (100)%), post-exertional fatigue (100%), sleep disorder (100%), frequent urination (98%), persistent headache (95%), cold extremities (94%), achiness/myalgia (92%), chills (89%), cognitive dysfunction (84%), sore throat (79%), irritability (78%), balance problems (60%), twitching (56%), nausea (51%) and depression (35%).

Dr. Jessop's statistics were somewhat different for those who had symptoms for greater than eight months. She also described many other past and present symptoms in her patients. And interestingly enough, enlarged lymph glands were present in only 20% of the acute group and 10% of the chronic group.

In describing this illness, the CFIDS Association said,

"It is a complex illness characterized by incapacitating fatigue, neurological and other symptoms . . . .These symptoms tend to

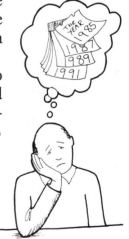

*Presentation at CFIDS Association Research Conference, P.O. Box 220398, Charlotte, NC, 28222, November 18, 1990.

wax and wane but are often severely debilitating and may last for many months or years. All segments of the population are at risk but adults under the age of 45 seem to be most susceptible and a majority of persons with CFIDS. . . .are women."*

According to the CFIDS Association,

"Research suggests that CFIDS results from a dysfunction of the immune system. The exact nature of this dysfunction has not yet been well defined, but it can be generally viewed as an 'up regulated' or overactive state (which is responsible for most of the symptoms). Ironically, there is also evidence of some immune suppression in CFIDS; patients exhibit certain 'down regulated' signs. For example, in many patients, there are functional deficiencies in 'natural killer cells' (an important component of the immune system responsible for protection against viruses and cancer)."

In describing this illness, which in England, Canada, Australia and New Zealand is called Myalgic Encephalomyelitis or M.E., Dr. Byron Hyde, Chairman, The Nightingale Research Foundation** said, "M.E. is a chronic viral illness that occurs in epidemics or after an apparently minor infection. This severe disease is characterized by:

- Muscle failure with marked fatigue, pain or exhaustion in the exercised muscle
- Inability to return to the normal state of mental and physical activity
- Marked variability and fluctuation of symptoms
- Major sleep disturbance
- Problems of dyslexia, memory loss, aphasia
- Severe malaise

*The *CFIDS Chronicle*, Spring/Summer 1990, page iii.
**The Nightingale Research Foundation was incorporated in Canada as a charitable association in 1988 to conduct and assist research into the cause and cure of Myalgic Encephalomyelitis (M.E.) and to serve as an educational institution for the Canadian public, physicians, nurses, teachers and their professional associates.

Professionals from many different disciplines, including immunology, toxicology, mycology, environmental medicine and dentistry have noted that some individuals may develop CFS (or an illness indistinguishable from it) in other ways. Here are a few of them:

- **After an acute nonepidemic viral illness.** Causes of such viral illness include the Epstein-Barr virus, the HHV6 virus, the Coxsackie virus, the hepatitis virus and the influenza virus.

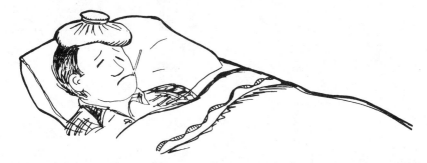

- **After working in an airtight office building loaded with pollutants, including:**
    building materials which "outgas" chemical odors
        (formaldehyde-containing wall board, carpet,
        foam rubber, paints, glues and waxes)
    tobacco smoke, perfumes, and other cosmetics
    floor cleaners, bathroom chemicals
    copy papers, marking pencils
    insecticides
    molds in the air conditioning system.*

Illness that develops in office workers exposed to these substances has been called the "sick building syndrome".

---

*Sherry Rogers, M.D., 2800 W. Genesee St., Syracuse, New York 13219, has described the improvement of patients with the Post Viral Syndrome following immunotherapy for mold sensitivity. (S. Rogers, "Indoor fungi as part of the cause of the recalcitrant symptoms of the tight building syndrome, *Environment International*, Vol. 17, pp 271-75, 1991.)

- **After living in a home polluted with environmental chemicals.**[*] These include cigarette smoke, cosmetics, pesticides, laundry and bathroom chemicals, gas cooking stoves, freshly dry-cleaned clothes and many of the same pollutants found in office buildings.

Nicholas Ashford, Ph.D., Claudia Miller, M.D., and other speakers at the January 1990 International Symposium in Dallas, Texas, on "Man and His Environment in Health and Disease" emphasized the hazards of indoor air pollution. And in a presentation at the American Lung Association's Second Annual Science Writer's Forum in Annapolis, Maryland, Lance A. Wallace, Ph.D. stated, "Personal activities and consumer products rather than exposure from living in an industrial area, account for the bulk of our exposures to most of the toxic chemicals we studied . . . . Our findings are so at odds with conventional wisdom that most people have not yet grasped their import."[**]

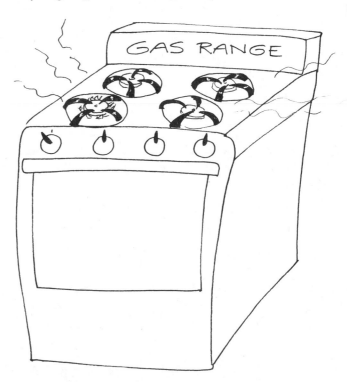

---

[*]See a further discussion of chemical pollutants in Section V.
[**]*JAMA*, 262, 3101-3102, December 1989.

• **After exposure to toxic chemicals in a factory.**

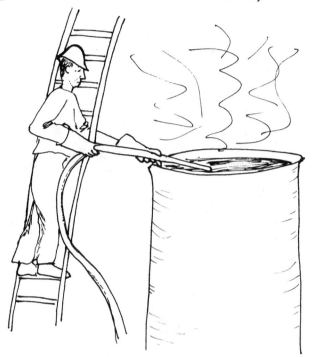

• **After living in the tropics and acquiring a parasitic infection.**

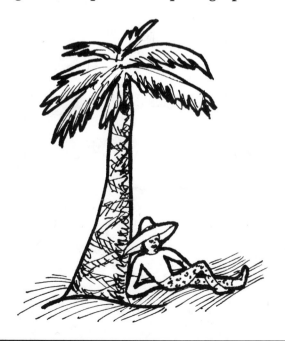

- Living in a damp, moldy home.

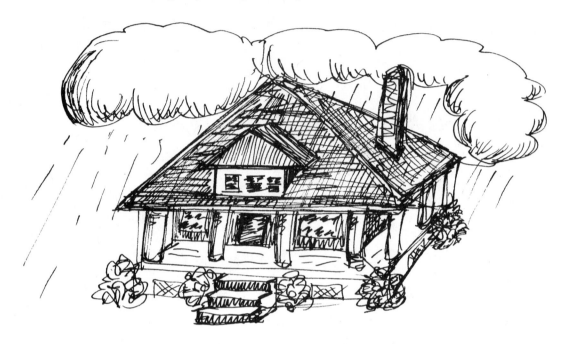

- Following the insertion of mercury/amalgam dental fillings.

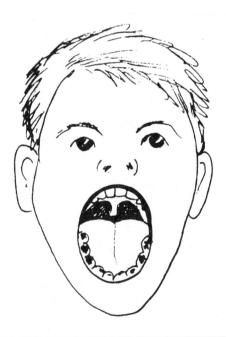

• **After taking long-term antibiotics.** *

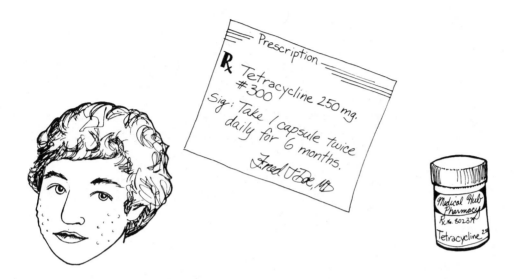

CFS can be compared to a forest fire.
Such a fire may start for several reasons:

• A careless tourist fails to extinguish a fire at his campsite.
• Lightning strikes.
• A lighted cigarette thrown by a passing motorist.
• Arson
• A volcanic eruption

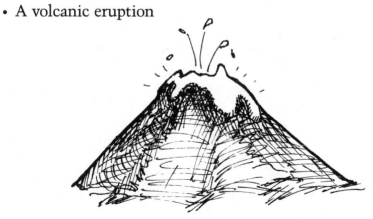

*Taking long term antibiotics for acne, recurrent respiratory, urinary or prostate infections leads to overgrowth of the common yeast *Candida albicans.*

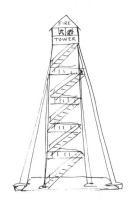

Whatever the triggering mechanism, once a blaze starts, it may spread because of:

- Preexisting drought
- High winds
- Inaccessibility of the area
- Failure of government authorities to allocate sufficient funds for firefighters and firefighting equipment

Like a forest fire, CFS can start in many ways. Once it gets started, the immune system is weakened. And when the immune system can't do its job viruses and bacteria begin to multiply and raise large families . . . .

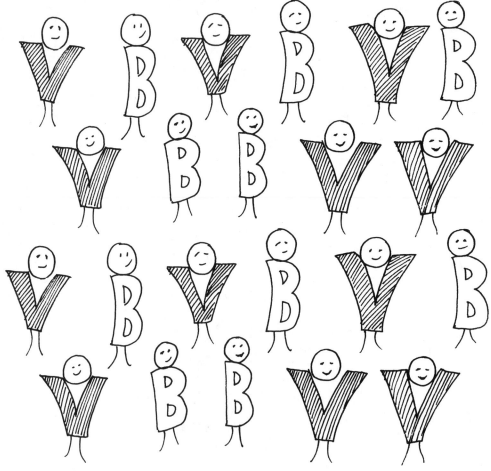

infections may then develop and make people sick.

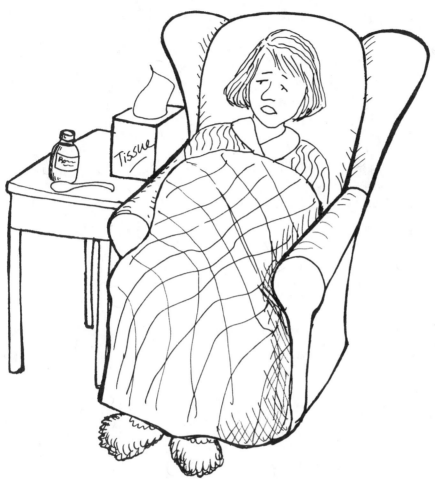

The person with an infection may be given broad spectrum antibiotic drugs.

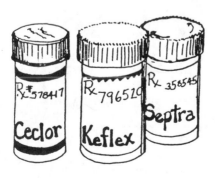

Such medications may cause vaginal yeast infections

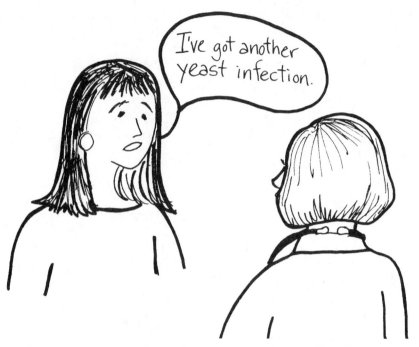

and yeast overgrowth in the gut—leading to diarrhea, constipation, abdominal pain and absorption of food allergens.

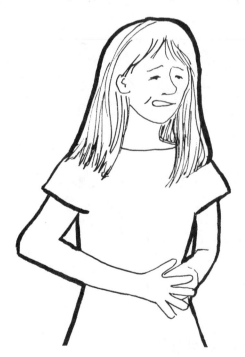

Yeast infections may cause further immunosuppression leading to . . .

• a vicious cycle of vaginal yeast infections*

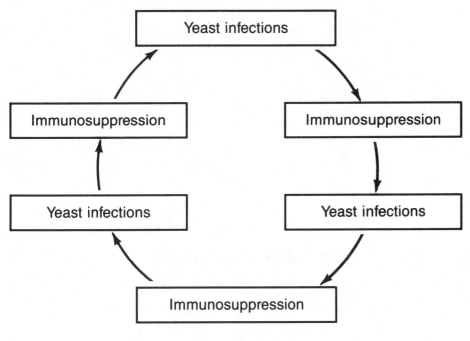

• more viral infections

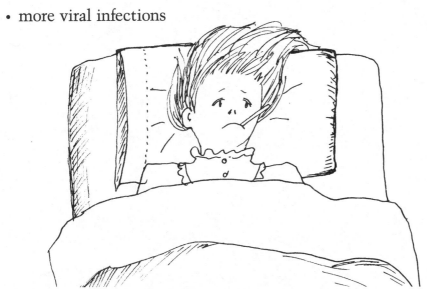

*For a further discussion, see Section V.

• a vicious cycle of bacterial infections

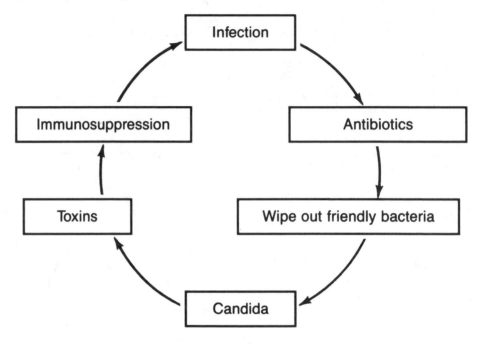

• Proliferation of giardia and other parasites*

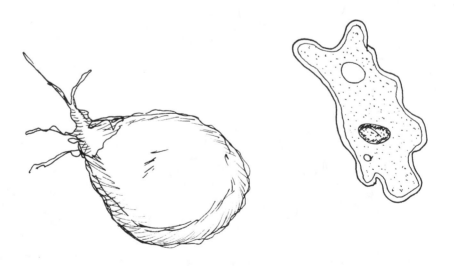

*L. Galland, R. Jenkins, J. Mowbray, *Post-viral Fatigue Syndrome*, John Wiley and Sons, Ltd., London, 1991.

- endocrine dysfunction

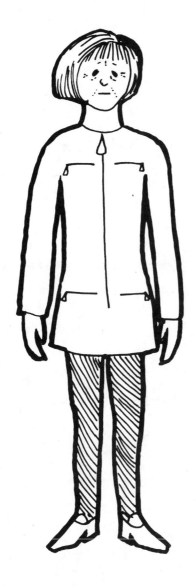

fatigue

sugar craving

dry skin

PMS

infertility

loss of libido

subnormal
temperature

irregular
menstruation

The illness cascade that then develops causes disturbances in many parts of the body.

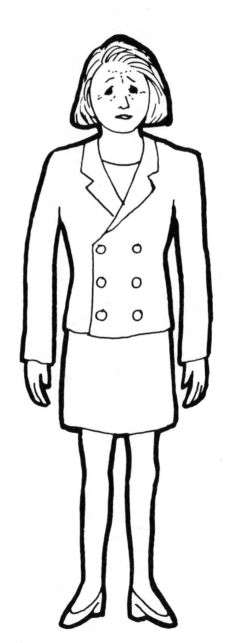

inability to
concentrate

nasal
congestion

cough

tingling

palpitation

insomnia

headache

poor
memory

abdominal
pain

urinary
symptoms

muscle
pain

numbness

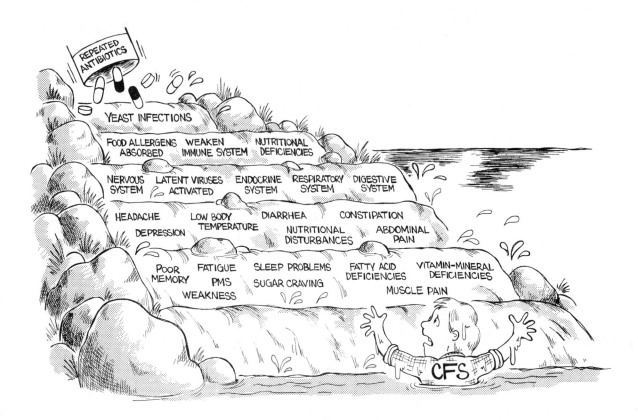

More About CFS—And Where I'm Coming From

As you look at and/or read this book (especially if you're a physician), you may ask, How many CFS patients has the author treated? Has he carried out research studies on viruses . . . or on the immune system? What are his qualifications?

I don't blame you for asking and before proceeding, I'd like to tell you where I'm coming from. I'm a 74-year-old pediatrician, allergist and medical writer. I'm a clinician—a practicing physician. Although I'm a Fellow of the American Academy of Pediatrics, the American College of Allergy and Immunology and the American Academy of Environmental Medicine, my knowledge of immunology and virology leaves much to be desired. Moreover, it is limited almost entirely to what I've heard in lectures and read in the scientific literature or in the lay press.

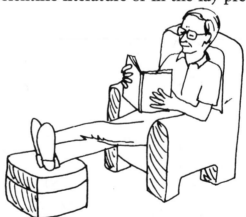

Yet, like all physicians in the United States during the past seven or eight years, I've read many reports in the medical literature about the Chronic Fatigue Syndrome (CFS). Then, in visits I made to Canada, England, Australia and New Zealand many people I met (including both professional and nonprofessionals) talked about "M.E.," a disorder that seemed identical to CFS.

My interest in CFS was also stimulated by the hundreds of people who had read *The Yeast Connection*, who wrote and called me saying, "I have CFS and your book has really helped me." As was the case with many professionals and nonprofessionals, my interest in CFS was stimulated by the increasing attention it was receiving in the press and media. For example, Dorothy (played by Bea Arthur), who is featured in the popular TV program *The Golden Girls* was affected by CFS.

To learn more about CFS, in October 1988 I attended the First Annual East Coast Symposium on CFS in Rhode Island sponsored by Governor Edward D. DiPrete, and cosponsored by the Rhode Island General Assembly, the Rhode Island Department of Health and Brown University Program in Medicine. In April 1989 I attended a second CFS conference sponsored by the San Francisco Department of Public Health, the San Francisco Medical Society, the University of California, San Francisco Department of Medicine and School of Nursing. Then I attended a third conference in Charlotte, North Carolina, in November 1990, sponsored by the CFIDS Association, Inc.

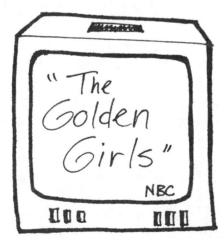

I agree 100% with the researchers and clinicians at these conferences who said, in effect, "People with devastating fatigue, muscle aching, memory loss, confused thinking, digestive problems, food allergies, chemical sensitivities and other symptoms are suffering from a true disease. Moreover, these symptoms may persist for months or years and interfere with a person's ability to work and carry on a normal home life."

These symptoms may persist for months or years and interfere with a person's ability to work and carry on a normal home life.

If you are such a person, and you feel "sick all over," I don't blame you for being annoyed, frustrated and angry if someone says, "Buck up, get back to work, your complaints are all in your head." Or, "Depression is the cause of your symptoms."

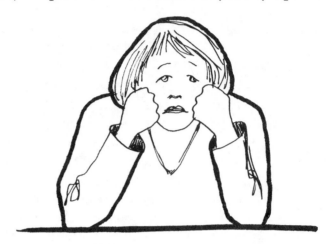

CFS "is for real." The symptoms *are* caused by organic changes that affect the immune system, the nervous system, the endocrine system, the musculoskeletal system and many other parts of the body. The brilliant observations of David Bell, Paul Cheney, Elaine DeFreitas, Jay Goldstein, Seymour Grufferman, William Hermann, Jr., Brendan Hilliard, Byron Hyde, James Jones, Nancy Klimas, Anthony Komaroff, Hilary Koprowski, Alan Landay, Jay Levy, John Martin, Daniel Peterson, Irina Rozovsky, Robert Suhadolnik, Dennis Wakefield and other investigators, show that viruses of various types appear to play a significant role in causing CFS. And they are working tirelessly to uncover more information and develop more effective methods of treatment.

Viruses of various types appear to play a significant role in causing CFS.

Much remains to be learned about the causes of CFS. Yet, professionals and nonprofessionals in the United States, Canada, Scotland, Australia and New Zealand have found that most people with this disorder can be helped by a comprehensive treatment program.

Different professionals emphasize different parts of such a program and no one claims to have all the answers. Certainly, I do not. Yet, in my pediatric and allergy practice, I've found that many people with chronic fatigue, headache, muscle aches, memory loss, digestive disorders and other symptoms can be helped when they . . .

Many people can be helped when they clean up their diet.

36

- clean up their diet. This means eating a lot more vegetables, fruits and whole grains and less meats.

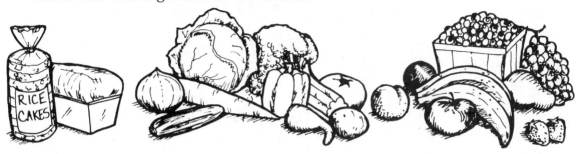

- avoid foods of low nutritional quality.

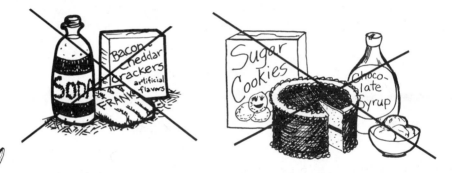

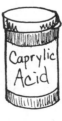

- search for and avoid foods that cause sensitivity reactions.
- take prescription and/or nonprescription antifungal medications including nystatin, Nizoral, Diflucan, *Lactobacillus acidophilus*, and/or other probiotics, caprylic acid, Tanalbit™, citrus seed extracts, Kyolic or other garlic products and/or other substances that curb the growth of *Candida albicans* in the digestive tract.

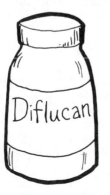

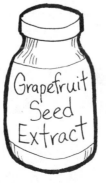

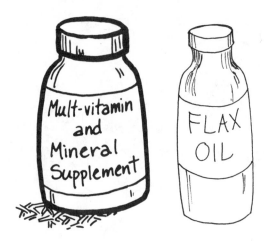

• take nutritional supplements, including yeast-
free vitamins, minerals
and essential fatty acids.

• receive psychological support.

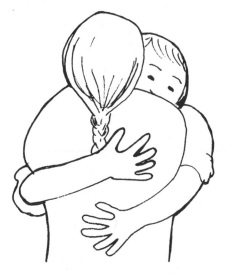

Because of my success in treating and helping so many patients using this program, I've emphasized the yeast connection to CFS. Yet, I fully realize that I may be like one of the six blind men of Indostan who went to see the elephant.

As you'll see when you read John Godfrey Saxe's classic poem, each blind man described the elephant according to what he had seen and each blind man had a different story.

In this book I describe the CFS "elephant" based on the part I've become most familiar with. Yet, I freely acknowledge that there are other parts that I know little about.

The Blind Men and the Elephant

It was six men of Indostan
    To learning much inclined,
Who went to see the elephant
    (Though all of them were blind),
That each by observation
    Might satisfy his mind.

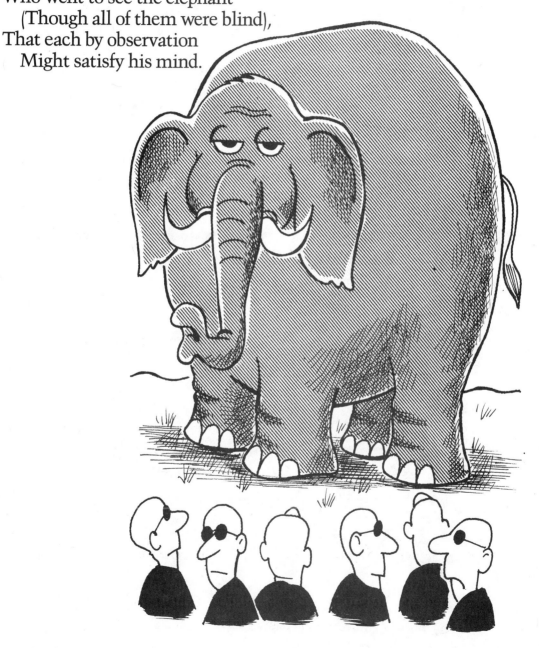

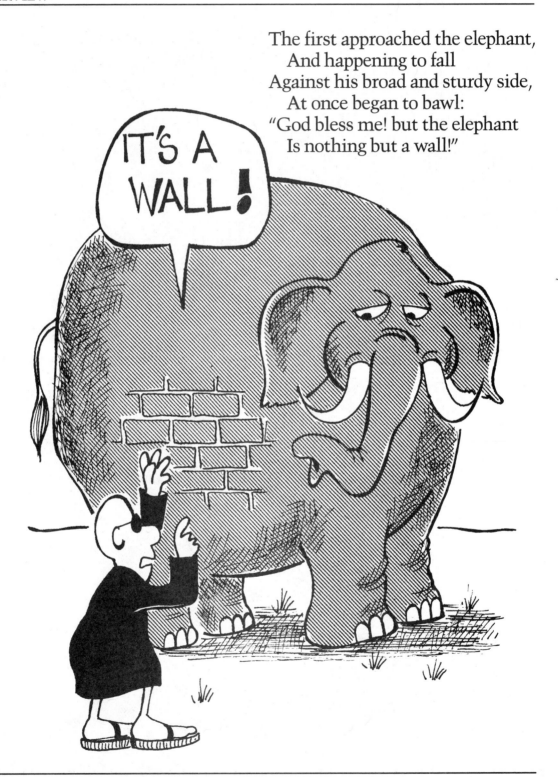

The second feeling of the tusk,
    Cried: "Ho! What have we here
So very round and smooth and sharp?
    To me 'tis mighty clear
This wonder of an elephant
    Is very like a spear!"

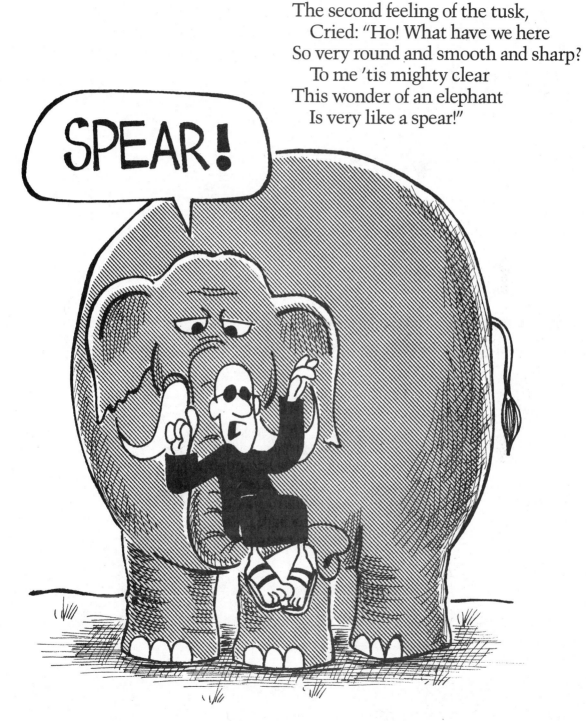

The third approached the animal,
  And, happening to take
The squirming trunk within his hands,
  Thus boldly up and spake:
"I see," quoth he, "the elephant
  Is very like a snake!"

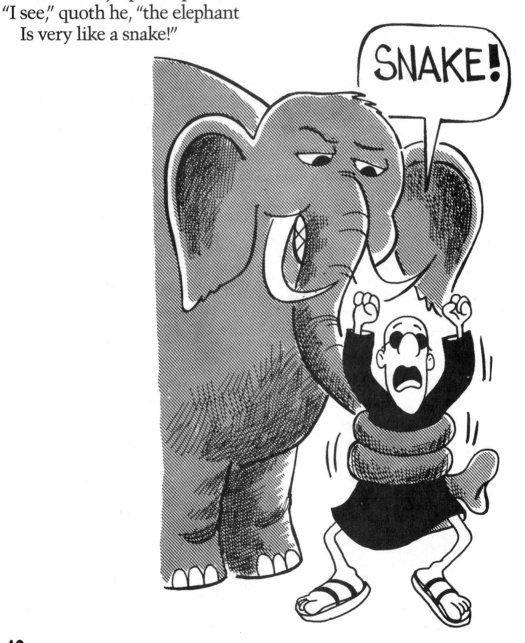

The fourth reached out his eager hand,
    And felt about the knee:
"What most this wondrous beast is like
    Is mighty plain," quote he;
" 'Tis clear enough, the elephant
    Is very like a tree."

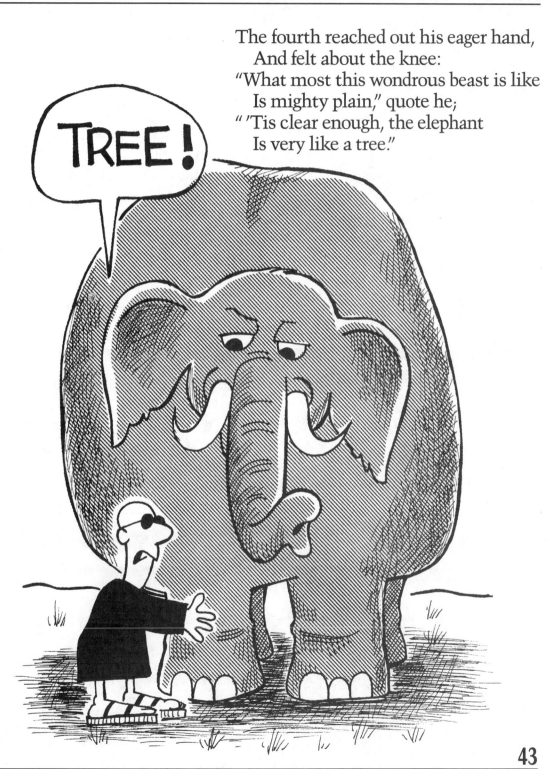

The fifth who chanced to touch the ear,
Said: "E'en the blindest man
Can tell what this resembles most;
Deny the fact who can
This marvel of an elephant
Is very like a fan!"

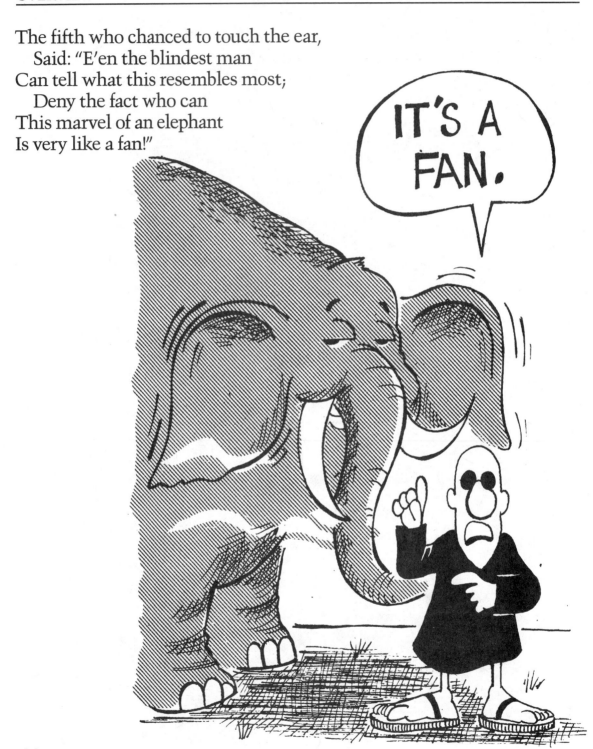

The sixth no sooner had begun
   About the beast to grope,
Than, seizing on the swinging tail
   That fell within his scope,
"I see," quoth he, "the elephant
   Is very like a rope!"

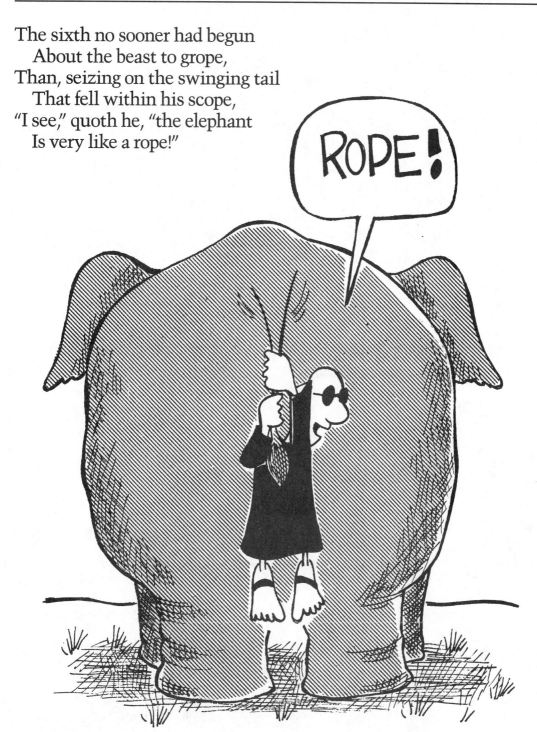

And so these men of Indostan
    Disputed loud and long.
Each of his own opinion
    Exceeding stiff and strong,
Though each was partly in the right,
    And all were in the wrong!

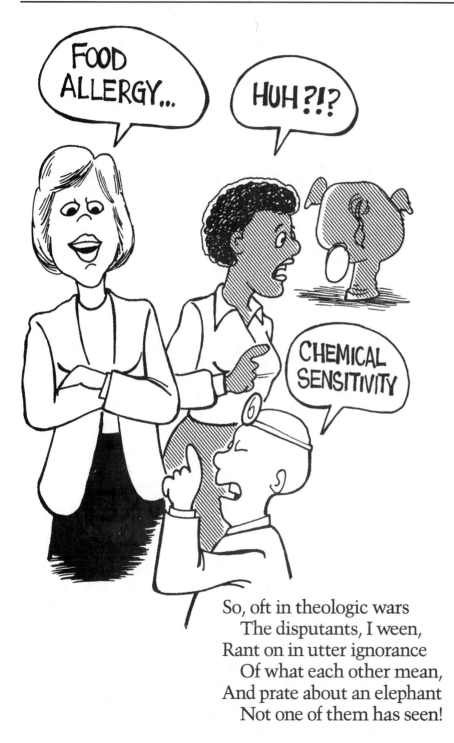

So, oft in theologic wars
   The disputants, I ween,
Rant on in utter ignorance
   Of what each other mean,
And prate about an elephant
   Not one of them has seen!

John Godfrey Saxe   **47**

Chronic Fatigue and Food Sensitivities

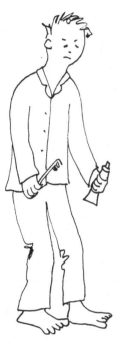

In 1949, I opened my pediatric office in my hometown of Jackson, Tennessee. And I saw children of all ages with many different types of problems. Although I was able to help many of these children and their parents, there were other children who puzzled me—children I failed to help. One such youngster (I'll call him Tom) came to see me four or five times during the year 1955. His complaints included fatigue, weakness and inability to get out of bed in the morning. He also complained of headache, irritability, abdominal pain and muscle aches.

I went over Tom with a fine tooth comb and put him through a battery of laboratory tests. All proved to be negative. Because I suspected a psychological problem, I took 12-year old Tom to breakfast at a nearby restaurant. I wanted to put him at ease and see if I could uncover an emotional stress at home or at school.

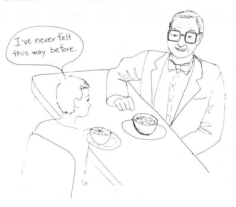

I came up empty-handed. Tom said, "My parents are getting along fine. My grades at school have been good—until recently. Now I'm so tired, I have trouble waking up and getting up in the morning. My mother and teachers think that I've suddenly gotten lazy. These problems began this fall—I've never felt this way before."

A few days later, Tom's mother came into my office for a visit. She said, "I have an idea—I wonder if Tom's symptoms could be caused by a sensitivity to cow's milk? Here's why I think so. During the past several months he's been drinking three or four glasses a day—trying to put on extra weight."

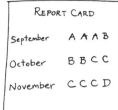

REPORT CARD	
September	A A A B
October	B B C C
November	C C C D

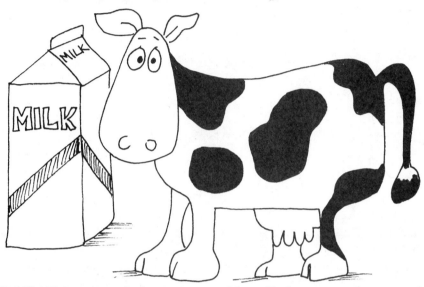

"Milk!?" I responded. "How could milk have anything to do with Tom's fatigue?"

Tom's mother replied, "When Tom was a baby, he was bothered with colic and a rash on his cheeks and in the bends of his elbows. His pediatrician removed milk from his diet and the rash went away. When he drank milk again, the rash returned. I tried him off and on milk three times and each time when I gave him milk his rash returned.

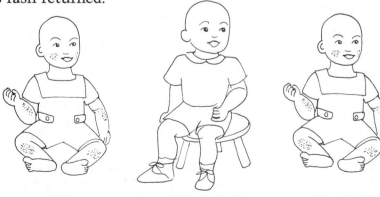

Milk   Milk eliminated   Milk added back

"Tom drank little milk during the ensuing years until about three months ago. Not long after he started drinking a lot of milk, he began to complain of headache and fatigue. He also looked pale and there were dark circles under his eyes. Based on Tom's problems when he was a baby, I think it makes sense to take him off milk now and see what happens."

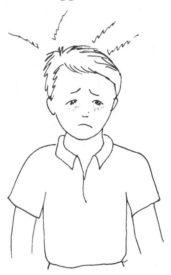

"Although I didn't understand how or why drinking milk could cause Tom's problems, I agreed with Tom's mother that experimenting with his diet made sense."

A week later, Tom's mother called and said, "Tom is like a different child. He bounced out of bed this morning whistling. No headache, muscle aches or belly aches." *I was astounded because I had learned something that I hadn't known about before— intolerance, allergies or sensitivities to common foods could provoke fatigue and other systemic and nervous symptoms.*

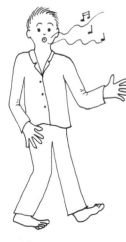

Not long after that, I happened to be thumbing through the November 1954 issue of *Pediatric Clinics of North America,* and I came across an article by a University of Kansas physician, Frederic Speer, entitled "The Allergic Tension-Fatigue Syndrome." In his article, Dr. Speer described a number of his patients with fatigue, irritability and other symptoms who improved dramatically when common foods were eliminated from their diet.

Much to my surprise, I found 21 references at the end of Speer's article. Among the reports he cited was an article by Albert Rowe,

Sr.,* of Oakland, California, who in 1930 described his experiences in studying and treating patients with fatigue, headache and other symptoms.

He noted that many of these patients improved—often dramatically—when they avoided wheat, corn, milk, egg and other common foods. Rowe called this disorder "allergic toxemia." And he continued to write and talk about food-related fatigue until his death in the early 1970s.

Many tired patients improved when they avoided wheat, corn, milk and other common foods.

Following in Rowe's footsteps, Albert Rowe, Jr., Herbert Rinkel and Theron Randolph in the 1940s described patients with food-related fatigue, depression and other symptoms which could be relieved using 5- to 10-day elimination diets.

As I read and reread the Speer article and the reports of other physicians who described food-related fatigue and other systemic and nervous symptoms, I was amazed. And I said to myself, "I wonder if a food sensitivity could be responsible for Marlene's drowsiness and fatigue . . . fatigue that makes her unable to sit at her desk at school, even though she's somehow able to keep up with her work. Or George's lethargy, which keeps him from going out and playing with the rest of the gang."

So I began putting a number of my tired, dreamy, irritable, inattentive patients on one-week trial diets. Although I didn't help all of them, I was excited because I began to receive reports from mothers who said, "Susie's like a different child. But when I give her chocolate milk, corn chips, wheat, or eggs, her symptoms return.

On the diet, Susie's like a different child. But when she drinks chocolate milk, her symptoms return.

I collected and summarized my findings on 23 of these patients and presented them at the Allergy Section of the American Academy of Pediatrics in October 1958, and I published my findings on 50 of these tired, irritable children in *Pediatrics* in 1961.

• diagnosis of food sensitivity was made in the following manner. Symptoms and signs were relieved by eliminating suspected foods from the diet for 5 to 12 days and then reproduced by giving the food back to the child.

During the '60s and '70s, I saw and helped hundreds of my patients using carefully designed and properly executed elimination

---

*A.H. Rowe, Sr., "Allergic Toxemia and Migraine Due to Food Allergy," *California and Western Medicine*, 33:785, 1930.

diets. Moreover, I found that food sensitivities could affect just about any and every part of the body. Common symptoms included fatigue, drowsiness and depression in some youngsters and irritability, short attention span and overactivity in others. And in some patients, these symptoms would alternate.

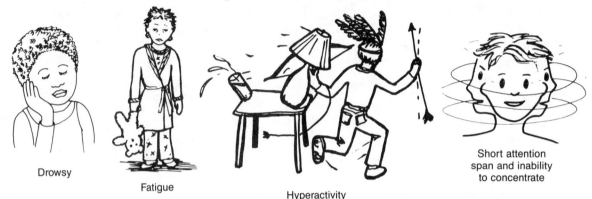

Drowsy

Fatigue

Hyperactivity

Short attention
span and inability
to concentrate

During the '60s, '70s and '80s, a number of physicians in practice and in academic centers described their findings on children with food-induced fatigue and other symptoms. Included among the academicians were William C. Deamer*, professor of pediatrics, University of California, San Francisco; John W. Gerrard, professor of pediatrics, University of Saskatchewan; Douglas Sandberg, professor of pediatrics, University of Miami; Frank A. Oski** and Walter Tunnessen, Jr.,*** professors of pediatrics at the Upstate Medical Center of New York, Syracuse.

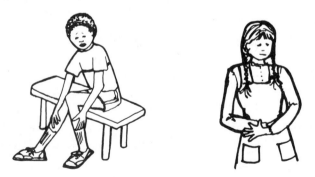

*W. C. Deamer, *Pediatrics*, 52:307, 1973.
**Now Chairman of the Department of Pediatrics, Johns Hopkins School of Medicine.
***Now Associate Chairman for Medical Education, Children's Hospital of Philadelphia (C.H.O.P.).

Dr. Deamer, a pediatric allergist, became interested in the Allergic Tension-Fatigue Syndrome in the early 1960s. In the next two decades he presented his observations in scientific exhibits and in articles and commentaries in the medical literature. In discussing recurrent abdominal pain, headache and limb pains he said,

Recurrent abdominal pain, headache, aching muscles and joints have been observed as symptoms of food allergies. William C. Deamer, M.D.

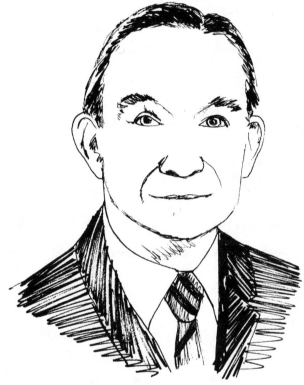

"In one series of 96 children with the Allergic Tension-Fatigue Syndrome seen in our Pediatric Allergy Clinic and privately, the six most common complaints—other than respiratory tract symptoms—were in order: headache, 61%; recurrent abdominal pain, 58%; pallor, 52%; fatigue or tiredness, 47%; limb pains, 36% . . .

"All 96 patients were successfully treated for the stated symptoms by elimination of specific food allergens . . . . Milk and chocolate in particular. In most instances, either a sibling or a parent had a history of similar symptoms attributable to food sensitivity."

In 1977, Frank A. Oski, M.D., who was at that time chairman of the department of pediatrics at the Upstate Medical Center at Syracuse, expressed concern over what he felt to be the excessive emphasis on milk in the diet of American children. He summarized his thoughts in a book entitled *Don't Drink Your Milk.*[*] Here are excerpts from this book:

> "Being against cow's milk is equated with being un-American. It's easy to understand this view which is inspired mainly by the advertising practices and political pressure of the American Dairy Industry. For many of us, our earliest memories of childhood include the plea, 'Hurry up and finish your milk.'"

In his book, Dr. Oski cited reports that showed that milk caused health problems for a variety of reasons, including excessive fat and lactose intolerance. He also reviewed and cited my article "Food Allergy, The Great Masquerader," which was published in the *Pediatric Clinics of North America* in February 1975. In a chapter of his book entitled "Milk and the Tension-Fatigue Syndrome" Dr. Oski commented,

The child may have to put his head down on the desk at school because he's feeling so tired.

> "Most people, including physicians, believe that allergies to food . . . produce only classical symptoms as skin rashes, respiratory symptoms, or gastrointestinal disorders. There is a growing body of evidence, however, to suggest that certain allergies may manifest themselves primarily as changes in personality, emotions, or in one's general sense of well-being. . . .
>
> "The child or adult with motor fatigue always seems to feel weak and tired. The child may interrupt his playing in order to rest or may even have to put his head down on the desk at school because he's feeling so tired. Excessive drowsiness and torpor are typical. These children are particularly listless in the morning. They're difficult to awaken and appear never to have a good night's sleep. . . .
>
> "Although the Tension-Fatigue Syndrome is the most common manifestation of food allergy, it is by no means the only one. Vague, recurrent abdominal pains, repeated headaches, aching muscles and joints and even bedwetting have been observed as symptoms of food allergy.

At a meeting of the American Academy of Pediatrics in the early 1970s, Dr. Deamer and his associate Dr. Oscar Lee Frick

---

[*]F.A. Oski, *Don't Drink Your Milk,* Molica Press, Ltd., 1914 Teall Ave., Syracuse, NY 13203, pp. 85-88, 1977, 1983.

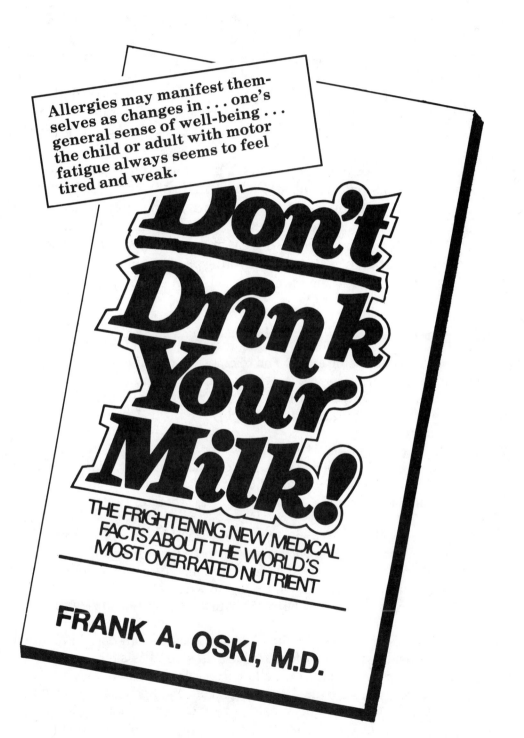

Allergies may manifest themselves as changes in . . . one's general sense of well-being . . . the child or adult with motor fatigue always seems to feel tired and weak.

Don't Drink Your Milk!

THE FRIGHTENING NEW MEDICAL FACTS ABOUT THE WORLD'S MOST OVERRATED NUTRIENT

FRANK A. OSKI, M.D.

presented a scientific exhibit on the Allergic Tension-Fatigue Syndrome. The exhibit featured a large color photograph of a tired-looking child with dark circles under her eyes. Mrs. Walter Tunnessen, Jr., the wife of one of Dr. Oski's associates, stopped at the exhibit. After looking at the picture and reviewing the symptoms of the Allergic/Tension/Fatigue Syndrome, she said to herself, "I believe that some of our child's symptoms are food-related."

During the next several years, Dr. Tunnessen found that he could help his own child and other tired, polysymptomatic patients by identifying foods that were triggering their symptoms and removing them from the diet. And in an article in *CLINI-PEARLS*, in presenting the history of an eight-year-old boy with lethargy and fatigue to a group of young pediatricians, Dr. Tunnessen made the following comments:

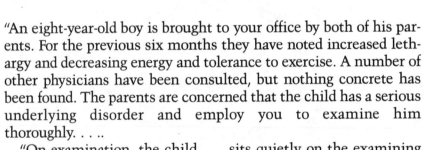

"An eight-year-old boy is brought to your office by both of his parents. For the previous six months they have noted increased lethargy and decreasing energy and tolerance to exercise. A number of other physicians have been consulted, but nothing concrete has been found. The parents are concerned that the child has a serious underlying disorder and employ you to examine him thoroughly. . . ..

"On examination, the child . . . sits quietly on the examining table and looks tired and pale. Dark circles rim his eyelids. Except for some shotty cervical adenopathy, the results of the physical examination are completely normal. . . . (Laboratory tests are also normal.)

"Whenever both parents accompany a child to the office, I know the index of parental concern has reached titanic proportions. The father extols his son's past performance in a recreational wrestling program. Now the boy is barely able to wrestle five minutes before becoming exhausted. The mother pipes in that *he rarely joins other children in after-school play.* . . ." [emphasis added]

"Where do we go from here? Maybe the problem does have an emotional basis, but before we label this child as such, consider the great masquerader, food allergy. . . . I cannot prove it with esoteric or even routine laboratory tests . . . the proof of the pudding . . . is in some simple dietary elimination . . . a benign procedure, most often painless, not requiring hospitalization and

Clini-Pearls®

Vol. 2 No. 6 July/August 1979

A Continuing Medical Education Publication for the Practicing Pediatrician

Editor
Walter W. Tunnessen, Jr. MD
State University of New York
Upstate Medical Center
Syracuse, NY 13210

> "Fatigue, tiredness and achiness are frequently overlooked manifestations of food allergies."

AN 8-YEAR-OLD BOY WITH LETHARGY AND FATIGUE

An 8-year-old boy is brought to your office by both of his parents. For the previous six months, they have noted increasing lethargy and decreasing energy and tolerance to exercise. A number of other physicians have been consulted, but nothing concrete has been found. The parents are concerned that their child has a serious underlying illness and implore you to examine him thoroughly.

The boy's appetite is excellent. There has been no weight loss, vomiting or diarrhea. He has not suffered from an unusual number of infections, nor has he had a persistent cough, or joint pains. Some recent concerns developed with a grandparent, and the parents realize that emotional problems may be playing a role.

On examination, the child is in the 75th percentile for height and weight. He sits hunched over quietly on the examining table and looks tired and pale. Dark circles rim his eyelids. Except for some shotty cervical adenopathy, the results of the physical examination are completely normal.

What should you consider?

Discussion

Whenever both parents accompany a child to the office, I know the index of parental concern has reached titanic proportions. The

father extols his son's past performance in a recreational wrestling program. Now the boy is barely able to wrestle five minutes before becoming exhausted. The mother pipes in that he rarely joins other children in afterschool play. Your examination is unrevealing except for the observation that the child appears tired out and has allergic shiners. Perhaps exercise-induced asthma? No history of wheezing is obtained, and, after a few minutes up and down, nothing is heard on auscultation, nor has a chronic [...] voiced concern [...] A complete [...] that [...] bin [...] and [...] rential [...] ulin test [...] Maybe the [...] d basis. But [...] such, consider [...] the great masquerader—food allergy. This just happens to be a favorite diagnosis of mine. Our new house staff winces in disbelief whenever I raise its hoary head. I cannot prove it with esoteric or even routine laboratory tests. There is usually no test-tube con-

> The culprits I find most common are milk, chocolate and egg, although cane sugar, corn and wheat should also be considered.

W[...]
An ES[...] subsequently[...]

Where do we [...] problem does have [...] before we label this chi[...]

Dista Products Company • Division of Eli Lilly and Company • Indianapolis, Indiana 46206
Published by Creative Medical Publications, Inc. for Dista Products Company. Division of Eli

Creative Medical Publica[...]
I Adler De[...]

> **The culprits I find most common are milk, chocolate and eggs, although cane sugar, corn and wheat should also be considered . . ..**

downright inexpensive. *The culprits I find most common are milk, chocolate and eggs, although cane sugar, corn and wheat should also be considered. Removing these foods from the diet a few at a time for a week or two is all that is necessary. Should the child improve—the eliminated foods are reintroduced . . . Relief of symptoms further supports the diagnosis."* [emphasis added]

"I, too had been a doubting Thomas until my son responded to dietary elimination . . . The boy presented in the case above was taken off milk, chocolate and eggs. Within a week he was a new person."

Like many pediatricians interested in allergy, in the 1970s I began to see more adult patients. These included not only men and women with hay fever, asthma and skin rashes, but also people with a variety of other complaints, including fatigue, headache, muscle aches and depression. I was delighted and excited when many of these patients improved when they eliminated common foods from their diets.

I was also able to help many tired, polysymptomatic adult patients by teaching them how to avoid tobacco smoke, insecticides and odorous chemicals. Others I helped by recommending lifestyle changes, nutritional supplements and using allergy extracts and vaccines. But I didn't help every person who came to see me, as you'll see in the following section.

The Yeast Connection to Chronic Fatigue Syndrome

In 1976, a 35-year-old woman (I'll call her Linda) came to my office seeking help. In fact, she was "sick all over." Although she showed some improvement when she changed her diet and cleaned up the chemical pollutants in her home, she continued to experience health problems of many sorts, including devastating fatigue.

I was unable to help Linda, and she moved away from West Tennessee. I lost contact with her; then in the fall of 1979, I learned from one of her former neighbors that Linda had moved back to West Tennessee and that she was healthy, active and energetic. So I called her up and said, "Linda I hear you're doing well. I'd love to know what you did to get your life and health back on track." And she replied, "I'll tell you, Dr. Crook, and I won't even charge you for an office visit!"

Dr. Crook, I won't even charge you for an office visit!

When Linda came to my office she handed me a copy of an article published in a little known Canadian medical journal.* It was written by C. Orian Truss, M.D., a Birmingham, Alabama specialist in internal medicine.** She said, "Dr. Crook read this paper. It contains information which will enable you to help some of your difficult, tired, irritable and depressed patients."

Dr. Truss' report told how the common yeast *Candida albicans*, growing on the warm interior membranes of the body (especially the gut and the vagina) could play an important role in causing problems in many parts of the body. Symptoms in patients with yeast-connected health problems included fatigue, PMS, depression and disorders of the immune, endocrine and nervous systems.

---

*C.O. Truss, "Tissue Injury Induced by *Candida albicans:* Mental and Neurologic Manifestations." *Journal of Orthomolecular Psychiatry,* 7:17-37, 1978
**See also Section III and VII.

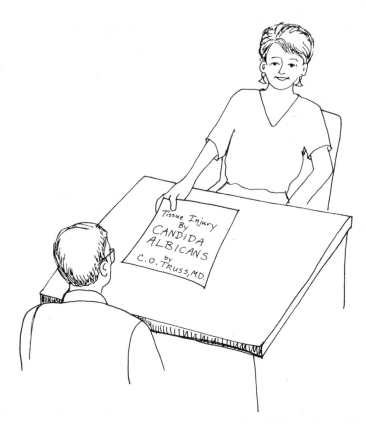

After reading the paper, I called Dr. Truss to obtain additional information. And I asked, "How do you make a diagnosis of a candida-related health problem? Are there tests that help?" Dr. Truss replied,

Yeast-connected health problems are suspected especially in persons who have received repeated courses of anti-biotic drugs.

"Since everyone has some yeast in the digestive tract, and most women have it in the vagina, smears and cultures do not help significantly in making the diagnosis. Instead it's suspected in any person who has received repeated courses of broad spectrum antibiotic drugs, such as the tetracyclines, ampicillin, amoxicillin, Keflex or Ceclor. Birth control pills and steroids also encourage the growth of candida.

"It is further suspected in the person with such a medical history who develops fatigue, headache, depression and other symptoms who has failed to respond to multiple diagnostic evaluations and therapies. Finally, it is confirmed by the response of such patients to a special diet and oral antifungal medication."

I was skeptical about some of the things Dr. Truss told me. Yet, because I had many patients who seemed to fit the category he described, I was interested. So I began to place a number of my tired, polysymptomatic patients on the treatment program recommended by Dr. Truss. Within about six months I had successfully treated 20 such patients and I was delighted and astounded at their response.

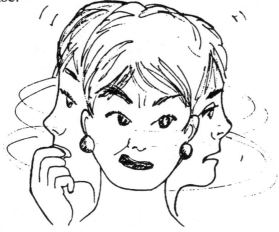

Because of the response of these patients I began to treat—and help—other patients (especially women between 25 and 45) who complained of fatigue, muscle aches, poor memory, mental confusion, depression, headache, digestive disorders, sexual dysfunction and other symptoms which made them feel "sick all over." My treatment program in working with these patients featured a sugar-free special diet and the antifungal medication nystatin.

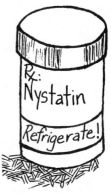

During the early 1980s, Truss' observations spread to other physicians in the United States, England, Australia and New Zealand. And hundreds of them found that a special diet and the antifungal medications nystatin and Nizoral (ketoconazole) helped their patients.

My ability to help these patients and the interest of dozens of physicians and their patients led me to write *The Yeast Connection*. The first and second editions of this book were published in hardback in late 1983 and the summer of 1984.

In 1985, many people who had read *The Yeast Connection* wrote to me and said that the Epstein-Barr virus (EBV) and other viruses were causing many people to develop an illness similar to those described in my book.

To get an additional opinion on the relationship of candida yeasts to viral infections, I consulted Elmer Cranton, M.D., a graduate of Harvard Medical School and editor (at that time) of the *Journal of Advancement in Medicine.* Here's an excerpt of his comments:

"In treating patients in my practice with yeast-related illness, I find that close to ¼ have viral disease. There is also no question that the health problems of the vast majority of these patients are primarily candida related. I feel that the chronic yeast condition weakens the immunity and causes EBV to occur and to become persistent . . .

"I'm not certain which comes first, the chicken or the egg. That is, did the EBV lower immunity and cause a person to become more susceptible to yeast or vice versa? I'm sure that it must occur in both directions."

Candida ◄───► Immunosuppression ◄───► Viral infection

I also sought the opinion of Sidney MacDonald Baker, M.D., who at that time was a member of the Clinical Faculty, Yale Medical School and he commented,

There are general trends toward something interfering with immune function in people in our population." Sidney M. Baker, M.D.

"I think it fairly likely that the yeast problem is more significant than the EBV problem in terms of an original etiologic factor. On the other hand, it is worth considering that there are general trends toward something interfering with immune function in people in our population and antibiotics may not be the whole answer."

Because of the new information I'd learned about the Candida-Related Complex, I wrote and published a much-expanded, updated and revised paperback, third edition in October 1986.

Included in this edition were the comments of Drs. Baker and Cranton and other information about CFS (which was at that time still being referred to as Chronic Epstein-Barr Virus infection, CEBV).

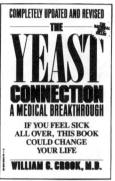

Along with my interest in yeast-connected health problems, my interest in food sensitivities continued. So did my interest in writing. Then in 1988, I completed and published a 220-page illustrated book, *Detecting Your Hidden Allergies*. This book contained simple instructions to carrying out elimination/challenge diets, along with an extensive review of articles in the medical and lay literature which described food-related fatigue, headache, muscle aches and other health problems.

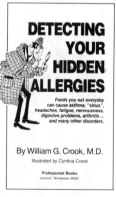

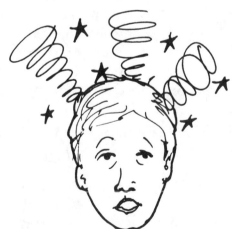

Included in *Detecting Your Hidden Allergies* was a reference to the first chapter of Daniel* in the Old Testament. Daniel and

---

*Daniel, 1:20, Good News Bible: The Bible in Today's English Version (New York); American Bible Society, 1976 pp. 954-55.

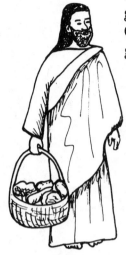

three of his young friends, Shadrach, Meshach and Abednego had been chosen to the court of King Nebuchadnezzar. The King also gave orders that they be given the food and wine of the Royal Court. Daniel, however, did not want the food so he went to the guard who was in charge of him and his three friends and he said,

"Test us for ten days—give us vegetables to eat and water to drink. Then compare us with the young men who are eating the food of the royal court, and base your decision on how we look. . . .

"When the time was up, they looked healthier and stronger than all those who had been eating the royal food. So from then on the guard let them continue to eat vegetables instead of what the king provided.

"At the end of three years, set by the king, Ashpenaz took all the young men to Nebuchadnezzar . . . No matter what question the king asked or what problem he raised, these four knew ten times more than any fortuneteller or magician in his whole kingdom."

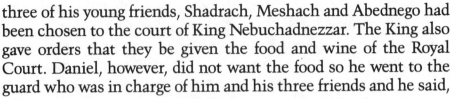

Another ancient reference to the relationship of food to mental and physical fatigue can be found in the writings of Hippocrates who said, "There are certain persons who cannot readily change their diet with impunity. . . . Such persons provided they take dinner when it is not their wont immediately become heavy and inactive both in body and mind."*

During 1987 and 1988, my own observations and those of dozens of other physicians, showed that people with candida-related health problems were sensitive to foods they were eating every day. Common offenders were yeast, milk (and other dairy products), wheat and corn. However, some people were sensitive to other foods, including eggs, legumes, citrus and potato. And also, almost without exception, symptoms were aggravated by

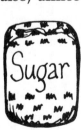 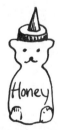 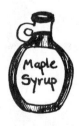 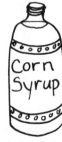

---

*Hippocrates, *On Ancient Medicine* (Adams 1886) as quoted by Iris R. Bell, M.D. Ph.D., Clinical Ecology, *New Medical Approach to Environmental Illness*. Common Knowledge Press, Bolinas, Calif, 1982, p. 7.

sugar, corn syrup, honey, maple syrup and other simple carbohydrates. In many individuals, fruits also caused problems.

Because of my growing awareness of the importance of food sensitivities in patients with the Candida Related Complex, in 1989, with the collaboration of Marjorie Hurt Jones, R.N.*, I wrote and published *The Yeast Connection Cookbook—A Guide to Good Nutrition and Better Health.* Included in this book was a discussion of the importance of diets containing more complex carbohydrates and less fat (especially "bad" fats) and less protein.

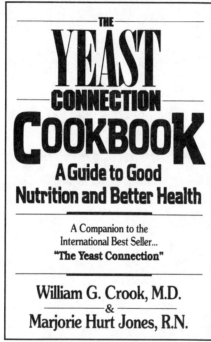

Although a special diet and antifungal medication does not provide a quick fix for every person with fatigue, muscle aches, poor memory and other symptoms which make him feel "sick all over," a comprehensive program featuring a special diet and antifungal medication will help many, and perhaps most, individuals with CFS.

---

*Jones also is the author of *The Allergy Self-Help Cookbook* (Rodale Press) and *Superfood—Allergy Recipes.* She also publishes a newsletter "Mastering Food Allergies." For more information write to MAST Enterprises, Inc., 2615 N. 4th St., Suite 677, Coeur d'Alene, ID 83814.

SECTION II

The Yeast Connection

Are Your Health Problems Yeast Connected?

The common yeast *Candida albicans* normally lives on the mucous membranes of the digestive tract and vagina. So do billions of friendly germs. When you're healthy, these yeasts cause no problems. But when you take antibiotics (especially if you take them repeatedly), birth control pills, the cortisone group of drugs and high sugar diets, yeasts multiply and raise large families.

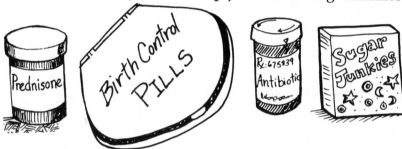

Symptoms that develop from candida overgrowth or infection include vaginal yeast infections, thrush, bloating, constipation, diarrhea and abdominal pain. These same yeasts may also cause other problems. Here are three probable mechanisms:

- You can develop allergic reactions to *Candida albicans*.
- Overgrowth of this yeast in the digestive tract may create what has been called an "intestinal dysbiosis" or a "leaky gut." As a result, more food allergens are absorbed.

 Nutrients

 Normal gut flora

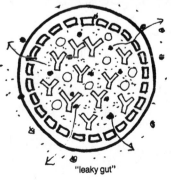
"leaky gut"

 Candida albicans

Toxins and/or food allergins

- Studies by the Japanese researcher, Kazuo Iwata, M.D. (Department of Microbiology, Faculty of Medicine, University of Tokyo), show that *Candida albicans* puts out high and low molecular weight toxins that can weaken your immune system.

Other studies cited by Steven S. Witkin, Ph.D. (Cornell University Medical College), indicate that candida can be involved in the induction of immunosuppression.*

A number of other reports in the medical literature provide support for the relationship of *Candida albicans* to a diverse group of health problems that affect people of all ages and both sexes.**

The possibility (or probability) that your CFS is yeast-connected is based mainly on your history and the response of your symptoms to a special diet and antifungal medication. However, elevation in candida-specific antibodies may provide your physician with additional support for the diagnosis of a candida-related disorder. A number of laboratories carry out these tests.***

More recently, other laboratories are carrying out special studies on the bowel contents obtained by purged stools or by an examination of the rectal mucus. For more information, send a stamped, self-addressed envelope to:

---

*See also Section III.
**Excerpts and abstracts of several of these reports can be obtained from the nonprofit International Health Foundation, Box 3494Y, Jackson, TN 38303. A SASE (two stamps) and a $3 donation is requested. You can also obtain a 263-page compendium entitled "Medical Support for the Candida/Human Interaction," from this foundation. A $15 donation is requested.
***1. Antibody Assay Labs, 805 W. La Veta #210, Orange, CA 92668 (Alan Broughton, M.D.) (714) 538- 3255.
   2. Biological Information Systems, Inc., 101 S. San Mateo Dr., #315, San Mateo, CA 94401 (415) 342-8323 (F.T. Guilford, M.D. and G. DerBalian, Ph.D.).
   3. Cerodex Laboratories, Inc., 2227 W. Lindsey #1401, Norman, OK 73069 (405) 288-2458 (Howard Hagglund, M.D. and David Bauman, Ph.D.) CEIA test is marketed by MEDI-TREND, Inc., Albuquerque, NM, 1-800-545-8900.
   4. Immunodiagnostic Laboratories, 400 29th St., #508, Oakland, CA 94609 (Edward Winger, M.D.) (415) 839-6477.
   5. Immuno Sciences Lab, Inc., 1801 La Cienaga Blvd., Suite 302, Los Angeles, CA 90035 (A. Wojdani, Ph.D.) (213) 287-1884.

Great Smokies Diagnostic Laboratory
18 Regent Park Blvd.
Asheville, NC 28806
800-522-4762
800-833-5524 (in Canada)

Dowell Laboratory
99 S. Hibbert
Mesa, AZ 85210
(602) 964-7151

To tell if your health problems are candida-related, you should:

1. Have a knowledgeable physician carefully review your medical history and carry out examinations and tests to rule out other causes of your symptoms.
2. Review your own history using the questionnaire on the following pages.
3. Follow the trial treatment program briefly outlined in this book.

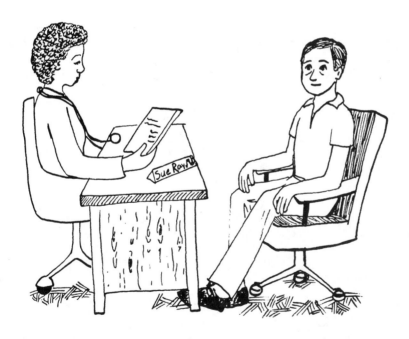

Here's a simple questionnaire that will help you and your physician evaluate the relationship of *Candida albicans* to your health problems. If your answer is "yes" to any question, circle the number in the right hand column. When you've completed the questionnaire, add up the points you've circled. Your score will help you determine the possibility (or probability) that your CFS is yeast connected.

Have you taken repeated or prolonged courses of antibacterial drugs?	4
Are you bothered by recurrent vaginal, prostate or urinary infections?	3
Do you feel worse on damp days or in musty, moldy places?	3
Are you bothered by hormone disturbances, including PMS, menstrual irregularities, sexual dysfunction, sugar craving or low body temperature?	2
Do some foods disagree with you or trigger your symptoms?	2
Have you taken repeated or prolonged courses of prednisone or other steroids?	2
Do you suffer with constipation, diarrhea, bloating or abdominal pain?	1
Are you unusually sensitive to tobacco smoke, perfume, colognes, fabric or odors?	1
Does your skin itch, tingle or burn; or is it unusually dry; or are you bothered by rashes?	1
Have you taken birth control pills for over three years?	1

Scoring for women:

If your score is 8 or more, your fatigue and other health problems are probably yeast connected.

If your score is 12 or more, your fatigue and other health problems are almost certainly yeast connected.

Scoring for men:

If your score is 6 or more, your fatigue and other health problems are probably yeast connected.

If your score is 10 or more, your fatigue and other health problems are almost certainly yeast connected.

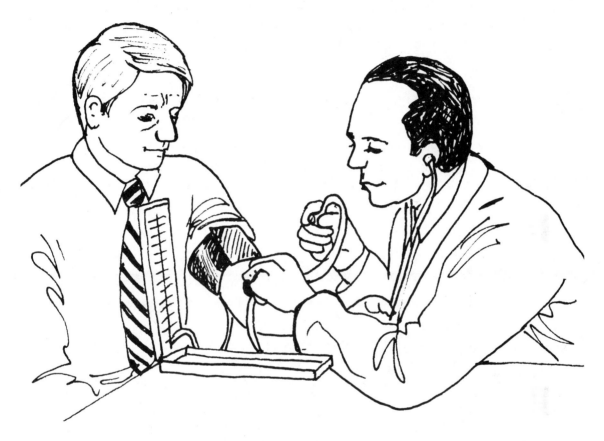

Note: Many of the symptoms listed in this questionnaire may be related to other causes. So, before concluding that your health problems are yeast connected, you should go to your physician for a careful physical examination and appropriate laboratory studies and/or other tests.

As pointed out by Ray C. Wunderlich, M.D. of St. Petersburg, Florida,

"Desirable at all times is a balanced approach that holds a healthy respect of *Candida albicans*. At the same time, one does not wish to overlook the many other health departures that invite the candida syndrome. Those who suspect that they have symptoms due to candida overgrowth must not plunge headlong into a quest for a 'magic bullet.' Best and most long lasting health will be fostered by careful inquiry into yeast, but also, into psychological, nutritional, allergic, degenerative and toxic factors."

Yeasts and How They Make You Sick

What are yeasts?

Yeasts are single-cell organisms that belong to the vegetable kingdom, and like their mold cousins, they live all around you. One family of yeasts, *Candida albicans*, normally lives in your body and, more especially, in your digestive tract. This yeast possesses a number of unique traits, including certain animal-like characteristics. And it must consume other substances such as sugar and fats in order to survive.

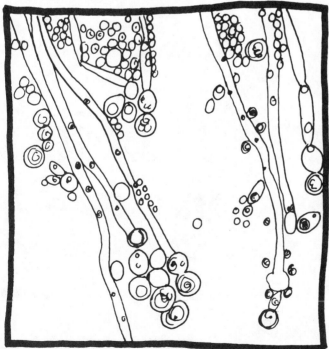

In addition, Candida has been referred to as a "Dr. Jekyll and Mr. Hyde" sort of a critter. Here's why: it can switch from a single-cell yeast form into a branching fungal form. This fungal form can burrow beneath the surfaces of mucous membranes.

Yeasts Normally Live in Your Body

Yeasts normally live on the mucous membranes of the digestive tract and vagina. So do billions of friendly germs. Unfriendly bacteria, viruses, allergens and other enemies also find their way into these and other membrane-lined passageways and cavities. But when your immunity system is strong, they aren't able to break through into your deeper tissues or bloodstream and make you sick.

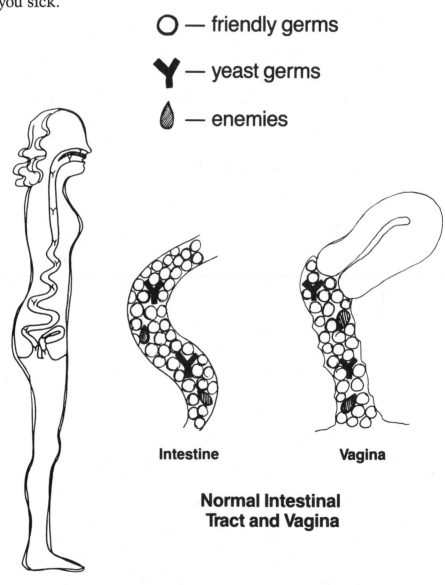

○ — friendly germs

Y — yeast germs

◖ — enemies

Intestine   **Vagina**

**Normal Intestinal
Tract and Vagina**

When Yeasts Multiply They Produce Toxins

When you take antibiotics, especially if you take them repeatedly, many of the friendly germs in your body (especially those in your digestive tract) are "wiped out." Since yeasts aren't harmed by these antibiotics, they spread out and raise large families (the medical term is "colonization").

When yeasts multiply, they produce toxins. Yeast overgrowth in the gut may also play a part in causing food allergies and nutritional deficiencies.

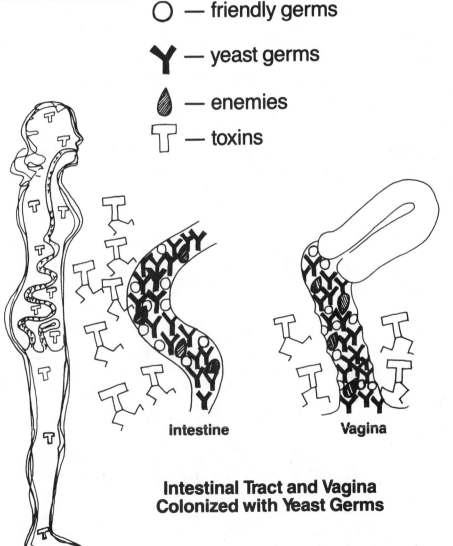

○ — friendly germs

Y — yeast germs

● — enemies

T — toxins

Intestine   **Vagina**

**Intestinal Tract and Vagina
Colonized with Yeast Germs**

About Your Immune System and How It Protects You

 — attackers (enemies)

 — defenders

— mucous membrane

Your immune system is composed of many different defenders, including white blood cells, antibodies and immunoglobulins. Some sit just under the surface of your mucous membranes*— ready to pounce on invaders.

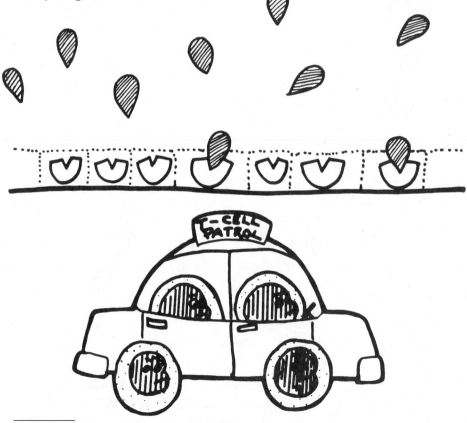

---

*Such a membrane forms the "skin" of the interior cavities of your body (mouth, nose, digestive tract, respiratory tract, vagina, etc.).

Others—including the lymphocytes (a special type of white blood cell)—circulate and patrol the deeper tissues and organs of the body a hundred or more times a day attacking and wiping out enemies that may have sneaked in.

Yeast Toxins Weaken Your Immune System

When your immune system is weak, you're apt to feel "sick all over" and develop yeast and/or fungous infections of the skin, nails or vagina.

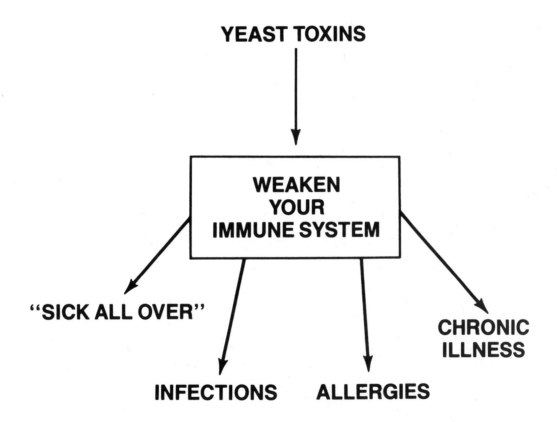

You may also become more susceptible to viral, bacterial and other infections, and develop mold, chemical, food and other allergies, intolerances and sensitivities.

You may also develop other health disorders, including CFS, hives, psoriasis, arthritis, Crohn's disease or multiple sclerosis.

Other Factors Also Weaken Your Immune System

A viral infection may weaken your immune system. Nutritional deficiencies (caused by inadequate intake and/or poor absorption of essential nutrients) may also weaken your immune system.

So does living or working in an environment loaded with chemical pollutants of many types.

A heavy load of environmental mold also adversely affects your immune system. So does emotional stress or deprivation.*

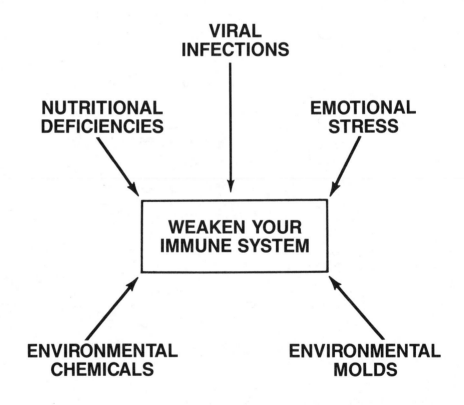

---

*As described by Ronald T. Glasser in his book *The Body Is the Hero*, 1976; Norman Cousins in his books *Anatomy of an Illness* and *The Healing Heart*; and Bernie Siegel in his books, *Love, Medicine and Miracles* and *Peace, Love and Healing*.

Yeast Toxins Make You "Sick All Over"

Yeast toxins affect your immune system, your nervous system, and your endocrine system.* Moreover, these systems are all connected.

So yeast toxins play a role in causing allergies, vaginal, bladder, prostate and other infections, as well as fatigue, headache, memory loss, depression, insomnia and other nervous symptoms. When your endocrine system is adversely affected you may develop menstrual irregularities, PMS, sexual dysfunction, infertility, sugar craving, anxiety, constipation, dry skin, low body temperature and fatigue.

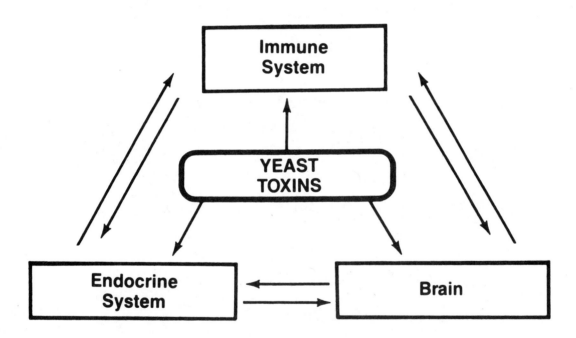

---

*Thyroid, pancreatic, adrenal and sex hormones.

Every Part of Your Body Is Connected to Every Other Part

Obviously (although we sometimes seem to forget it), every part of your body is connected to every other part. So when yeast toxins and allergens affect one part of the body, they're also causing changes in other parts.

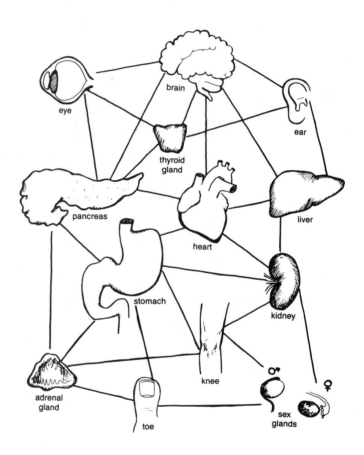

Support For The Yeast Connection to CFS

Searching for the Yeast Connection

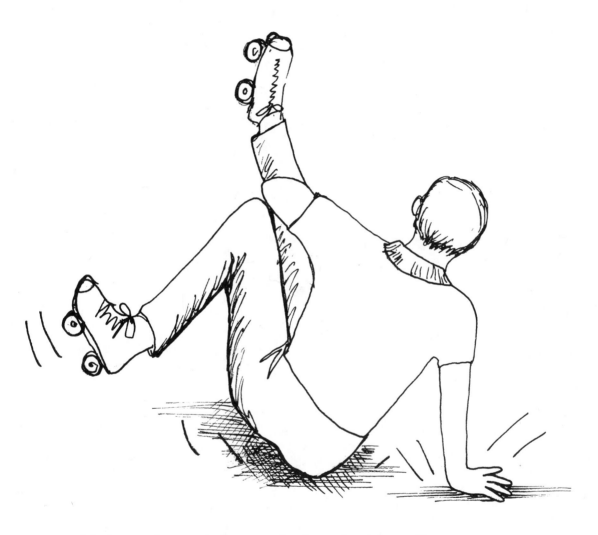

In establishing a diagnosis for a medical condition, you'll sometimes be able to do it easily and quickly. Here are examples: A person falls while roller skating and catches his weight on his hand. He immediately develops pain and swelling just above his wrist and an X-ray shows a fracture. In such a person the diagnosis is made easily.

A similar situation may exist in a person who develops abdominal pain and nausea. Six hours after the pain starts, it moves down to the right lower side of the abdomen. The person goes to a physician, who examines him and finds localized tenderness in the painful area. Simple laboratory studies show that the patient's urine specimen is normal and the white blood count is elevated. In such a patient, the diagnosis of acute appendicitis is easy to make.

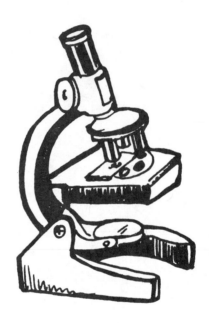

There are many other examples, including the person with a sore throat who shows a positive test for Group A streptococci. And so on.

Yet, sometimes, the trail of events that lead up to a disorder isn't as easy to follow. And in thinking about CFS and the yeast connection, I like to compare the situation to Angela Lansbury's popular television series "Murder, She Wrote."

On these programs you never see the villain killing his victim in the presence of witnesses. Instead, he sneaks up when no one is looking, does the evil deed and steals away. And when Angela tracks down the guilty party, she does a lot of sleuthing.

Clues I've seen her use include mud on shoes, juice stains on a shirt, peculiar tire tracks, rose petals on the floor and lipstick on the collar. *And so it is in tracking down the yeast connection to CFS—you must search for and uncover clues in many different places.* On the following pages, you'll find some of them.

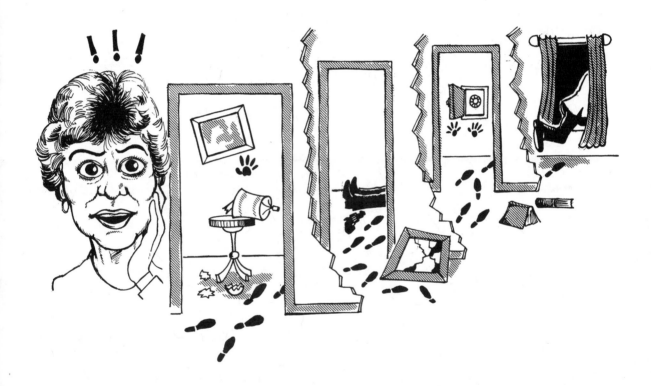

CFS and the Yeast Connection

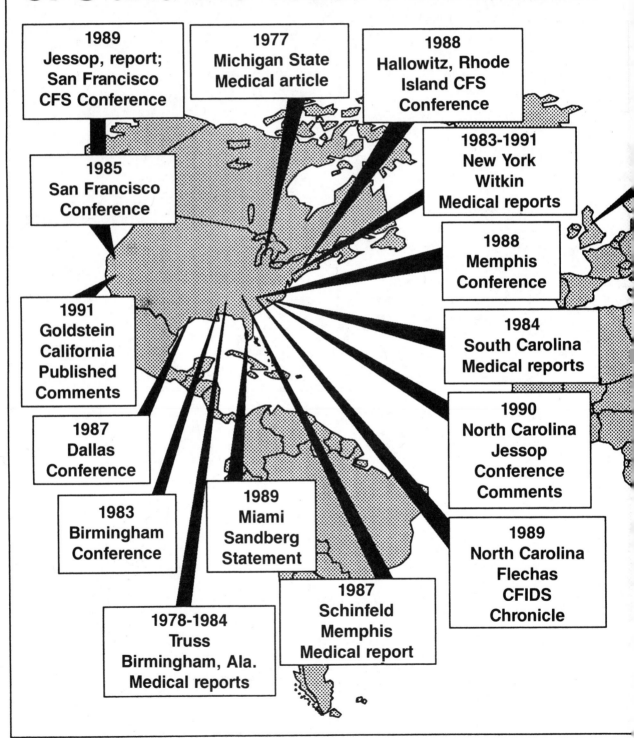

1989
Jessop, report;
San Francisco
CFS Conference

1977
Michigan State
Medical article

1988
Hallowitz, Rhode
Island CFS
Conference

1985
San Francisco
Conference

1983-1991
New York
Witkin
Medical reports

1991
Goldstein
California
Published
Comments

1988
Memphis
Conference

1984
South Carolina
Medical reports

1987
Dallas
Conference

1990
North Carolina
Jessop
Conference
Comments

1983
Birmingham
Conference

1989
Miami
Sandberg
Statement

1989
North Carolina
Flechas
CFIDS
Chronicle

1978-1984
Truss
Birmingham, Ala.
Medical reports

1987
Schinfeld
Memphis
Medical report

A number of people, reports and conferences have described the relationship of *Candida albicans* to CFS and related disorders.

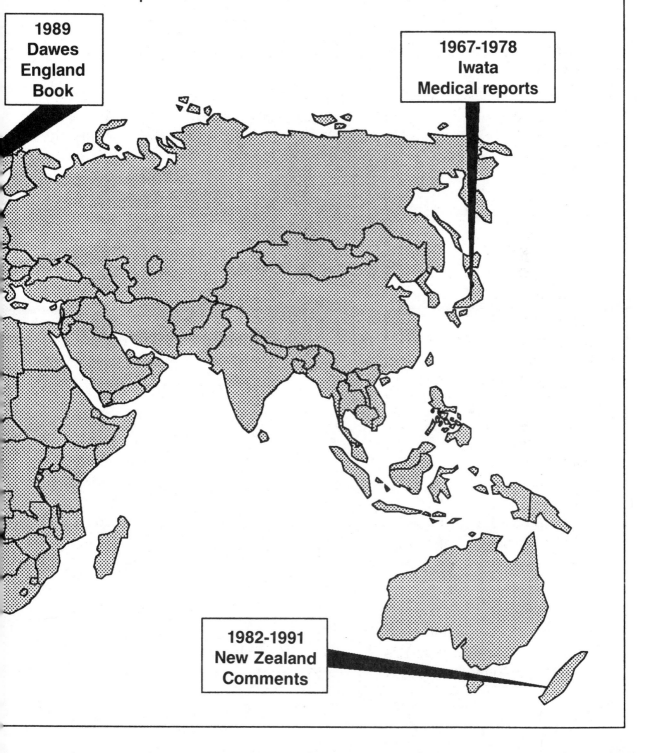

1989
Dawes
England
Book

1967-1978
Iwata
Medical reports

1982-1991
New Zealand
Comments

Candida albicans and The Immune System

Observations of Kazuo Iwata, M.D.

In the late 1960s, a Japanese bacteriologist, Kazuo Iwata, M.D., began studying *Candida albicans*. And in 1967, along with his co-workers, he isolated a potent lethal toxin, *canditoxin*, from a virulent strain of *C. albicans*.* He and his colleagues published their observations on this toxin and its effect on the immune system on several occasions.

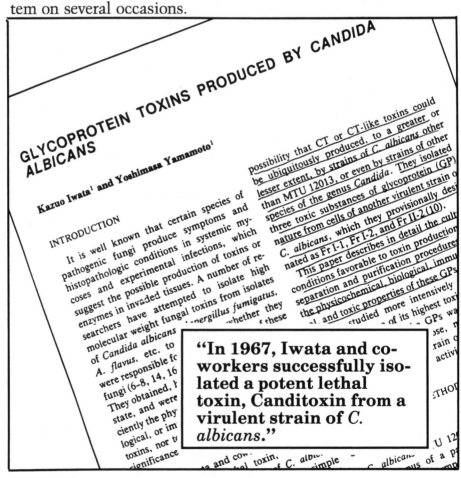

> "In 1967, Iwata and co-workers successfully isolated a potent lethal toxin, Canditoxin from a virulent strain of *C. albicans.*"

*K. Iwata and Y. Yamamoto, Proceedings of the Fourth International Conference on the Mycoses, June 1977, PAHO, Scientific Publication No. 356.

> In case of infection with a virulent strain of *Candida albicans*, a selective decrease in the number of T cells was characteristically noted.

Symposium *Medical Mycology*
Flims, January 1977

mykosen, Suppl. 1, 72 – 81 (1978)
© Grosse Verlag 1978

Department of Microbiology, Faculty of Medicine, University of Tokyo, Japan
(Director: Prof. Dr. K. Iwata)

Cellular Immunity in Experimental Fungus Infections in Mice: The Influence of Infections and Treatment with a Candida Toxin on Spleen Lymphoid Cells

K. Iwata and K. Uchida

Summary

Mice whose cellular immunity was congenitally deficient (athymic nude mice) or artificially lowered by treatment with anti-thymocyte serum or cyclophosphamide were much more susceptible to lethal infections with *Candida albicans*, *Histoplasma capsulatum* and *Fonsecae (Phialophora) pedrosoi* than were untreated normal mice. Germfree mice were susceptible lethal infection with *Histoplasma capsulatum*, but rather resistant to that with *Candida al cans* or *Fonsecaea pedrosoi*.

When normal specific pathogen-free mice were infected with each of these pathogenic fu there occured a marked change in the fractions of certain subpopulations of spleen lymp cells during the course of infection; in the case of infection with a virulent strain of *Can albicans*, a selective decrease in the number of T cells was characteristical.... *In vit* sponsiveness to mitogens of spleen lymphoid cells isolated from ... s varia extent, depending on species of mitogens tested and ... m m canavalin A than comparable ... iven also caused decrease ... gal

When injected ... phoid cells simila This indicates the invaded tissues ma ing cellular immun tion with such toxi

> " ...Upon *Candida albicans* infection the toxin produced in the invaded tissues may act as an immunosuppressant to impair host defense mechanisms involving cellular immunity..."

Résumé

Chez les souris aya... chez celles présentant ... antithymocyte ou cyclo... toplasma capsulatum et . ... normales, non traitées. L... tions léthales à *Histoplas.* *Candida albicans* ou à *Fonsecaea pedrosoi*.

Lorsqu'on a inoculé des champignons pathogènes à des souris normales, i tions spécifiques, il y a eu un changement notable dans une fraction de certa tions des cellules lymphoides de la rate; ceci au cours de l'évolution de l'infe... Après inoculation d'une souche virulente de *Candida albicans* on a r... ... et sélective du nombre de cellules T. Les cellules lym ...

...ns à Candida ...osoi, est plus grande que ... de toute affection ont été plus sens ... ...ulatum, mais ont par contre mieux résisté ...de souris infe

Observations of C. Orian Truss, M.D.

In 1978, C. Orian Truss, M.D., reported in the first of a series of publications that mental and neurologic manifestations could be related to *Candida albicans*. (You'll find a further discussion of Dr. Truss' observations in Section VII.)

In his book *The Missing Diagnosis*,* Dr. C. Orian Truss, describes the histories of a number of his patients with autoimmune diseases who responded to a special diet and anti-yeast medication, nystatin. One of these patients was a 41-year old woman with systemic lupus erythematosus, who was troubled by symptoms which affected many parts of the body. *These included severe fatigue, skin rashes, neurological and musculoskeletal symptoms.* Her ANA (anti-nuclear antibody) fluctuated between 1:80 and 1:320. Here are excerpts from Dr. Truss' report.

"Significantly she had a history of much yeast vaginitis starting at age 19 years, aggravated by antibiotics and by pregnancy . . . constipation and bloating had been present since childhood and she complained bitterly of the loss of memory and concentration so common with chronic yeast infection. Thus, chronic candidiasis had preceded the onset of the lupus by many years . . .

Her response to diet and nystatin can only be described as dramatic.

"Her response to diet and nystatin can only be described as dramatic. In two days her bowel movements were normal and the bloating had cleared. She also described immediate 'clearing of my head', i.e. improvement in memory and concentration. In the first week she lost 7 lbs. of retained fluid, energy was described as 'much better', the arthritis and muscle soreness as 'better but not gone.'

"Two weeks later she reported, 'I'm doing super.' *Energy was described as 'much better' and she told of marked intellectual improvement; 'I can talk and stay on a subject'* . . . The only setback came following antibiotic therapy in association with movement of a kidney stone."

---

*C.O. Truss, *The Missing Diagnosis*, pages 89-90.

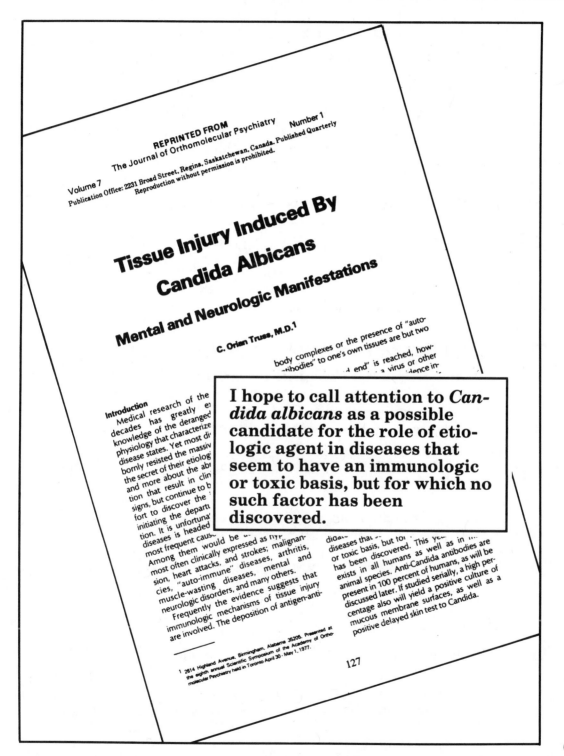

REPRINTED FROM
The Journal of Orthomolecular Psychiatry   Number 1
Volume 7
Publication Office: 2231 Broad Street, Regina, Saskatchewan, Canada. Published Quarterly
Reproduction without permission is prohibited.

Tissue Injury Induced By Candida Albicans

Mental and Neurologic Manifestations

C. Orian Truss, M.D.[1]

...body complexes or the presence of "auto-...ibodies" to one's own tissues are but two ...d end" is reached, how-... a virus or other ...dence in-...

I hope to call attention to *Candida albicans* as a possible candidate for the role of etiologic agent in diseases that seem to have an immunologic or toxic basis, but for which no such factor has been discovered.

Introduction

Medical research of the ... decades has greatly e... knowledge of the derange... physiology that characterize ... disease states. Yet most di... bornly resisted the massiv... the secret of their etiologi... and more about the ab... tion that result in clin... signs, but continue to b... fort to discover the ... initiating the depart... tion. It is unfortuna... diseases is headed ...

Among them would be ... most often clinically expressed as hy... sion, heart attacks, and strokes; malignan-... cies, "auto-immune" diseases, arthritis, muscle-wasting diseases, mental and neurologic disorders, and many others.

Frequently the evidence suggests that immunologic mechanisms of tissue injury are involved. The deposition of antigen-anti-

dise... that ... or toxic basis, but for... has been discovered. This ye... exists in all humans as well as in ... animal species. Anti-Candida antibodies are present in 100 percent of humans, as will be discussed later. If studied serially, a high percentage also will yield a positive culture of mucous membrane surfaces, as well as a positive delayed skin test to Candida.

1 2614 Highland Avenue, Birmingham, Alabama 35205. Presented at the eighth annual Scientific Symposium of the Academy of Orthomolecular Psychiatry held in Toronto April 30 - May 1, 1977.

127

Observations of Steven S. Witkin, Ph.D.

Further observations on the relationship of *Candida albicans* to the immune system were made by Steven S. Witkin, Ph.D., Director, Immunology Division, Department of Obstetrics and Gynecology, Cornell University Medical School, New York. During the past decade Dr. Witkin and his associates have studied many women with recurrent vaginal yeast infections.

In a recent letter to me, Witkin stated,

The evidence is now very good that candida can be involved in the induction of immunosuppression. Steven S. Witkin, Ph.D.

"I think the evidence is now very good that candida can be involved in the induction of immunosuppression, especially in allergic individuals. . . . My studies, dealing solely with vaginal infections have demonstrated that exposure to *Candida albicans*, in some, but not all women, leads to a localized suppression of cell-mediated immunity. This will subsequently increase the woman's susceptibility to candida and other infections.

"Furthermore, if *Candida albicans* is present at the time and location of an allergic response, the symptoms may be more severe due to the ability of candida to synergize with histamine. Treatments aimed at eliminating residual candida, inhibiting the synthesis of Prostaglandin E-2 or preventing allergic responses in susceptible women will sometimes end the cycle of immune suppression and allow the person's immune system to prevent the future growth of candida."

Here's a list of some of the publications on candida vaginal infections by Witkin and his associates:

S.S. Witkin, I.R. Yu, W.J. Ledger, "Inhibition of *Candida albicans*—Induced Lymphocyte Proliferation By Lymphocytes And Sera From Women With Recurrent Vaginitis." *AMJ Obstet. Gynecol.* 1983; 147:809-11.

S.S. Witkin, "Defective Immune Responses In Patients With Recurrent Candidiasis," *Infections In Medicine*, May/June 1985; Pages 129-32.

S.S. Witkin, J. Hirsch, and W.J. Ledger, "A Macrophage Defect In Women With Recurrent Candida Vaginitis And Its Reversal In Vitro By Prostaglandin Inhibitors", *AMJ, Obstet. Gynecol.*, 1986; 155:790-95.

S.S. Witkin, "Immunology Of Recurrent Vaginitis", *AMJ, Reprod. Immunol. Microbiol.,* 1987; 15:34-7.

S.S. Witkin, J. Jeremiah, W.J. Ledger, "A Localized Vaginal Allergic Response In Women With Recurrent Vaginitis," *J. Allergy, Clin., Immunol.,* 1988; 81:412-16.

S.S. Witkin, "Immunologic Factors Influencing Susceptibility To Recurrent Candidal Vaginitis," *Clinical Obstet. & Gyncol.,* Vol. 34, September, 1991.

Women And Chronic Fatigue Syndrome

Why Women Are More Apt to Develop CFS Than Men

CFS is especially apt to affect women between the ages of 20 and 45.

Almost without exception researchers and practicing physicians have found that CFS affects women more often than men. And women between the ages of 20 and 45 seem especially apt to develop this disorder.

Why is there such a gender difference? *Candida albicans* may provide a part of the answer.

- Hormonal changes associated with the normal menstrual cycle encourage yeast colonization.

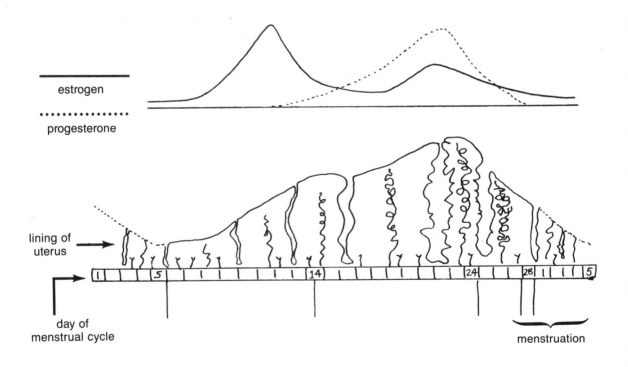

estrogen

••••••••••••••• progesterone

lining of uterus →

day of menstrual cycle

menstruation

• Birth control pills and pregnancy promote yeast overgrowth.

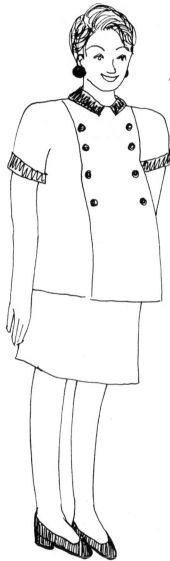

• Yeasts thrive on the warm interior membranes of the body, including the vagina.

• The anatomy of the female urinary tract makes women much more apt to develop urinary infections. Antibiotics (which promote yeast growth) are usually used in treating such infections.

• Women are more apt to establish a relationship with the physician. This may make them more apt to receive antibiotic drugs for respiratory infections.

Vaginal Yeast Infections and CFS

According to recent reports in the press and advertisements on TV and in women's magazines, 22 million American women are affected by recurrent vaginal yeast infections. Moreover, the incidence of these infections appears to be increasing.

The number of people with CFS—especially young women—is also increasing. Is there a connection?

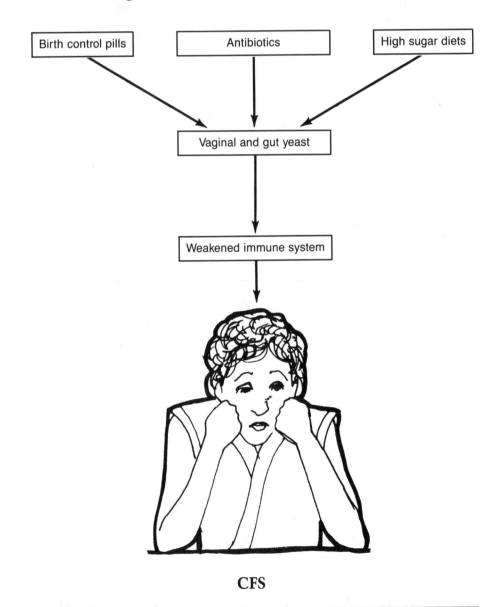

CFS

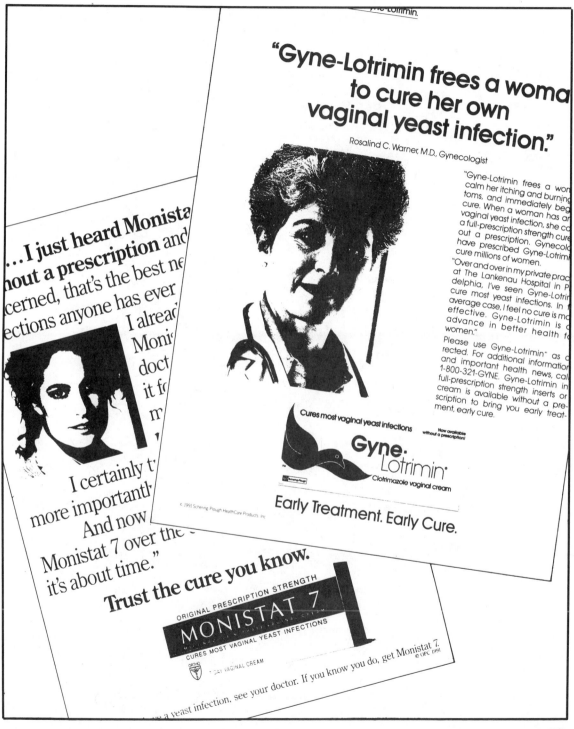

"THINK YEAST" — THE EXPANDING SPECTRUM OF CANDIDIASIS

MARTIN H. ZWERLING, M.D.*
KENNETH N. OWENS, M.D.**
NANCY H. RUTH, R.N., B.S.*

"There are no such things as incurables, there are only things for which man has not found a cure."

Consider the following "i
who is being treated by sev
gynecologist is treating her
and irregular menstrual per
yngologist is trying to cont
and chronic rhinitis. At the
nist is unsuccessfully attem
toms of bloating, indigesti
and a dermatologist is str
rashes, hives and psoriasi
has been unable to con
"nerves" are the cause of her
inability to concentrate and depression.

We have all been guilty of labeling such patients as "psychosomatic" and since there is "nothing physically wrong," conclude we can not cure
them.

Incurable? Not if you THINK YEAST
This patient and thousand
ing from ch

been thought of, or found to be the case of serious
systemic illness.

To Dr. C. Orian Truss[1] must go the credit for
discovering the relationship of the supposedly in-
yeast organism to many chronic
published in 1978, Dr.
every-

into the bloo
is an example of candida ca
dist part of the body.

the last forty years, new advances in med-
e permitted the candida to proliferate in
atients. These recent medical develop-

biotics by prescription and also in our
y can upset the normal gastrointestinal
avor the growth of yeast within us.
ds and *immune-suppressant drugs*
e growth of *Candida albicans.*
ontraceptives as well as *frequent*
can cause an imbalance of hormones
vergrowth of Candida.
edical advances should be added the
recent increased consumption of yeasty foods
such as bread, wine, cheeses and mushrooms,
which add to the imbalance in favor of yeasts.

SYMPTOMS

Most of the symptoms of chronic candidiasis
affect three main parts of the body.

candida.
candida is a common yeast infec-
of the vagina, mucosa and skin, it has rarely

> **Consider the following incurable patient who is being treated by several specialists. Symptoms include recurrent vaginitis ... irritability, inability to concentrate and depression.**

> **We have all been guilty of labeling such patients as "psychosomatic" and since there is "nothing physically wrong," conclude we cannot cure them.**

* Aiken Ear, Nose, Throat and Allergy, P.O. Box 2456, Aiken, S. C. 29801 (address correspondence to Dr. Zwerling).
** 148 Waterloo Street, SW, Aiken, S. C. 29801.

454

The South Carolina Report

In a three-page clinical report in the September 1984 issue of the *Journal of the South Carolina Medical Association*, Martin H. Zwerling, M.D., Kenneth M. Owens, M.D. and Nancy H. Ruth, R.N., B.S., described their experiences in treating 79 private patients with yeast-related health problems. There were 53 women and 26 men, and all were patients from the private practice of the authors. Seventy of these patients had good to excellent results. Four dropped out of the study and were lost to followup, and five showed no improvement.

In introducing their report, these authors emphasized yeast-connected health problems in women, and they stated,

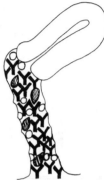

Vagina colonized with yeast germs

"Consider the following 'incurable' patient who has been treated by several specialists. A gynecologist is treating her recurrent vaginitis and irregular menstrual periods while an otolaryngologist is trying to control her external otitis and chronic rhinitis.

"At the same time an internist is unsuccessfully attempting to manage symptoms of bloating, indigestion and abdominal pain and a dermatologist is struggling with bizarre skin rashes, hives and psoriasis.

"Lastly, her psychiatrist has been unable to convince the patient that her 'nerves' are the cause of her extreme irritability, inability to concentrate and depression.

"We have all been guilty of labeling such patients as 'psychosomatic' and since 'there is nothing physically wrong' conclude we cannot cure them.

"Incurable? Not if you THINK YEAST. *This patient and thousands like her are suffering from chronic candidiasis.*"

In discussing yeast-related problems, the authors stated:

Incurable? Not if you THINK YEAST. This patient and thousands like her are suffering from chronic candidiasis.

"Normally the yeast lives in quiet balance with its human host and the usual bacteria inhabiting the mucosal skin and GI tracts and causes no symptoms or apparent harm. However, when this delicate balance is disturbed, the yeasts are free to . . . release their toxins into the blood stream.

"Over the last forty years new advances in medicine have permitted the candida to proliferate in certain patients. These recent developments are:

1. *Antibiotics* by prescription and also in our food supply can upset the normal gastrointestinal flora and favor the growth of yeast within us.

2. *Steroids* and *immunosuppressant* drugs stimulate the growth of *Candida albicans*.

3. *Oral contraceptives*, as well as frequent pregnancies, can cause an imbalance of hormones which favor overgrowth of candida.

The Michigan State University Study

While vaginal suppositories may relieve the symptoms of vaginitis, in many women the problem returns. And a study carried out at Michigan State University on 98 young women who complained of recurrent vaginitis appears to provide an explanation.*

Here's an abstract of the Michigan State Study published in the *Journal of the American Medical Association*:

"To test the hypothesis that all cases of vaginal candidiasis are associated with a 'reservoir' of this organism in the bowel, paired specimens of feces and vaginal material were cultured for *Candida albicans* simultaneously. Ninety-eight young women who complained of recurrent vaginitis were selected in sequence. The results showed that if *C.albicans* was cultured from the vagina, it was always found in the stool.

"Conversely, if it was not isolated from the stool, it was never found in the vagina. These data are presented as an explanation for the recurrent nature of *candida* vaginitis. And thus a cure for vaginitis would not be possible without prior eradication of *C. albicans* from the gut. The gut reservoir concept may well apply to other forms of candidiasis.

In their concluding comments, the authors of this article stated,

Gut yeasts may explain . . . immunological phenomena found in some people.

"Of economic importance is the knowledge that candida vaginitis cannot be cured by vigorously treating the vagina. Millions of consumer dollars are spent yearly in vain in hope of accomplishing this. . . . *Extending the gut reservoir concept may explain other forms of candidiasis and the immunological phenomena found in some people.*" [emphasis added]

---

*M.R. Miles, L. Olsen, and A. Rogers, "Recurrent Vaginal Candidiasis: Importance of an Intestinal Reservoir," *JAMA*, 238:1836-1837, October 28, 1977.

102

159

Recurrent Vaginal Candidiasis

Importance of an Intestinal Reservoir

Mary Ryan Miles, MD; Linda Olsen, MS; Alvin Rogers, PhD

• To test the hypothesis that all cases of vaginal candidiasi~
ated with a "reservoir" of this organism in the bowel. ~~
feces and vaginal material were cultured for ~
neously. Ninety-eight young women who
were selected in sequence. The results s~
tured from the vagina, it was always found
not isolated from the stool, it was never fou
presented as an explanation for the recurre
and thus a cure of vaginitis would not be pos
of C albicans from the gut. The gut-reservoir c~
forms of candidiasis.
(JAMA 238:1836-1837, 1977)

> **Extending the gut reservoir concept, may explain other forms of candidiasis and the immunological phenomena found in some people.**

CANDI~ A ALBICANS is found so
frequer~   ~he gut (stools) of
health   ~~t its presence
in th'   ~ccepted ~~
as ~   ~~
ing
tb
v

> **When C. albicans was cultured from the vagina it was always found in the stool.**

a~~
Vagin~~
become one o~ ~~
forms of vaginitis be~~
quently a recurrent problem~~
sons that some persons present ~~
repeated episodes of vaginitis and
other forms of mucocutaneous candidiasis are not known although precipitating events are known. Cellular
and humoral immunological data are
rapidly accumulating,~~ but as yet,
~~ntributed little knowledge in
~~ ~~genesis or

This pap~~   ~ evidence that
the intestin~ ~cts as a reservoir for C
albicans, where it may live in har-
mony with the rest of the host's fecal
flora. Minor alterations in the milieu
~f the host (ie, pregnancy and inges-
~ broad-spectrum antibiotics)
~~ve from commensal to
~cutaneous sur-
~ites of in-
~s, ie,
per or
results
at vagi-
~ur natu-
~tant pres-
~ the large
is not likely
remains the
bowe~
as long as ~
only treatment ta~~

~~n was used for
~ C albicans. This me-
~esignated to inhibit the growth
~ost micro-organisms but to allow the
growth of Candida species. Yeast growth
is evident as early as 24 hours after inoculation, but optimal growth may be expected between five and seven days when
incubated at 24 C. Approximately 1 gm of
fecal material and swabs containing vaginal specimens were inoculated direc~~y into
the media. Chlamydospore formation on
cornmeal plus polysorbate-80 agar was
used for positive identification of C albicans.

RESULTS

Ninety-eight patients were involved in the study. Fifty-one (52%)
were found to harbor C albicans in
both vagina and fecal material; 46
(47%) were Candida free in both sites
(Table 1). Thus, there was 100% correlation between the presence or absence of C albicans in the feces and
vagina of this population (Table 2).

A review of the patient's clinical
records supported the recurrent nature of candidiasis. In approximately
one third of the patients, there had
been no prior laboratory confirmation

PATIENTS AND METHODS

Patients.—Healthy, nonpregnant, female
patients, 18 to 20 years of age, who pre-

~ Incidence of C Albicans Isolation From Stool and Vagina

		Vagina No. (%)
~~	~~	~~ (52)

The Yeast Connection to PMS

The trail linking *Candida albicans* to PMS, depression and other symptoms leads next to Jay Schinfeld, M.D., Chief, Division of Reproductive Endocrinology and Associate Professor, Department of Obstetrics and Gynecology, Temple University School of Medicine.

In 1984, along with obstetrician/gynecologist John Curlin of Jackson, I paid a visit to Dr. Schinfeld who, at that time, was a member of the faculty of the University of Tennessee School of Medicine. During our visit with Dr. Schinfeld, we told him that we'd seen numerous patients who gave a history of recurrent or persistent vaginitis who then developed fatigue, depression and PMS.

Many of these women developed these symptoms after taking repeated or prolonged course of antibiotic drugs or following the use of birth control pills.

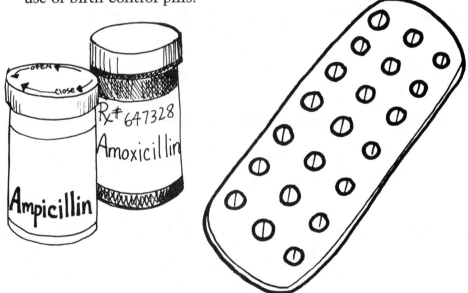

And in our discussions with him we said, "We do not claim to possess a 'quick fix' for all of these patients but we've been delighted at their response to a special diet and the oral antifungal medication, nystatin." Dr. Schinfeld was courteous, but skeptical. And he didn't seem especially interested in what we had to say. Then in the next year, several of his patients with PMS, including two with infertility responded to a special diet and nystatin.

So Dr. Schinfeld began a study on patients in the University of Tennessee PMS Clinic. He published his observations in July 1987* and presented them at the Candida Update Conference in Memphis in September 1988.**

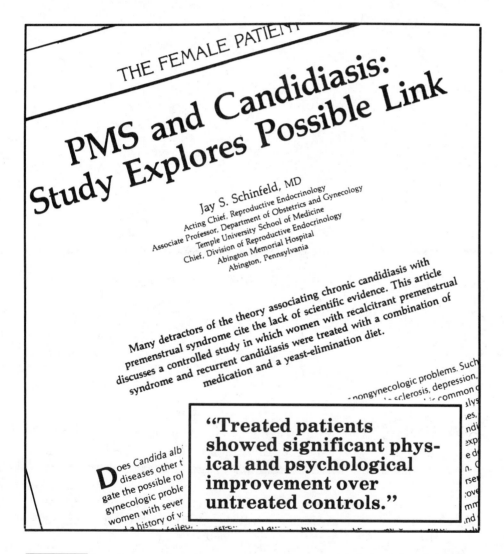

THE FEMALE PATIENT

PMS and Candidiasis: Study Explores Possible Link

Jay S. Schinfeld, MD
Acting Chief, Reproductive Endocrinology
Associate Professor, Department of Obstetrics and Gynecology
Temple University School of Medicine
Chief, Division of Reproductive Endocrinology
Abington Memorial Hospital
Abington, Pennsylvania

Many detractors of the theory associating chronic candidiasis with premenstrual syndrome cite the lack of scientific evidence. This article discusses a controlled study in which women with recalcitrant premenstrual syndrome and recurrent candidiasis were treated with a combination of medication and a yeast-elimination diet.

"Treated patients showed significant physical and psychological improvement over untreated controls."

*J. Schinfeld, "Possible Links of Chronic Candidiasis to PMS and Infertility," *The Female Patient*, pp. 66-73, July 1987.
**This conference was sponsored by the nonprofit International Health Foundation. A 263-page compendium, "Medical Support for the Candida/Human Interaction" (which contains abstracts of all the presentations at this conference, plus reprints, articles and commentaries from the medical literature) is available from this foundation. To order send a check for $20 to IHF, Box 3494, Jackson, TN 38303.

Symptoms present in Dr. Schinfeld's patients included depression, migraine, fatigue, anxiety, anger, loss of libido, mood swings, bloating and food cravings.

Here's a summary of Dr. Schinfeld's observations:

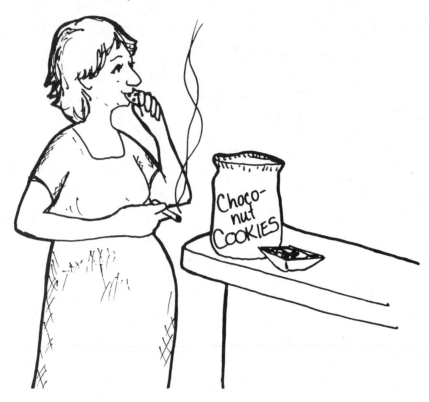

All women in the study had premenstrual syndrome and had not responsed to previous medical or psychological therapy.

"We performed a study at the University of Tennessee in which 32 women with severe premenstrual syndrome and a history of vaginal candidiasis for whom prior standardized therapy had failed were treated with oral anti-candida agents and yeast elimination diets.

"Treated patients showed significant physical and psychological improvement over untreated controls, although the mechanism for this improvement and the role of yeast in this disorder remained controversial."

"Further anecdotal reports have suggested that treatment of chronic candidiasis has resulted in prompt cessation of infertility. In addition to the obvious relief of local vaginal soreness, a discussion of possible alterations in immune mechanisms that might result in improved conception rates were discussed."

Conferences for Professionals on the Yeast/Human Interaction

Research studies and clinical reports presented at conferences in Alabama, California, Tennessee and Texas have provided support for the relationship of *Candida albicans* to a diverse group of health problems.

The Birmingham Conference

In December 1983, the Critical Illness Research Foundation, Birmingham, Alabama, sponsored a symposium to exchange ideas about the chemistry, immunology, microbiology, diagnosis and therapy of imbalances in the relationship between humans and the yeast—of their flora, food and environment.

Faculty members included John Rippon, Ph.D., University of Chicago, who discussed the ecology of yeasts and other fungi; E. W. Rosenberg, M.D., University of Tennessee, who discussed skin flora and inflammation; Kazuo Iwata, M.D., who discussed yeast toxins and the chemotherapy of yeast infections.

C. Orian Truss, M.D., discussed the laboratory assessment of chronic candidiasis, and Max D. Cooper, M.D., University of Alabama, discussed T-lymphocytes and yeast flora—Friends or Foes? A number of other physicians also made presentations. Sidney M. Baker, M.D., provided an overall summary of the conference.

The San Francisco Conference

A second conference on the yeast/human interaction was held in San Francisco in March 1985. Like the Birmingham conference, it was sponsored by the Critical Illness Research Foundation. Participants included Truss, Rosenberg, Baker and a number of other professionals, including Steven S. Witkin, Ph.D., of Cornell Medical School, who spoke on endocrine antibodies in patients with candidiasis and lymphocyte inhibition in patients with candidiasis. Sidney M. Baker, M.D., again served as conference moderator.

The Dallas and Memphis Conferences

A third conference, sponsored by the International Health Foundation, Inc., was held in Dallas in February 1987. And a fourth conference, sponsored by this Foundation was held in Memphis in September 1988. Here's a brief review of some of the presentations: Robert Skinner, M.D., University of Tennessee, discussed the role of yeast in seborrheic dermatitis and psoriasis; Jean Monro, M.D., London, England, described the role of candida in the post-viral syndrome; Jay Schinfeld, M.D., Temple University discussed the possible link of chronic candidiasis to PMS and infertility.

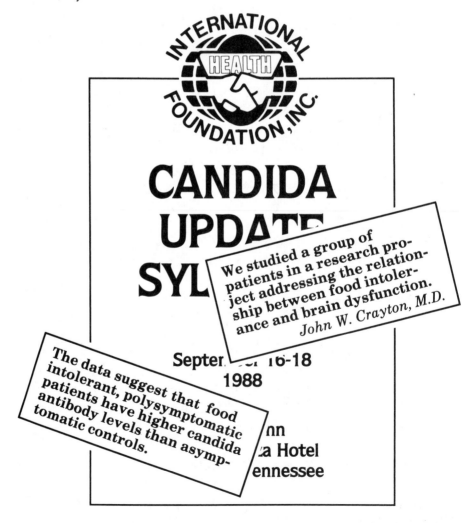

INTERNATIONAL HEALTH FOUNDATION, INC.

CANDIDA UPDATE SYL

We studied a group of patients in a research project addressing the relationship between food intolerance and brain dysfunction.
John W. Crayton, M.D.

September 16-18
1988

The data suggest that food intolerant, polysymptomatic patients have higher candida antibody levels than asymptomatic controls.

nn
a Hotel
ennessee

A number of conference participants presented clinical observations and others described laboratory studies in patients with candidiasis. George Kroker, M.D., suggested the term Candida Related Complex to describe patients with this common disorder.

One of the speakers, John W. Crayton, M.D., Professor of Psychiatry, Loyola Medical School, presented clinical and laboratory observations which provided support for the relationship of *Candida albicans* to fatigue, headache, depression and other symptoms. Here are excerpts from the abstract of Dr. Crayton's presentation:

"Reports have emerged which associate adverse reactions to foods with the presence of an overgrowth of *Candida albicans*. The diagnosis is usually made on the basis of a clinical picture characterized by fatigue, weakness, depression and a variety of somatic problems which may involve every organ system . . . We studied a group of patients recruited for a research project addressing the relationship between food intolerance and brain dysfunction. The 28 subjects ranged in age from 18 to 45; 20 were women and 8 were men.

"For inclusion in the study, all subjects had to report a significant history of psychological and neurological dysfunction, as well as a convincing history of exacerbations of symptoms following ingestion of food.

"Antibody responses to *Candida albicans* were determined for three antibody classes, IgG, IgA and IgM in an ELISA system. *Symptomatic subjects had significantly higher anti-candida antibodies of the IgG and IgA classes compared with controls.* . . The data suggest that food-intolerant, polysymptomatic subjects have higher antibody levels to candida antibodies than asymptomatic controls. These findings could indicate an enhanced immunologic reactivity to candida."

I was excited to hear the Crayton presentation because his studies provided laboratory confirmation for the relationship of candida to fatigue, weakness, depression and other symptoms. They also provided further support for the role food sensitivities contribute to CFS.*

Chronic Epstein-Barr Virus Syndrome (CEBV)
Chronic Fatigue Syndrome (CFS)
Chronic Fatigue and Immune Dysfunction Syndrome (CFIDS)

RHODE ISLAND PRESENTS

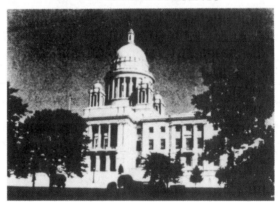

Governor's First Annual East Coast Symposium
EDWARD D. DiPRETE, GOVERNOR

October 22, 1988
Newport Marriott
25 America's Cup Avenue
Newport, R.I.

Co-Sponsored By:
R.I. General Assembly
R.I. Department of Health
Brown University Program
*   in Medicine*

*For a further discussion of food sensitivities and chronic fatigue, see Sections I and V.

Support from Other Professionals

Observations by Robert Hallowitz, M.D.

The next step in the CFS/yeast connection trail came in September 1988. At that time, Agnes Jonas, a "networking friend" from Connecticut, called and said, "Dr. Crook, a CFS conference is being held in Rhode Island. I think you'll be interested in this conference for many reasons. Here's one of them. Robert Hallowitz, one of the conference participants, will make a presentation which provides support for the yeast connection to CFS."

After talking to Agnes, I decided to attended the conference. Other speakers at the conference included Drs. Anthony L. Komaroff, James F. Jones and Paul E. Cheney. These speakers presented their clinical and research findings and the observations of others in dealing with CFS. In general, emphasis was placed on the role of viruses, including the Epstein-Barr and HHV6 viruses.

Dr. Hallowitz presented a different point of view. He said,

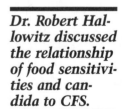

"There are at least four areas of immune hyperresponsiveness which are responsible for the emergence of the 'viral dimension.'

- *"Hidden food sensitivities*. Such sensitivities differ from true allergies and must be identified by elimination diets. Food related symptoms include fatigue, attention deficits, mood swings, joint and muscle aches and migraine.

- *"Overgrowth of the common yeast Candida albicans* which is encouraged by repeated or prolonged courses of antibiotic drugs, steroids or birth control pills. While this hypothesis is 'controversial', many people with CFS will respond to nystatin, acidophilus and the dietary restriction of sugar, white starch and alcohol.

Dr. Robert Hallowitz discussed the relationship of food sensitivities and candida to CFS.

111

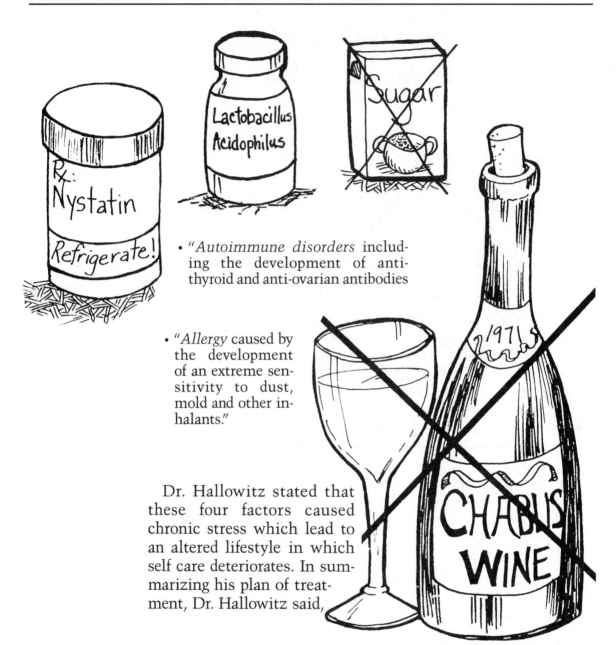

• "*Autoimmune disorders* including the development of anti-thyroid and anti-ovarian antibodies

• "*Allergy* caused by the development of an extreme sensitivity to dust, mold and other inhalants."

Dr. Hallowitz stated that these four factors caused chronic stress which lead to an altered lifestyle in which self care deteriorates. In summarizing his plan of treatment, Dr. Hallowitz said,

CFS is very manageable in the majority of cases.

"I employ a wide diversity of therapeutic programs individually tailored to the patient's needs. Using such a program . . . about 70% of my patients return to at least 75% to 80% of normal. It is my firm belief that this syndrome is very manageable in the majority of cases."

The San Francisco Chronic Fatigue Conference

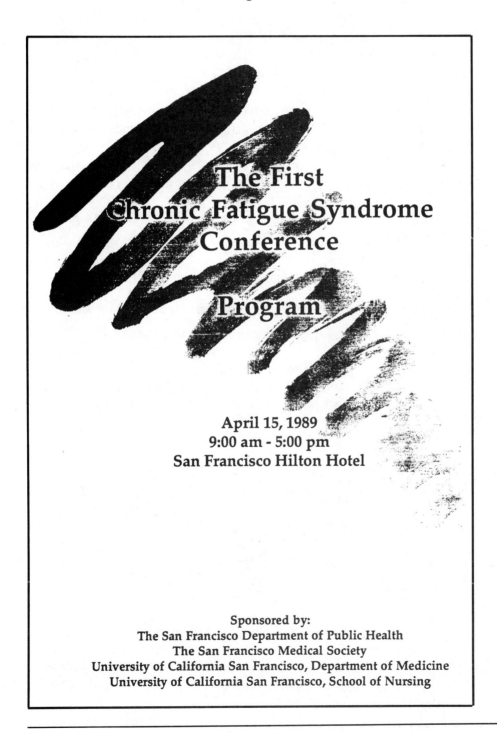

The First
Chronic Fatigue Syndrome
Conference

Program

April 15, 1989
9:00 am - 5:00 pm
San Francisco Hilton Hotel

Sponsored by:
The San Francisco Department of Public Health
The San Francisco Medical Society
University of California San Francisco, Department of Medicine
University of California San Francisco, School of Nursing

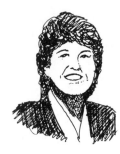

Observations of Carol Jessop, M.D.

The CFS/yeast connection trail next led to California. A couple of months after the Rhode Island conference, the late Phyllis Saifer, M.D., of Berkeley, California, called and said, "A CFS conference will be held in San Francisco in April. I think you'll be especially interested in this conference because a friend of mine, Dr. Carol Jessop, will be presenting exciting information about the response of her CFS patients to a sugar-free special diet and Nizoral (ketoconazole).

I attended this conference on April 15, 1989, along with 500 professionals and nonprofessionals. Conference speakers (in addition to Dr. Jessop) included Paul Cheney, M.D., Ph.D.; James F. Jones, M.D.; Anthony Komaroff, M.D.; Jay A. Levy, M.D.; and other professionals who have been on the cutting edge in studying and treating CFS.

In her presentation, Dr. Jessop, an assistant clinical professor, UCSF, and an internist in private practice in El Cerrito, California, described her findings in 1,100 patients with CFS.

Here's a report of Dr. Jessop's presentation:*

"Internist Carol Jessop, a private practitioner in El Cerrito, California, who is following 1100 patients with CFS, believes the illness would be more aptly called 'chronic devastation syndrome.'"

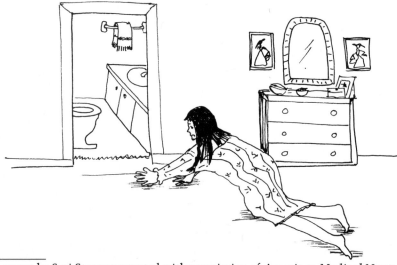

---

*A report by Sari Staver excerpted with permission of *American Medical News*, copyright 1989, American Medical Association.

"In many instances, said Dr. Jessop, CFS patients became so ill that they had to crawl to the bathroom.

"According to Dr. Jessop, 80% of her patients had recurrent ear, nose and throat infections as children; had acne as adolescents; had recurrent hives, anxiety attacks, headaches and bowel problems; and had to stop drinking alcohol because it didn't agree with them. Ninety percent had cholesterol levels higher than 225.

"Beginning last year, Dr. Jessop treated 900 of her CFS patients with ketoconazole, a drug used to treat candidiasis, and placed them on a sugar-free diet. Since then, 529 have returned to their previous health and another 232 have shown improvement.

"Dr. Jessop said that her patients have taught her about CFS. She said, 'I didn't learn it in medical school. She urged more physicians to listen to complaints from fatigued patients. It's important that the patients feel they're in control.'

Dr. Jessop urged physicians to listen to their patient's complaints.

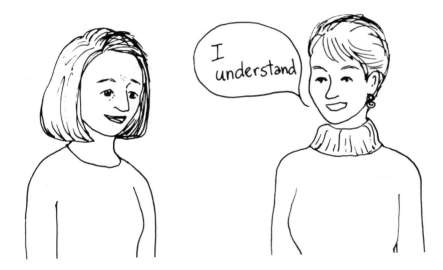

"If patients are also seeking help from alternative health practitioners, such as body workers or acupuncturists', Dr. Jessop says she doesn't discourage them.

"Often she says such patients 'feel abandoned' by the traditional medical community. 'Keep up a dialogue with your patients', Dr. Jessop urged.'"

Observations by Jorge Flechas, M.D.

The CFS/yeast connection trail next led to North Carolina. After the San Francisco conference, I became more and more interested in CFS. And I began to receive the *CFIDS Chronicle,* the publication of the CFIDS Association, Inc., (P.O. Box 220398, Charlotte, NC 22228-0398). In the Summer/Fall 1989 issue of the *CFIDS Chronicle* (pages 40-42), Jorge D. Flechas, M.D., M.P.H., Hendersonville, North Carolina, in an article, "Yeast and the CFIDS Patient" said, "In our CFIDS population we've found overgrowth of *Candida albicans* on the mucous tissues of the body to be a common occurrence. This overgrowth is seen primarily as a yeast infection of the mouth (oral thrush), recurrent vaginal yeast infections and mycotic enteritis, with irritable bowel syndrome."

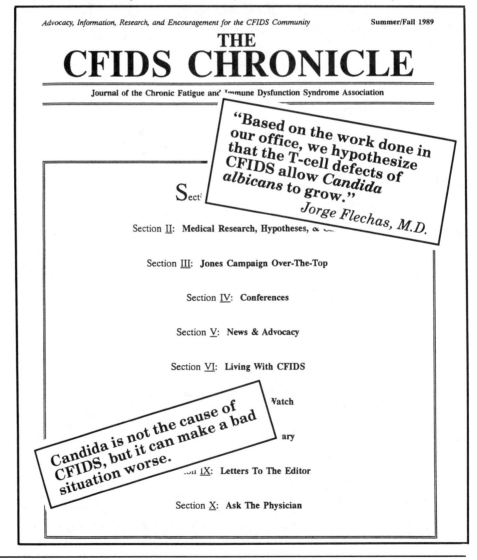

Advocacy, Information, Research, and Encouragement for the CFIDS Community   Summer/Fall 1989

THE
CFIDS CHRONICLE

Journal of the Chronic Fatigue and Immune Dysfunction Syndrome Association

"Based on the work done in our office, we hypothesize that the T-cell defects of CFIDS allow *Candida albicans* to grow."
— *Jorge Flechas, M.D.*

Section I:

Section II: Medical Research, Hypotheses, & ...

Section III: Jones Campaign Over-The-Top

Section IV: Conferences

Section V: News & Advocacy

Section VI: Living With CFIDS

Candida is not the cause of CFIDS, but it can make a bad situation worse.

Watch

ary

Section IX: Letters To The Editor

Section X: Ask The Physician

In his continuing discussion, Dr. Flechas pointed out that it is mainly the T-cells that are responsible for viral and fungal surveillance, and he said, "Based on the work done in our office, we hypothesize that the T-cell defects of CFIDS allow *Candida albicans* to grow."

In discussing treatment, Dr. Flechas emphasized the importance of limiting access of the yeast to refined carbohydrates because they're known to increase the adhesion of the yeast cell to the epithelial cells of the body. He also discussed the various antifungal drugs, including nystatin and Nizoral, and he concluded his 2½ page commentary with these remarks: "Candida is not the cause of CFIDS, but it can make a bad situation worse. It is important that an aggressive anti-yeast program be in place for the CFIDS patient until his/her immune system returns to its normal state."

Observations by Douglas H. Sandberg, M.D.

Interest in and support for the relationship of *Candida albicans* to a diverse group of health problems was expressed by Douglas H. Sandberg, M.D., Professor of Pediatrics, University of Miami, in a statement dated September 22, 1989.

Here are excerpts from Dr. Sandberg's statement:

"The association of a wide range of systemic clinical manifestations with an unusual degree of colonization by *Candida albicans* was suggested first by Truss in 1978. . . . The concept appealed to a variety of groups of medical practitioners . . . who began to look for this problem and to treat patients according to the methods developed by Truss. . . .

"As treatment of this putative entity became more prevalent, the relative lack of scientific data supporting the concept has provoked controversy regarding its validity. Those physicians who began to recognize and treat patients with this disorder began to confirm through their own experiences the validity of this diagnosis. . . . For them it would be very difficult to forego treatment of the disorder until further investigations provide further scientific support for existence of this illness.

". . . Confirmation of the diagnosis remains difficult, evaluation of efficacy of therapeutic measures incomplete; and tools for monitoring of therapeutic response below standard we have come to expect in modern medical practice. . . .

It is important that an aggressive anti-yeast program be in place for the CFIDS patient until his/her immune system returns to its normal state. Jorge D. Flechas, M.D., MPH

117

"In spite of these shortcomings, I am convinced that this disorder exists and that it is important. It must be considered in differential diagnosis of patients with a variety of chronic complaints. Since diagnosis at times can be made only through determining response to a therapeutic trial some patients will have to be treated without a firm diagnosis prior to institution of therapy.

"It is vitally important that this concept not be used to casually treat for 'Chronic Candidiasis' any patient with a poorly defined medical problem. It is essential that other important diagnoses be considered before diagnosis of candida-related illness is made . . . . The potential importance of candida-related illness demands intensive research into all aspects of its diagnosis and treatment."

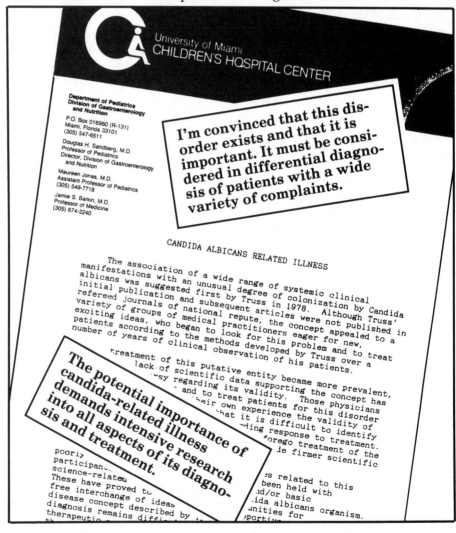

Support from Other Countries

Even before CEBV (Chronic Epstein-Barr Virus Infection), CFS and CFIDS were widely publicized in the United States, professionals and nonprofessionals in the United Kingdom, Canada, Australia and New Zealand were concerned about "M.E." and had noted a yeast connection to this illness.

Comments from New Zealand*

In 1982, Toni Jeffreys discussed the relationship of *Candida albicans* to M.E. In her commentary she included quotations from Orian Truss' article in the *Journal of Orthomolecular Psychiatry* in which he discussed the effects of candida on the immune system. She also briefly reviewed the treatment measures recommended by Dr. Truss:

- A diet low in carbohydrates and yeasty foods
- The avoidance of antibiotics and contraceptive hormones
- The avoidance of environments high in mold and mildew
- Oral nystatin

And she said that such a treatment program "offers hope for some of us, as it is much easier to chase and kill off a fungal infection than a virus."

> *It is much easier to kill off a fungal infection than a virus.*

In a subsequent article in *Meeting-Place* entitled "A Trial Use of Nystatin for Presumed Gastrointestinal Candidiasis,"** the author in discussing antiyeast therapy stated, "By 1983, several chronically ill members of ANZMES had tried it with highly successful results and it was *the first treatment they had tried which gave a relatively simple and rapid improvement.*"

During the past several years other articles, commentaries and letters published in the New Zealand journal, *Meeting-Place* have provided support for the yeast connection to CFS. Yet, the editor Jim Brook also presented both sides of the candida controversy on

---

*From Mediate 11, December, 1982 as cited in *Meeting-Place 35,* January 1991, page 10.
**You'll find a further discussion of this journal in Section IX.

a number of occasions, including a comprehensive 34-page discussion in *Meeting-Place 35*, January 1991.

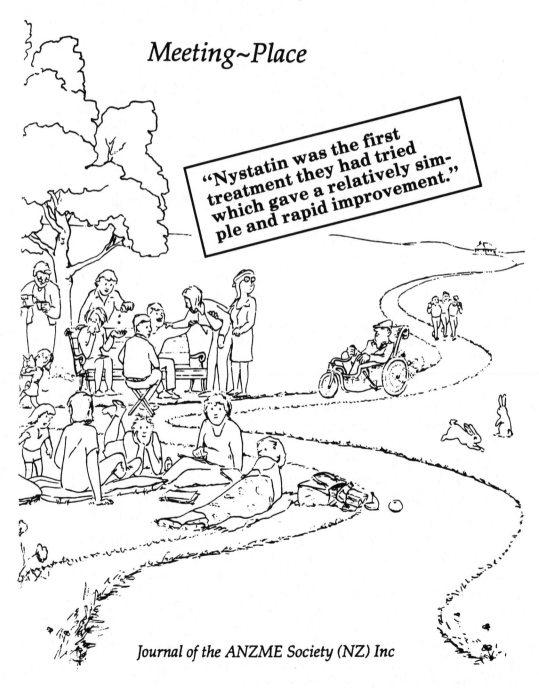

Meeting~Place

"Nystatin was the first treatment they had tried which gave a relatively simple and rapid improvement."

Journal of the ANZME Society (NZ) Inc

In February 1988, another New Zealander, Dianne M. Gunn, in her 90-page book, *Out of the Maze—A Holistic Approach to the M.E. Syndrome** discussed the relationship of *Candida albicans* to M.E. In the preface to her book she said, "My initial experience of M.E. was like being in a maze of pain, depression and despair—a maze from which there was no escape. During a second horrific relapse, I have explored the many pathways and know there can be a way out. This book is an attempt to share my experience with you."

In her book, Ms. Gunn describes the typical history of the person afflicted with M.E. and then describes the multiple treatment measures which had helped her and others regain their health. Included in her book was a chapter entitled *"Candida albicans in Illness."* In it she said,

> "Why a chapter on candida in a book on M.E.? Dr. E. W. Goringe says that recent research points more and more to the involvement of candida in M.E. A conservative estimate has put it at 50% of M.E. patients having a candida problem, but it is possibly a lot more . . . . My own experience and those of other M.E. sufferers suggest that candida should be considered a possibility . . . . By dealing with the candida problem you will be unloading the immune system and enabling it to better recover its vital function in fighting M.E."

By dealing with the candida problem, your immune system will be better able to fight M.E.

Comments from Canada

Some thirty years ago, John W. Gerrard, M.D., professor of pediatrics, University of Saskatchewan, noted that many of his patients showed adverse reactions to common foods. And in his 1973 book *Understanding Allergies*, he described children with bedwetting, migraine, recurrent abdominal pain and other problems which were relieved following the elimination of one or more common foods from the child's diet.

He also talked about the relationship of foods to reactions involving the nervous system, including hyperactivity, irritability, fatigue and drowsiness. Here are excerpts from his book,

> "At first I found it hard to believe that harmless foods could so change a child's personality; but many parents have made confir-

*D.M. Gunn, *Out of the Maze*, Bay of Plenty M.E. Support Group, Inc., Bay of Plenty MS Society, Inc. combined, 13 Tynan St., Te Puke, New Zealand, 3071.

121

matory or unsolicited observations, and I am now fully convinced that in ways we do not yet understand, the allergic child's, and adult's too, behavior can be altered and modified as dramatically by foods as it can be altered by drugs. The following examples indicate the bizarre nature of these problems. A medical student . . . has to avoid food containing corn because corn makes him so drowsy he can hardly keep his eyes open."

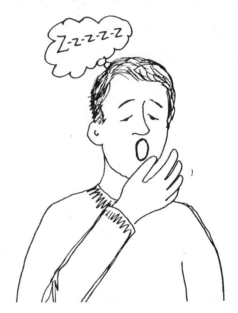

Dr. Gerrard also told about "an internist who has found that he has to avoid foods containing egg and wheat because these two foods make him irritable." Another example was a 9-year old who behaved normally on a restricted diet. But when this child ate chocolate, she developed nose bleeds, tantrums, insomnia, bed-wetting, dark circles under her eyes, stomach ache, headache and fatigue.

During the past decade, Dr. Gerrard has developed an interest in the Chronic Fatigue Syndrome. And with some of his colleagues at the University of Saskatchean, he has sought to obtain funds to study patients with CFS using nystatin and a special diet. Here are comments he made recently:

Patients with the chronic fatigue syndrome and the yeast connection have many symptoms in common.

"Patients with the chronic fatigue syndrome and the yeast connection have many symptoms in common. They also have this in common, that there is no single test or series of tests to prove that the patient has either of these disorders.

"I think that fatigue in the normal individual is triggered when the patient needs to rest if he is to recover from his illness. It is the body's way of telling him to take things easy if he wants to get better. Treatment of his primary disease leads to recovery and to a return of his vitality.

"The person with the Chronic Fatigue Syndrome and the yeast connection seems to be unnecessarily fatigued. Fatigue seems to be hindering his recovery. In the absence of any wonder drug to restore his vitality, we must set about finding the cause of as many of his symptoms as we can.

"With a little careful sleuthing, we can find out what is causing his nasal stuffiness, his headaches, his spells of bloating, his diarrhea, his constipation and his muscle and joint pains. Foods, environmental chemicals and candida are often to blame. By sorting out these problems, we can at least put him on the road to recovery."

By sorting out these problems, we can at least put him on the road to recovery.

Comments from England

During the mid-1980s while in London, I met Belinda Dawes, a physician who had been educated in Australia. The following year my wife Betsy, my daughter Cynthia and I saw Belinda in New York. During our visit, we discussed medical topics of mutual interest including food sensitivities, environmental illness and the Candida-Related Complex. Subsequently, Belinda began recommending *The Yeast Connection* and several of my other publications to her patients.

About two years later, during another visit to London, I saw Belinda again. And she said,

"I'm seeing dozens of patients with M.E . . . . so many that I'm writing a book on the subject which will be published later this year. Moreover, I'm now the assistant medical advisor to the M.E. Association and medical advisor to the M.E. Action Campaign. I also run two clinics in London for M.E. patients."

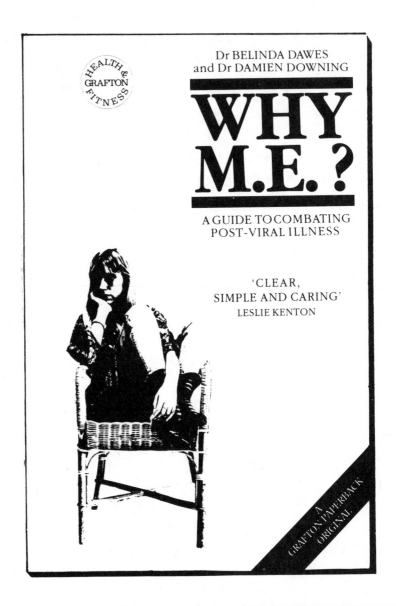

Dr BELINDA DAWES
and Dr DAMIEN DOWNING

HEALTH & FITNESS
GRAFTON

WHY M.E. ?

A GUIDE TO COMBATING
POST-VIRAL ILLNESS

'CLEAR,
SIMPLE AND CARING'
LESLIE KENTON

A GRAFTON PAPERBACK ORIGINAL

Late in 1989 I received a copy of *Why M.E.?* by Drs. Belinda Dawes and Damien Downing. Included in this interesting book were chapters on Immune Dysfunction, Food Allergies, Nutritional Therapy, The World We Live In, Parasites and Candida, Candida, The Losing Battle, Winning the Candida Battle and Live to Recover.

I was, of course, delighted to see that Belinda discussed the yeast connection to M.E. Here's an excerpt of her comments.

"I have been treating candida for about 5 years now and have seen over a thousand patients suffering from various candida-related illnesses. When I first heard about the role of Candida infections in humans from Dr. Billy Crook . . . I was fairly skeptical but quite excited about it in the hope that I might find a patient for whom this treatment was relevant and whom I was able to help.

"I remember Billy saying to me that once you start to treat candida, 90% of your patients will have it. I looked at him rather amusedly and thought that it might be the case for him but would not be for me; However, I would now say that *without doubt, candida infection plays a role in the ill health of almost all patients I see. Although their illness may not be directly related to the candida problem, eliminating candida from their body and its related consequences has certainly been one of the factors in their recovery."*

> *Without doubt, candida infection plays a role in the ill health of almost all patients I see.*

I received a letter from Belinda in November 1991 just as the manuscript of this book was going to the typesetter. She said,

"Thank you very much for the information on your new book . . . It looks very interesting. The only piece of information I would add is that I have been using Diflucan for the last few months in treating candida and have exceptional results. I have also found no side effects."

More Support from England

In a September 3, 1991, letter to me, Dr. David Dowson, Hampshire, England, said,

"As far as candida is concerned I am now of the opinion that probably 60% of patients with Chronic Fatigue Syndrome have candida to some extent. Our approach to candida is now multiple with both dietary, orthodox medication and homeopathic medication combined. We have found that amphotericin is the antifungal treatment of choice, but I believe that it is not readily available in America."

Other Comments About CFS and the Yeast Connection

Comments by David S. Bell, M.D.

In his book, *The Disease of a Thousand Names*, * David S. Bell, M.D., F.A.A.P, reviewed the many complex factors that affect the immune system in individuals with CFIDS. And he pointed out that viruses of different types are present in larger than normal amounts . . . not because they are causing the illness but because the immune system is suppressed, allowing them more freedom to replicate than they would otherwise have.

And in a discussion entitled "Other Agent Reactivation," he said,

"For years, some clinicians and researchers have been maintaining that the common yeast, *Candida albicans*, is the cause of symptoms associated with CFIDS. A very popular book, *The Yeast Connection* by Dr. Crook describes this in detail and it has been a common experience to many clinicians that patients with CFIDS have an unnatural overgrowth of the yeast, candida. In my own experience, at least 20% of patients will have some history of oral candidiasis. Dr. Carol Jessop has reported that over 80% of CFIDS patients will have some evidence of candida by stainings and scrapings taken from their mouth.

> *. . .it has been a common experience to many clinicians that patients with CFIDS have an unnatural overgrowth of the yeast, candida. David S. Bell, M.D.*

"Some studies have pointed out higher levels of antibodies to candida than should be expected in the general population. Like EBV, candida is ubiquitous . . . the presence of candidiasis is a sign of poor immune functioning, not just infection with candida. This appears to be the case with CFIDS; while candida is present, it is not the cause, but instead another innocent bystander drawn into the battle."

---

*Pollard Publications, P.O. Box 180, Lyndonville, NY 14098

Additional Remarks by Carol Jessop, M.D.

On November 17-18, 1990, the CFIDS Association, Inc., in conjunction with the Charlotte Area Health Education Center (AHEC), the New Mecklenburg County Health Department and the Mecklenburg County Medical Society sponsored a two-day conference, *"Chronic Fatigue and Immune Dysfunction Syndrome (CFIDS), Unraveling The Mystery."*

This conference featured 32 researchers, clinicians and persons with CFIDS (PWC's) who presented a broad spectrum of views about the disease. This conference provided a forum for the dissemination and discussion of the latest and most compelling CFIDS research findings. A deliberate attempt was made to address as many topics as practical in one weekend.

Participants at the conference included Dr. Carol Jessop, who discussed her findings in working with 1,324 patients with CFIDS seen between 1984 and 1990. In analyzing her patients, she reviewed the symptoms at the time of initial examination, the past histories, the physical and lab findings and their treatment, which featured the use of antifungal medications and a restricted diet (no alcohol, sugar, fruit or fruit juice). In summarizing her results, she said,

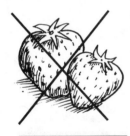

I don't believe we are going to find one single virus that causes this disease. Bacterial, fungal and parasitic agents (are) possible contributors. Carol Jessop, M.D.

"I don't believe we are going to find one single virus that causes this illness. However, I do think that genetic predisposition and environmental factors, such as antibiotics, birth control pills, toxins in the environment and infections all have to be considered. The whole group . . . bacterial, viral, fungal and parasitic agents need to be examined as possible contributors to this disease.

"84% of patients have recovered to a level at which they can remain working 30-40 hours a week. And, 30% have fully recovered. Yet, 44% of the patients experienced some recurrence of their symptoms with premenstrual stress, surgery or other infections."

Following her presentation, during a question and answer session, in discussing medications Dr. Jessop said,

"I try to evaluate every patient individually. I don't treat all of my patients with antiparasitics or antifungals because sometimes

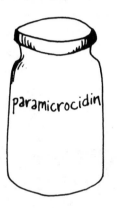

they don't have that condition. If they have a yeast overgrowth, my treatment of choice is three weeks of fluconazole (Diflucan), 100 mg. daily.

"I then re-evaluate the patient and may extend this protocol for another three weeks. Fluconazole is very, very effective. It also, interestingly enough, gets into the central nervous system and my patients report improvement of their cognitive dysfunction with fluconazole that I don't find with nystatin or Nizoral. These other agents would work but it may require a longer period of time."

If they have a yeast overgrowth, my treatment of choice is fluconazole.

"Again, I'm also using citric acid, grapefruit seed extract or ParaMicrocidin. There are other generics of this type that are *very active* against viruses, fungi and parasites. . . . Their length of treatment may be anywhere from five to nine months."

Comments by Jay A. Goldstein, M.D.

In the *Physician's Forum, The CFIDS Chronicle,* Vol. 1, Issue 1, March 1991, Dr. Goldstein, author of the book *The Chronic Fatigue Syndrome: The Struggle for Health,* stated that contrary to popular belief, there are a vast number of useful treatments of CFIDS, although they have to be carefully and intelligently employed case by case. And in a paragraph entitled "Battling Yeast," he made the following comments,

"I am still unclear about the role of the Candida Hypersensitivity Syndrome. Techniques used in its diagnosis are unsatisfactory in my experience, yet I am impressed with the sincerity of certain clinicians who believe in the entity, some of whom are conducting research about the effectiveness of its diagnosis and treatment.

"The usual anti-yeast diet is too restrictive for most patients. Avoidance of refined carbohydrates, alcohol, caffeine and perhaps certain fruits and dairy products should be sufficient. Although fluconazole (Diflucan) is quite expensive, it is also quite safe and a quick trial of this agent may help to make the diagnosis and establish a treatment. It is especially useful if the patient complains of

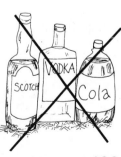

intestinal bloating which is not non-ulcer dyspepsia. I have had success with this approach in only a few patients but they have been resistant to almost every other treatment."*

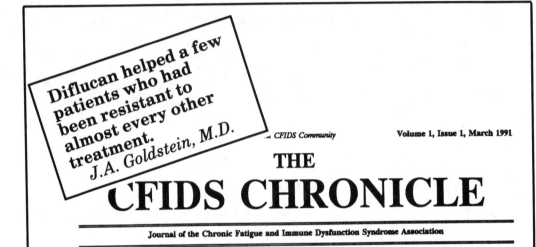

Diflucan helped a few patients who had been resistant to almost every other treatment.
J.A. Goldstein, M.D.

CFIDS Community   **Volume 1, Issue 1, March 1991**

THE
CFIDS CHRONICLE

Journal of the Chronic Fatigue and Immune Dysfunction Syndrome Association

Physicians' Forum

Given the complexities and diversity of symptoms of CFIDS, how do you approach the treatment of CFIDS patients?

FEATURING RESPONSES FROM:

David S. Bell, MD; Paul R. Cheney, MD, PhD;
Jay A. Goldstein, MD; and Charles W. Lapp, MD

PAGES 1 - 17

*The _CFIDS Chronicle,_ Spring 1991 conference issue, page 69.

SECTION **IV**

Regaining Your Health

If you suffer from CFS, you resemble an overloaded camel. To regain your health, look good, feel good and enjoy life, you'll need to unload "many bundles of straw." This may take months—even a year or more. But then your camel will be off and running.

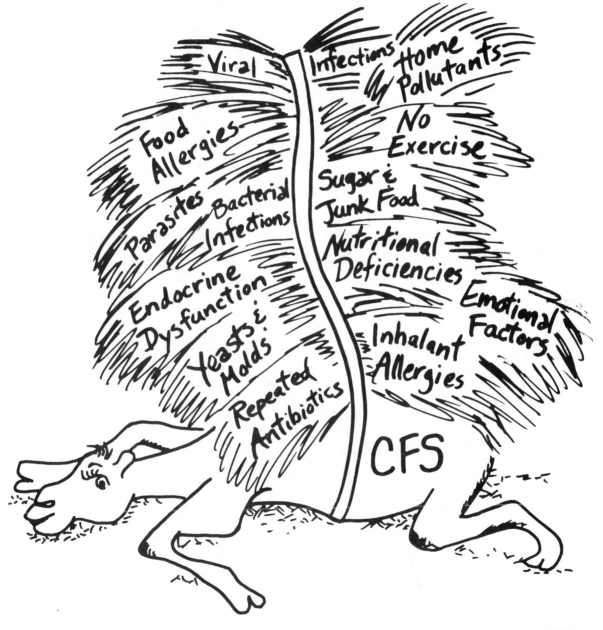

The first step in regaining your health is cleaning up your diet and getting rid of junk food. While you're doing this, get rid of the pollutants in your home. You'll, of course, need to make lifestyle changes, obtain sufficient rest and work with your physician. Then, do simple detective work which will enable you to track down and avoid foods that cause allergic reactions.

Next, because the pesky yeast *Candida albicans* gets out of control in people with weakened immune systems, take steps to control candida. These include avoiding sugar and other simple carbohydrates and taking prescription and nonprescription anti-yeast medication. You'll also need psychological support, essential fatty acids, magnesium, zinc and other nutritional supplements. And as your strength returns, you'll need to take gradually increasing amounts of exercise.

The pictures and notes in this section will help you get started.*

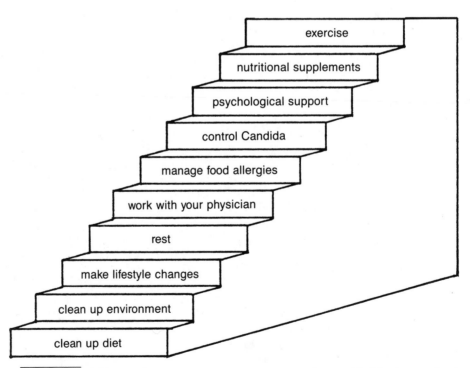

*If in spite of this treatment program you continue to be troubled by insomnia, depression and muscle pains, your physician may prescribe medications which will help relieve these and other symptoms.

Clean Up Your Diet

The diet of Americans during the last several decades has changed dramatically since pioneer days. We live in a "fast-food" society and eat processed and packaged foods which contain sugar, food coloring, flavors, chemicals, additives and pesticides. We drink beverages that are loaded with sugar, phosphates, caffeine, food colors, aspartame and other additives.

Changing your diet won't be easy, yet, many people will improve significantly—even dramatically—when you make changes suggested on the next few pages.

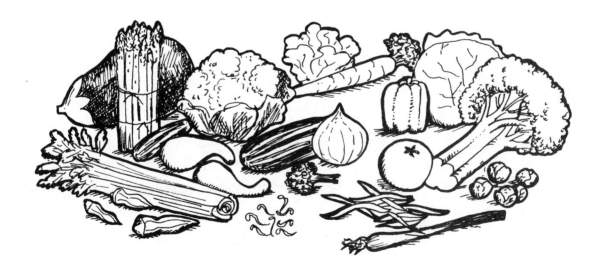

Cut down—better still avoid—foods and drinks containing sugar . . .

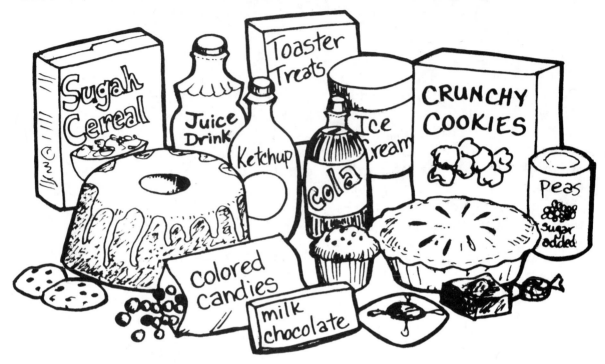

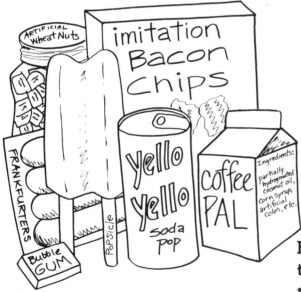

And those containing food colors, phosphates, aspartame and other additives and flavors.

Processed and packaged foods containing the "bad fats"—coconut oil, palm oil, other and hydrogenated or partially hydrogenated vegetable oils.

Offer more . . .   potatoes, peas, beans, sweet potatoes, tomatoes, carrots, onions and
celery.

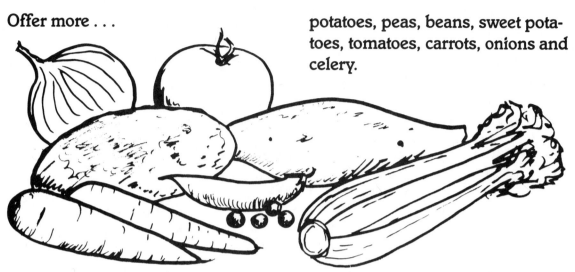

Also try some other vegetables:
asparagus, beets, broccoli, brussels
sprouts, cabbage, cauliflower, egg-
plant, kale, jicama, peppers, rad-
ishes, snow peas, squash and
turnips.

Offer more . . .

Fruits

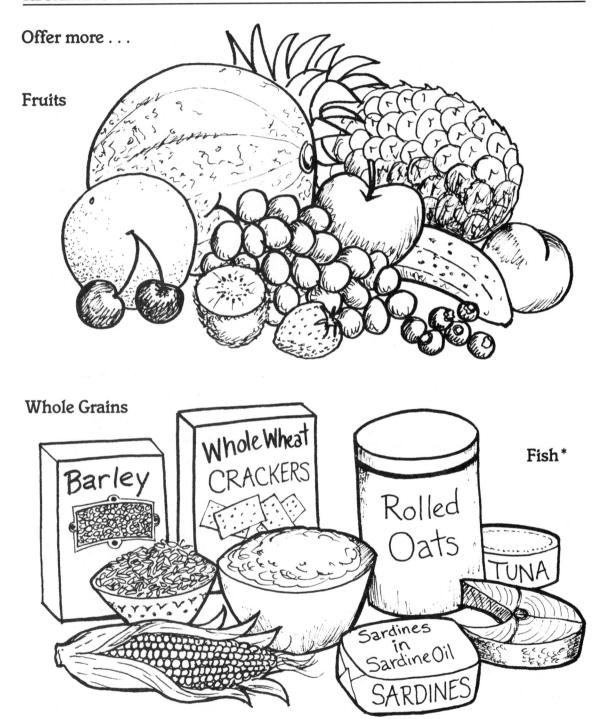

Whole Grains

Fish*

*Choose those low in fat. Cod, haddock, flounder, grouper, pollock, snapper and tuna are relatively safe *if* caught offshore.

Buy special vegetable oils*

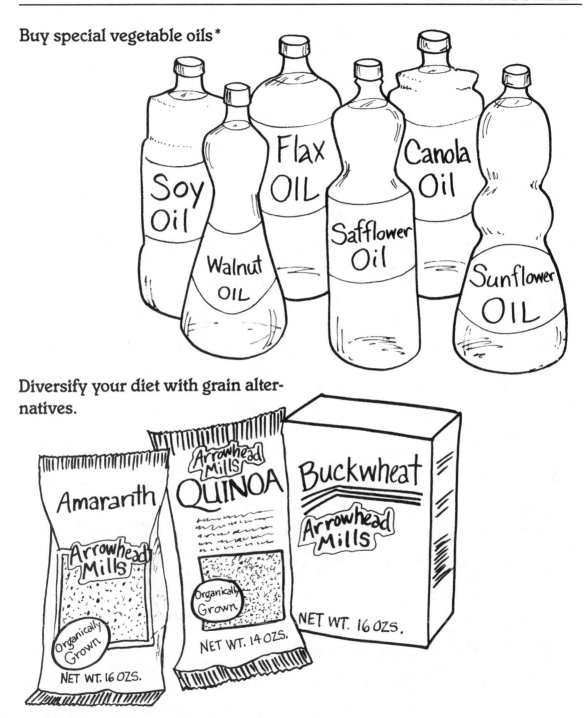

Diversify your diet with grain alternatives.

---

*Organically grown, unrefined or "expeller pressed." Available in health food stores and in some supermarkets.

Look for chemically uncontaminated
foods.

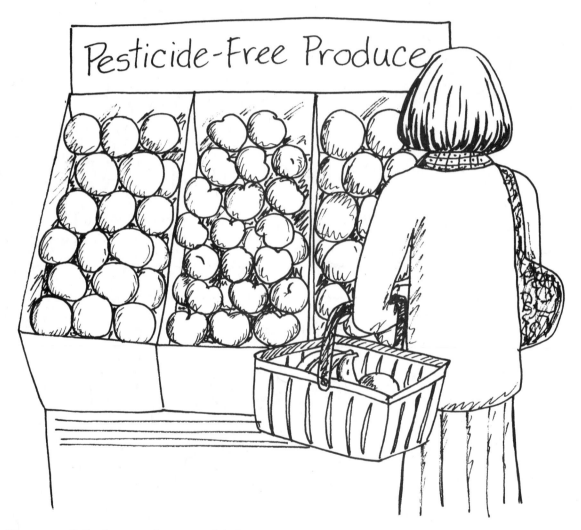

Become label-conscious and join
others who are working for healthier
foods. *

---

*Michael Jacobson, Ph.D., Center for Science in the Public Interest, 1875 Connecticut
Ave., N.W., Washington, DC 20009. 202-332-9110.

Become an informed
consumer.
Read:

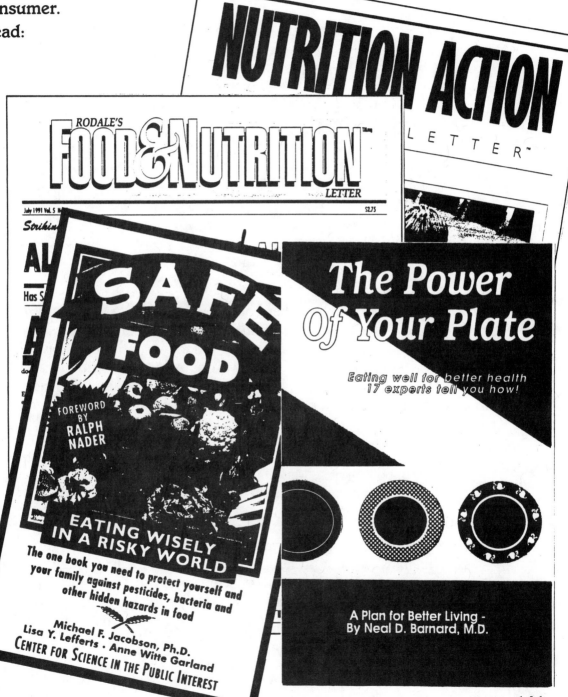

Clean Up Your Home Environment

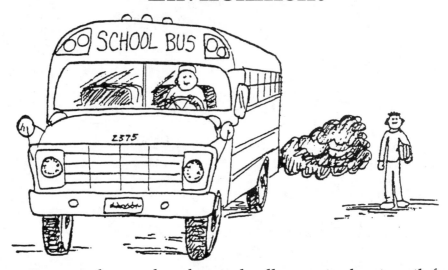

Everyone knows that chemical pollutants in the air, soil, food and water are adversely affecting us and our families. Yet, you may be surprised to learn that indoor air pollutants may be bothering you more than those you're exposed to outdoors.

Some years ago Theron Randolph,* a pioneer Chicago internist, allergist and specialist in environmental medicine, warned:

> "While it is true that outdoor air pollution is a significant source of exposure, a far greater threat is posed by the presence of indoor . . . air pollution. . . . Many household products give off noxious fumes. Indoor air pollution is particularly dangerous because exposure is so constant."

During the past 25 years, Randolph and several hundred physicians and other professionals in the American Academy of Environmental Medicine have been studying and treating patients with chronic health disorders related to chemical overload. And they have found that by lightening this load, many patients with puzzling and persistent health problems improve.

Indoor air pollution is particularly dangerous because exposure is so constant. Theron Randolph, M.D.

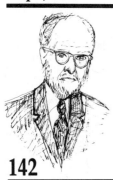

---

*T.G. Randolph, R.W. Moss, *An Alternative Approach to Allergies*, New York: Harper and Row, 1989, p. 50.

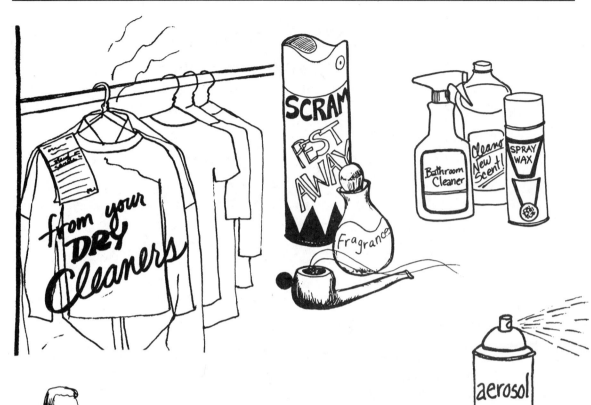

The person with environmentally induced illness (EI) or multiple chemical sensitivity (MCS) and their physicians who are working to help them, have faced much of the same sorts of skepticism and hostility as those who have been working to bring CFS into the medical mainstream. Yet, happily, the situation seems to be changing.* Organizations who are leading the battle to gain credibility for EI and MCS include the American Academy of Environmental Medicine (Box 16106, Denver, Colorado 80216) and the Human Ecology Action League (HEAL), P.O. Box 41926, Atlanta, GA 30359-1126, with chapters throughout the country.

---

*A 17-page special report, "Multiple Chemical Sensitivity," presents both sides of this controversial subject. Copies may be obtained by writing to American Chemical Society, Distribution, Room 210, 1155 16th St., N.W., Washington, DC 20036. Price $10.

One such individual, Agnes Jonas, a Connecticut woman, has written thousands of letters and knocked on the doors of the senators and representatives in her state saying, "Please stop, look and listen. Countless people are being made ill by environmental pollutants."

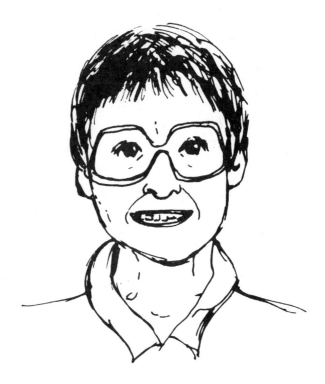

Indoor air pollution is especially dangerous for you and other family members because exposure is so constant. Here are a few suggestions for reducing it:

1. Don't smoke, and don't let people smoke in your home. People in homes where others are smoking experience *twice* as many respiratory infections as individuals in smoke-free homes, and such infections set up a vicious cycle of other health problems.
2. Don't spray insecticides inside of your home.
3. Don't use odorous, toxic or potentially toxic substances in your home.

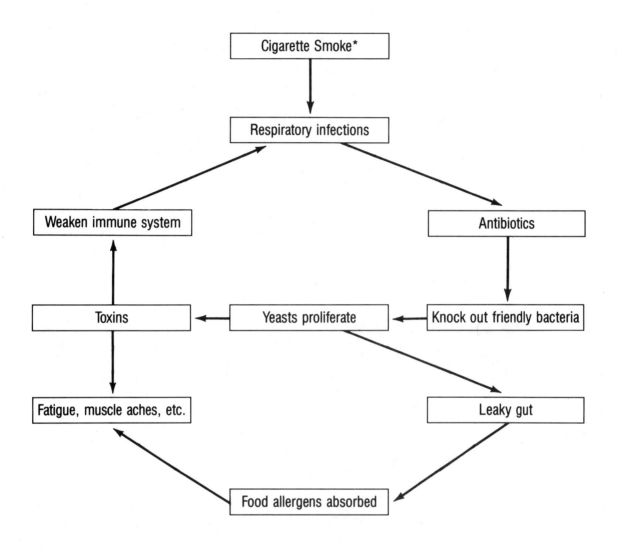

Your resistance resembles a rain barrel and chemicals in your environment are like pipes draining into the barrel. When you're exposed to many chemicals, your barrel overflows and symptoms develop.

---

*Exposure to other chemical pollutants also increases the chances of developing respiratory infections and other health problems.

145

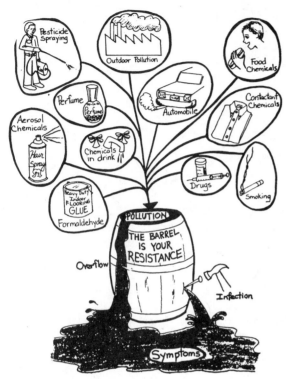

Adapted from William Rea M.D.
Used with permission.

Sources of information about chemical pollutants in our air, soil and water.

Environ—A magazine for ecologic living and health. Wary Canary Press, Box 2204, Ft. Collins, CO 80522. (303) 224-0083. One year subscription (4 issues) $15.

The Allergy and Environmental Health Association, Box 871, Cambridge, Ontario, Canada M1R 5X9. Annual membership and subscription to *AEHA Quarterly*, $25.

Environmental Action, 6930 Carroll Ave., 6th Floor, Tacoma Park, MD 20912. This national political lobbying and education organization publishes a bimonthly magazine. Membership is $25 a year (includes cost of the magazine).

Human Ecology Action League, Inc., P.O. Box 41926, Atlanta, GA 30359-1126. This volunteer organization publishes a quarterly magazine, *The Human Ecologist*. Local chapters in various parts of the country provide information for people with chemical sensitivities.

The Delicate Balance, the publication of the Environmental Health Association of New Jersey, 1100 Rural Avenue, Voorhees, NJ 08043.

Citizens Clearing House for Hazardous Waste, Inc., P.O. Box 6806, Falls Church, VA 22040.

Environmental Health Association of Dallas, P.O. Box 226811, Dallas, TX 75222. This organization publishes a bimonthly newsletter. Subscription rate, $25.

The National Foundation for the Chemically Hypersensitive, P.O. Box 9, Wrightsville Beach, NC 28480.

Foundation for Advancement in Science and Education (FASE), 4801 Wilshire Blvd., Suite 215, Los Angeles, CA 90010.

Track Down Hidden Food Allergies

Systemic and nervous symptoms caused by food allergies* have been described by dozens of professionals during the past several decades. Yet, this relationship is often overlooked by physicians and other professionals. Here's why: *Most food allergies (and/or adverse food reactions) cannot be determined by allergy skin tests or laboratory tests. Instead, they must be identified by a carefully designed, properly executed elimination diet.* Any dietary ingredient can provoke nervous symptoms, including milk, food colors, additives, sugar, wheat, corn, egg, chocolate, yeast and citrus.

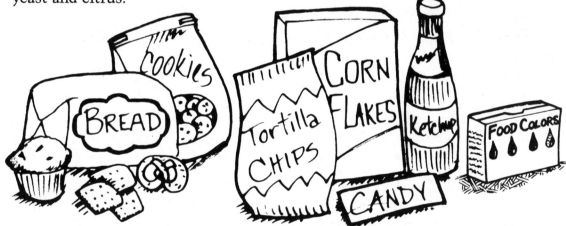

---

*Four types of allergic reactions have been identified and classified. One of these (Type I) is mediated through a blood fraction called "IgE." Reactions of this type produce positive scratch tests and positive RAST tests in individuals sensitive to pollens and other inhalants, and much less commonly in individuals sensitive to food. However, many and perhaps most individuals who show adverse food reactions discussed in this book will not show positive scratch or RAST tests. However, tests of other types may provide helpful clues.

At this time (1992), in spite of studies by many investigators during the past few years, many of the mechanisms and explanations for these food reactions remain obscure. Since they may not involve antigen and antibody reactions, many immunologists and other physicians prefer to call these food reactions "intolerances," "hypersensitivities," "adverse reactions" or "sensitivities."

How do I find out if my fatigue and other symptoms are caused by something I'm eating?

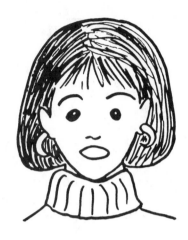

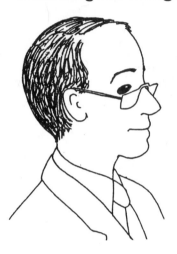

You carry out an elimination diet* avoiding many of your favorite foods.

What will I look for? How will I know these foods bother me?

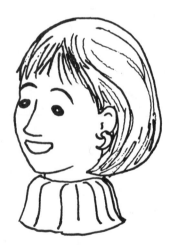

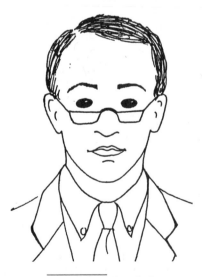

If you're sensitive to the foods you avoid, your symptoms will improve or disappear when you stop eating them. And they'll return when you eat them again.**

*You'll find detailed instructions for carrying out this diet in Section V.
**If you have had asthma or experienced swelling or other serious allergic reactions, get the help and consultation of your physicians before carrying out this diet.

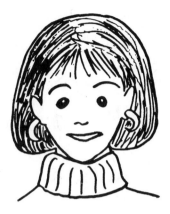

What do I do first?

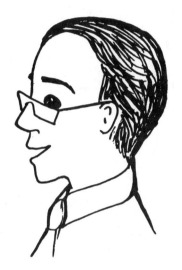

Discuss the diet with other family members.
Ask for their cooperation.

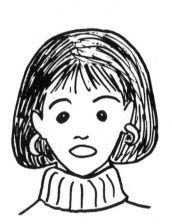

How long does it take to do the diet?

The elimination part of the diet lasts about a week, or until you show a convincing improvement in your symptoms.

Then, the second week, eat the foods you've eliminated—one food per day—and see if your symptoms return.

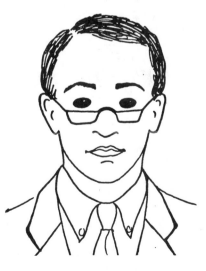

149

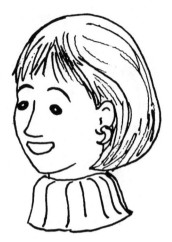

Please tell me more about the diet.

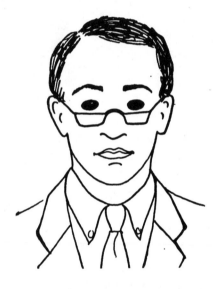

Pick a convenient time.

Don't try it during a holiday or when you're visiting.

Before beginning the diet keep a symptom and food diary for three days.

Continue the diary while you're eliminating foods and while you're eating them again.

If you eat away from home, take your food with you.

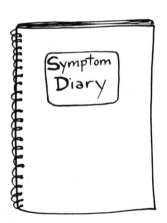

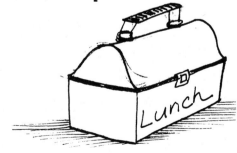

What You Can Eat or Drink

Any vegetable but corn and any fruit
but citrus.

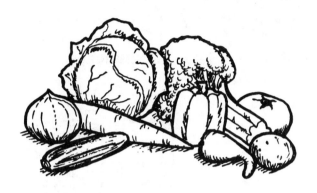

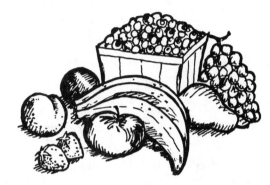

Any meat but bacon, sausage, hot
dogs and luncheon meat.

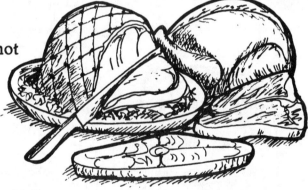

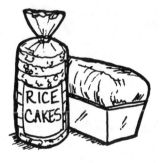

Oats, rice, barley, and the grain
alternatives, amaranth, quinoa and
buckwheat.

Unprocessed nuts.

Water (preferably bottled or filtered).

What You'll Need to Avoid

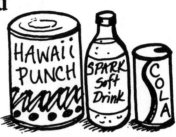

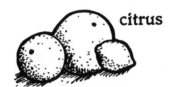
citrus

soft drinks, Kool-Aid, punches

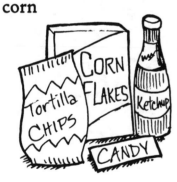
wheat

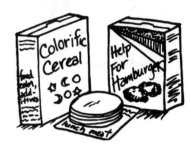

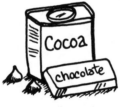
chocolate

corn

food colors, additives and flavors

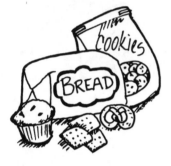

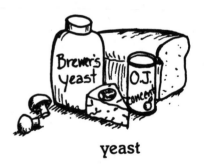
sugar

yeast

milk

processed and packaged foods

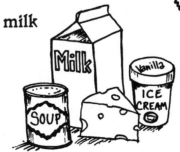

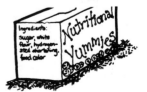

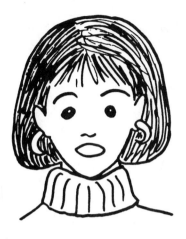

Suppose I identify several foods that bother me, yet I'm continuing to experience symptoms from something I'm eating.

You'll have to do more detective work. Here are my suggestions:

1. Consider the possibility that chemical contaminants in or on your foods are causing problems.

2. Remember that any food can cause symptoms, including beef, apple, chicken, potatoes, peanuts and/or other foods.

To identify sensitivity to these foods try the Caveman Diet* for a week.

On this diet, you avoid any food you eat more than once a week.

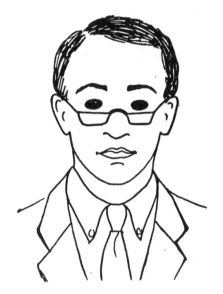

*You'll find a further discussion of this diet in Section V.

Here's good news. As you control yeasts in your digestive tract and your immune system improves, your food sensitivities will lessen and may disappear.

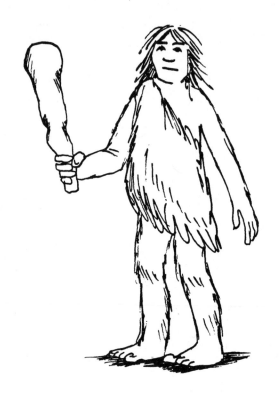

Control Candida

Studies carried out in Japan* show that *Candida albicans* produces high and low molecular weight toxins and that the toxin produced in the invaded tissues may act as an immunosuppressant.

On the next few pages you'll see how antibiotics may contribute to yeast overgrowth, a weakened immune system, repeated infections and food sensitivities.

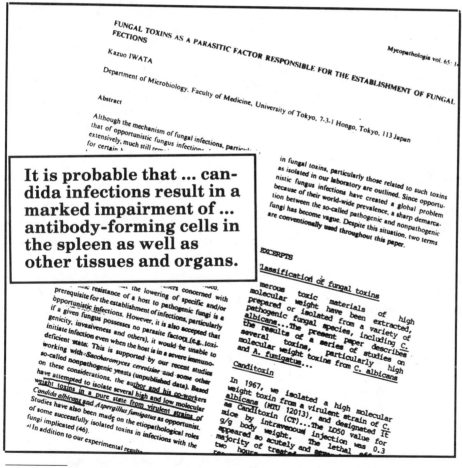

FUNGAL TOXINS AS A PARASITIC FACTOR RESPONSIBLE FOR THE ESTABLISHMENT OF FUNGAL INFECTIONS

Mycopathologia vol. 65: 1

Kazuo IWATA

Department of Microbiology, Faculty of Medicine, University of Tokyo, 7-3-1 Hongo, Tokyo, 113 Japan

Abstract

Although the mechanism of fungal infections, particul... that of opportunistic fungus infection... extensively, much still rem... for certain b...

> **It is probable that ... candida infections result in a marked impairment of ... antibody-forming cells in the spleen as well as other tissues and organs.**

in fungal toxins, particularly those related to such toxins as isolated in our laboratory are outlined. Since opportunistic fungus infections have created a global problem because of their world-wide prevalence, a sharp demarcation between the so-called pathogenic and nonpathogenic fungi has become vague. Despite this situation, two terms are conventionally used throughout this paper.

EXCERPTS

Classification of fungal toxins

...the resistance of a host to pathogenic and/or opportunistic infections. However, it is also accepted that if a given fungus possesses no parasite factor (e.g. toxigenicity, invasiveness and others), it would be unable to initiate infection even when the host is in a severe immunodeficient state. This is supported by our recent studies working with *Saccharomyces cerevisiae* and some other so-called nonpathogenic yeasts (unpublished data). Based on these considerations, the author and his co-workers have attempted to isolate several high and low molecular weight toxins in a pure state from virulent strains of *Candida albicans* and *Aspergillus fumigatus* as opportunist. Studies have also been made on the etiopathological roles of some successfully isolated toxins in infections with the fungi implicated (46).

In addition to our experimental results...

numerous toxic materials of high molecular weight have been extracted, prepared or isolated from a variety of pathogenic fungal species, including *C. albicans*...The present paper describes the results of a series of studies on several molecular toxins, particularly high molecular weight toxins from *C. albicans* and *A. fumigatus*...

Canditoxin

In 1967, we isolated a high molecular weight toxin from a virulent strain of *C. albicans* (MTU 12013), and designated it as Canditoxin (CT)...The LD50 value for mice by intravenous injection was 0.3 g/g body weight. The lethal appeared so acutely and sev... majority of treated... two hours...

*K. Iwata, "Fungal Toxins as a Parasitic Factor Responsible for the Establishment of Fungal Infections," *Mycopathologia*, 65:141-54.

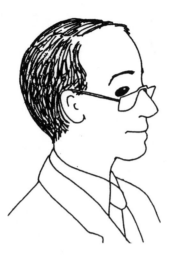

Repeated sinus (or other) infections may play a role in causing the Chronic Fatigue Syndrome.

How and why could they be related?

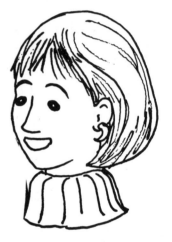

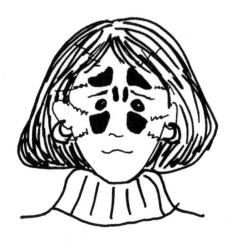

When you developed such infections

you were often treated with broad-spectrum antibiotic drugs.*

* As a child, adolescent or adult.

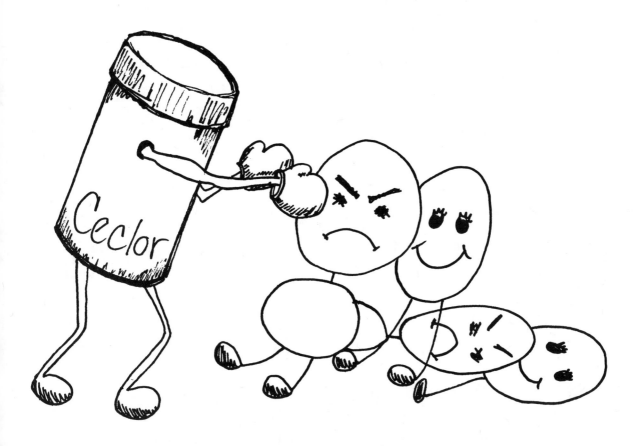

These drugs knock out friendly
germs while they're knocking out
enemies

Candida yeasts aren't affected by antibiotics.

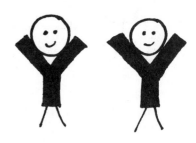

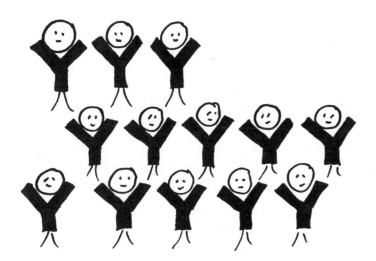

So they multiply and raise large families.

These candida yeasts put out toxins

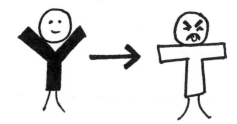

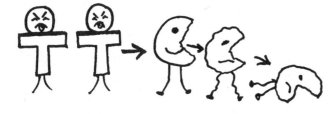

that weaken the immune system.

So you may experience repeated infections.

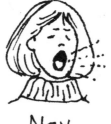 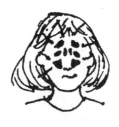 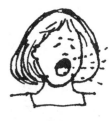

NOV   DEC   JAN

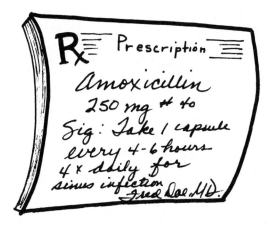

Each infection is treated with antibiotics.

So a vicious cycle develops.

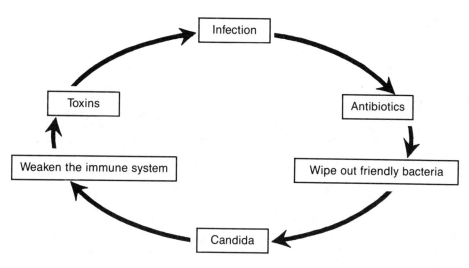

Infection

Antibiotics

Wipe out friendly bacteria

Candida

Weaken the immune system

Toxins

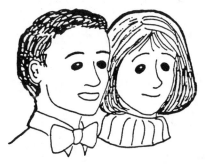

Candida overgrowth in your gut may also increase your chances of developing food allergies. *

What makes this happen?

*See also pages 199–202, and 317–321.

Candida may weaken the normal
intestinal membrane, creating what
has been described as a "leaky gut."

Toxins and food allergens may then
pass through this membrane and go to
other parts of the body.

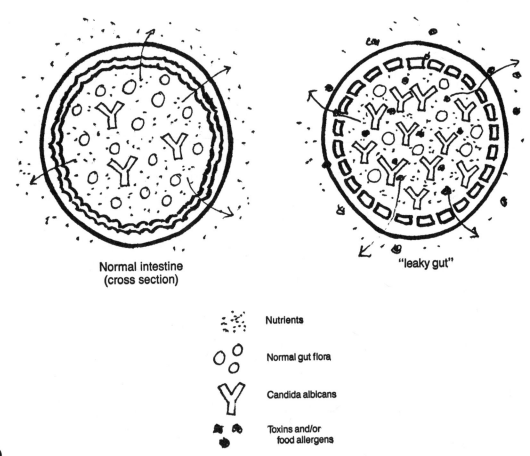

Normal intestine
(cross section)

"leaky gut"

Nutrients

Normal gut flora

Candida albicans

Toxins and/or
food allergens

Food allergens may also cause many other systemic and nervous symptoms.

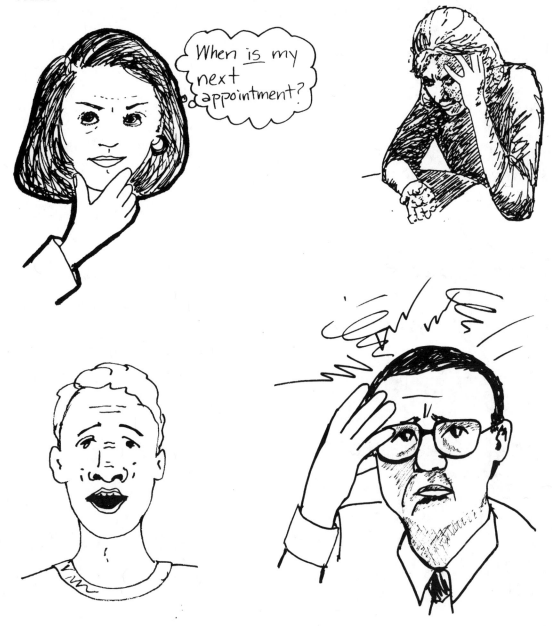

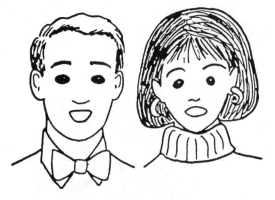

If my health problems are candida related, what do you advise?

You should avoid alcohol and foods and beverages that promote yeast growth, especially sugar . . .

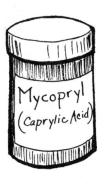

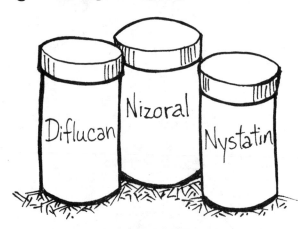

and take nystatin, Nizoral or Diflucan . . .

plus other substances that discourage yeast growth.

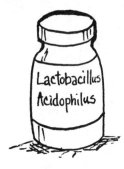

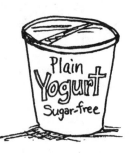

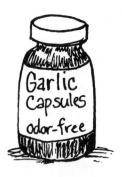

Psychological Support

Every person needs love, praise, smiles, encouragement, understanding and other psychological nutrients, even when she is enjoying good physical, mental and emotional health. I call these nutrients "psychological vitamins." Many recent scientific studies show conclusively that these nutrients strengthen the immune system.

When you're a person with CFS and you feel tired and spaced out and your head, stomach, arms, legs and back hurt, you understandably are apt to feel discouraged and depressed . . . .

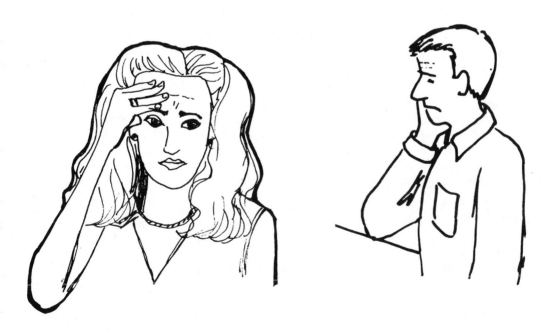

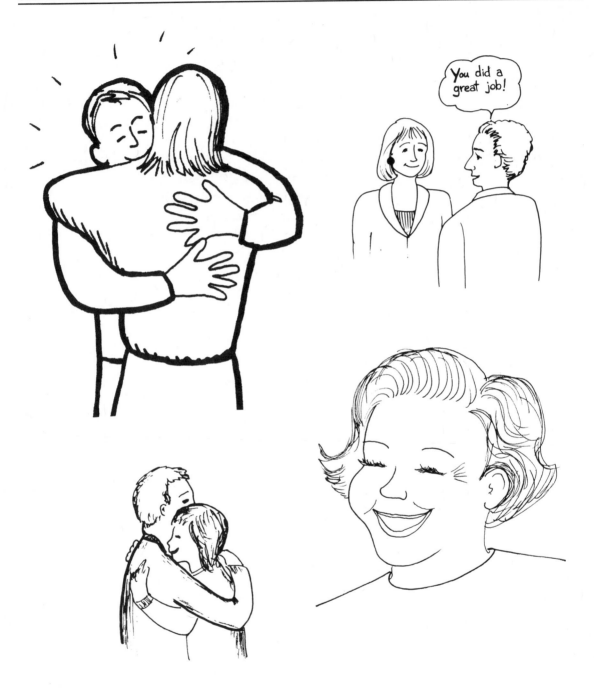

And love, praise, laughter, understanding and support will help you get well.

Nutritional Supplements

Many of the foods and beverages you and your family consume today are loaded with sugar, saturated fats and partially hydrogenated fats and oils. They also contain phosphates, artificial coloring, additives, insecticides and chemicals of many sorts. These foods are usually deficient in important nutrients and micronutrients, including zinc, calcium, magnesium, B vitamins and the essential fatty acids.

Cleaning up your diet, cutting out sugar, soft drinks and packaged and processed foods will help you obtain many of the nutrients you need. I also recommend nutritional supplements.* Moreover, a number of authorities are now supporting the use of such supplements to fortify the body's immune system and provide "nutritional insurance."

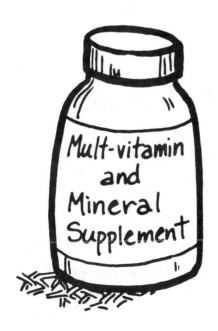

---

*For a further discussion of nutritional supplements, see pages 360-73 of *The Yeast Connection*, 3rd Edition.

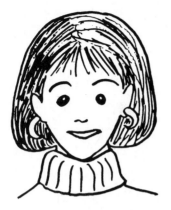

Do I need to take nutritional supplements?

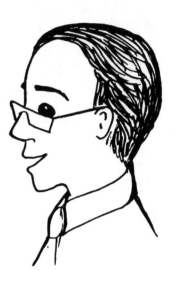

Yes. Here's why:

Many of the foods and beverages you've been consuming are deficient in important nutrients and micronutrients.

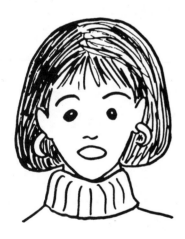

What are some of them?

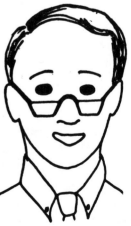

Vitamins, minerals and the essential fatty acids (EFAs).

What do they do? How do they help?

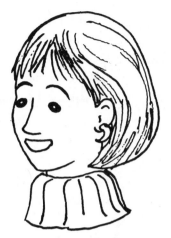

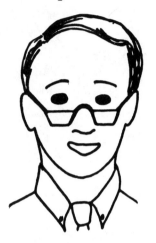

Like different members of a football team, they play important roles in keeping you healthy.

Give us some examples.

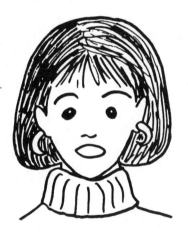

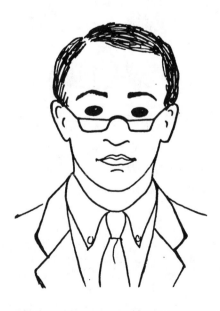

Zinc increases your resistance to infection. Supplemental iron is needed by women to help them build red blood cells.

Antioxidants, including selenium and vitamins A, C, and E, help protect you from environmental pollutants.

167

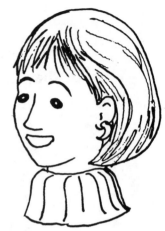

Are there still other nutrients that
help, and what do they do?

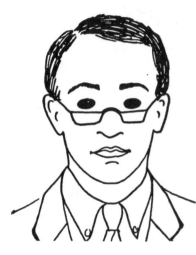

Yes, magnesium, calcium and vitamin B$_6$ help reduce nervous system
irritability.
Vitamin C strengthens the immune
system.
Other vitamins and minerals are
also important.

I've heard people talk about essential fatty acids. Could you tell me
about them?

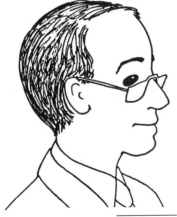

They're "good oils." We call them
EFAs, and like vitamins and minerals, they're also important members
of the nutrient team. *

*See Section VI for a further discussion of magnesium, essential fatty acids and other
nutritional supplements.

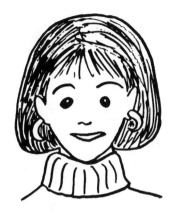

What are some of the symptoms of
an EFA deficiency?

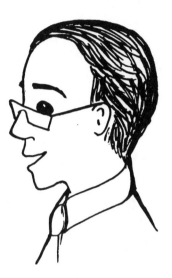

Dry, flaky skin or "chicken skin"
(bumps on arms, legs and cheeks).

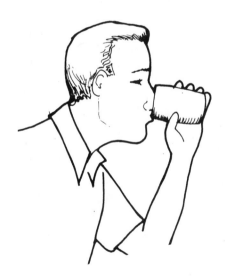

Dry hair.
Excessive thirst.
Muscle pain.
Allergies.

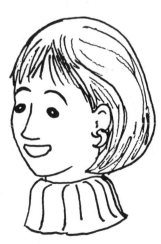

I have all of these symptoms. What
can I do to overcome my EFA deficiency?

Cut down on processed foods, especially those containing white flour and sugar.

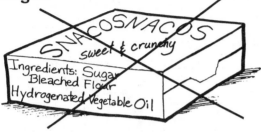

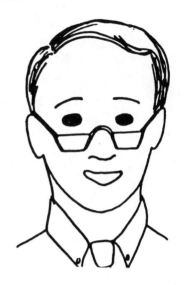

Avoid margarine and foods containing partially hydrogenated oils.

Eat salmon or sardines packed in sardine oil at least once a week.

Take EFA supplements.

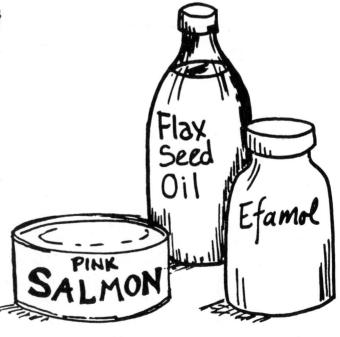

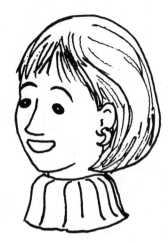

What vitamins and minerals do you recommend for your patients?

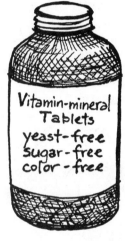

Yeast-free, sugar-free, color-free vitamin-mineral tablets or capsules.

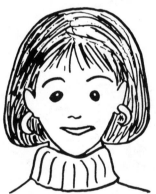

Do they help every person with CFS?

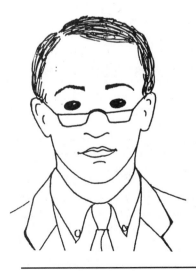

Most, but not all, persons with CFS benefit from these supplements.

171

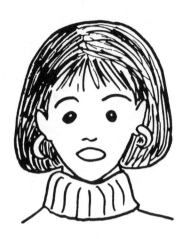

If they don't seem to help, what should I do?

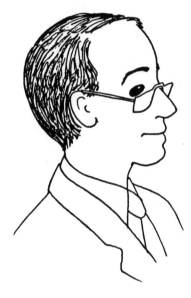

Continue them unless they disagree.

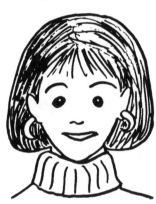

Any other suggestions?

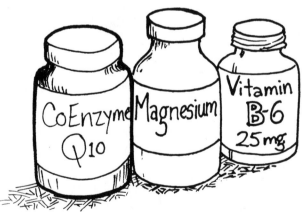

Many persons with CFS have been helped by extra magnesium, larger doses of B vitamins and Coenzyme Q_{10}*

---

*See Section VI for a further discussion of magnesium, vitamin B_{12} and Co-Q_{10}.

Exercise

In her superb book *Hope and Help for Chronic Fatigue Syndrome,* in a section titled "Take a Rational Approach to Exercise," Karen Feiden commented,

"When dragging yourself from the bedroom to the bathroom is exhausting, you don't need to be reminded to cut back on your vigorous tennis game or to drop out of aerobics class. The athletic accomplishments that may have once been a source of pride to you are obviously out of the question for now.

"Remember, though, that total bed rest can be very deleterious to your health. After a few days, you lose vital nutrients, blood circulation is affected and fewer gastric juices are secreted. To avoid further health problems, a minimal level of physical activity is recommended . . . .

"Seek a level of exercise that you can readily tolerate, but bear in mind that a therapeutic level for one person can exhaust another or cause flaring discomfort."

What sort of exercise do you recommend?

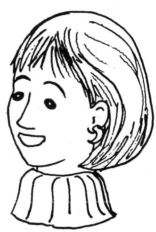

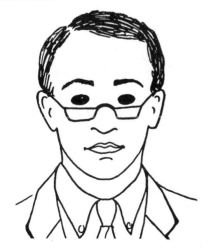

Begin with gentle stretching and slow walks.

And then—??

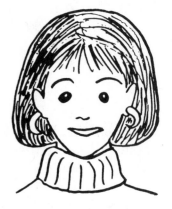

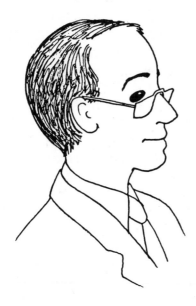

Gradually increase the duration and type of exercise. Don't overdo!

Summary

Causes of CFS

If you're involved in an earthquake, fire or automobile accident, your ensuing health problems develop suddenly and from a single cause. By contrast, if you have CFS, symptoms nearly always develop (and/or persist) because of multiple factors that weaken your immune system.

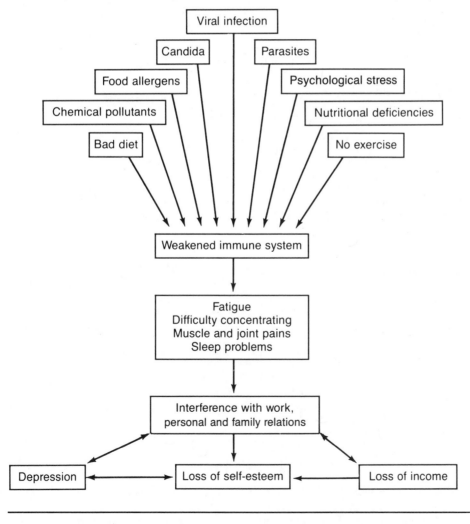

175

Regaining Your Health

Although there's no "magic bullet" or "quick fix" you can get well! On the pages that follow you'll find more information.

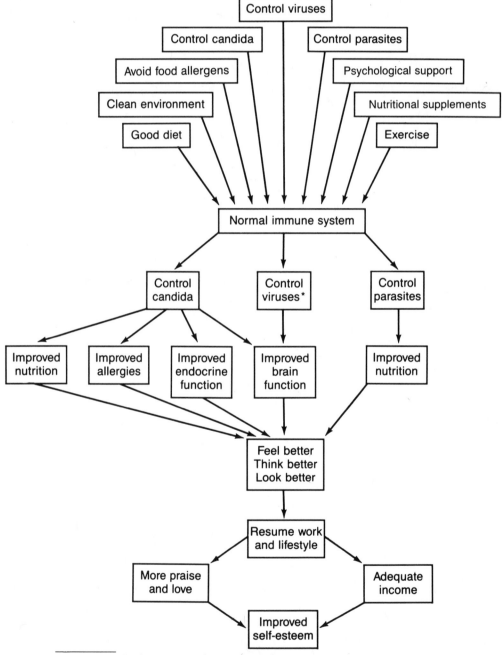

*Bacteria and other microorganisms may also cause problems.

SECTION **V**

More Information About ...

Diet

To fulfill your requirements for energy and to build, maintain and repair your body tissues, you need to eat a variety of foods. Good foods promote good health, and poor foods play an important role in causing disease. All foods contain proteins, fats or carbohydrates. And many foods are composed of combinations of all three of these sources of calories. If you take in more calories than you use up, you'll gain weight, and if you consume too few calories, you'll lose weight.

Beginning after World War I, North Americans and Europeans fell in love with meat, dairy products and eggs because they were "high-protein" foods. We somehow came to feel that protein was especially good for us even though these animal foods contained more calories from fat than from protein. Along with what might be called "protein mania," many of us believed that plant foods (such as potatoes, bread and beans) should be avoided or eaten in limited quantities. Here's why: We thought they were too "starchy" and "fattening."

After World War I we fell in love with meat and high protein foods.

The Influence of Nathan Pritikin

During the past 20 years, beginning with the observations of the late Nathan Pritikin, Americans have learned that high- protein, high-fat diets play a part in contributing to chronic diseases and that diets which feature complex carbohydrates promote good health.

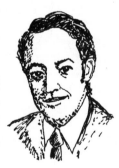

At first, this dietary advice was resisted by many members of the medical establishment who said in effect, "What right does Pritikin have to give people advice about diets? He isn't a doctor or a nutritionist." Yet, word of the success of the Pritikin high-complex-carbohydrate, low-fat, low-protein diets spread to people all over America. And ten years ago, CBS's "60 Minutes" featured people with heart disease, diabetes and other chronic disorders whose lives had been "turned around" while following the Pritikin program.

179

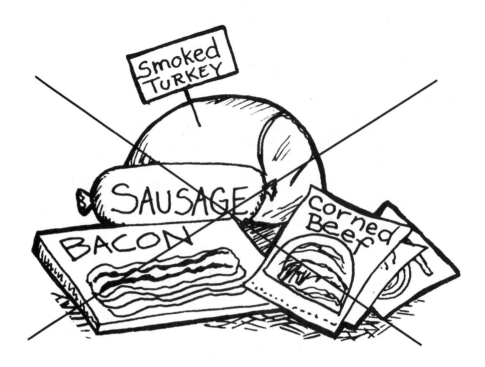

By chance, I sat next to Pritikin during dinner at a medical conference in the early 1970s. I was impressed by what he had to say about the importance of high-complex-carbohydrate diets. Because of my own interest in the relationship of diet to disease, we began to correspond. Subsequently, Pritikin invited me to serve as a member of the Advisory Board of his Longevity Research Institute.

In the late 1970s I attended a conference in Santa Barbara, California sponsored at Pritikin's Institute. There I heard a scientific presentation that should interest you (and others) with CFS, especially if you've been bothered by memory and concentration problems. Here's a brief summary of this study:

Significant improvement in intellectual performance on individuals who follow the Pritikin program.

"Intellectual tests were given to people who came to the Longevity Research Institute before they started on a treatment program which featured exercise and a diet containing 80% complex carbohydrates and 10% protein and 10% fat. The studies were repeated four weeks later (after those tested had been following the Pritikin program). *Their findings: Significant improvement in intellectual performance and test scores.*" [emphasis added]

180

At the same conference I learned for the first time that high-protein diets promote osteoporosis. And in a presentation on the subject, Robert E. Morrow, M.D., a Utah orthopedic surgeon said in effect,

"Protein foods produce an acid urine, and calcium is released from the bones to neutralize this acid. By contrast, vegetables and fruits produce an alkaline urine. Accordingly, people who eat less protein do not lose calcium in the urine."

Protein foods produce an acid urine, calcium loss . . . and osteoporosis.

Just about everyone during the 1980s began to eat less protein, and the idea of less fat and more complex carbohydrates has gained greater acceptance and popularity each year. Here are examples: In the March 1987 issue of *Nutrition Action Health Letter*, in her article "Overdosing on Protein," Elaine Blume commented,

"Long seen as the epitome of nutritional goodness, protein is beginning to lose its glow. . . . Evidence is growing that consuming large amounts of protein could contribute to osteoporosis, heart disease and certain cancers. A high protein intake is also harmful to individuals who suffer kidney disease."

New York Times health columnist Jane Brody,* in discussing the typical American dinner containing five to eight ounces of red meat, ¼ of a chicken or ½ pound of fish said,

"You don't have to be rich to eat such a dinner. Millions of Americans eat it almost every night thinking they're meeting their nutritional requirement . . . . The amount of protein is double, triple, even quadruple the amount needed in a single meal. . . . Since protein is an essential nutrient . . . and since . . . more must be better, Americans took to protein with such a vengeance that now the average person in this country, rich and poor alike, eats at least two times more protein than is really needed for good nutrition. High fat diets aren't good for you either."*

Americans eat at least two times more protein than is needed for good nutrition. Jane Brody.

Diets that are high in protein are usually high in fat. Here's why: Protein rich meats, whole milk, cheeses, eggs and nuts all

---

*Jane Brody's *Good Food Book*, New York, Bantam Books Edition, 1987.

contain a lot of fat. So when you reduce your protein intake, you'll cut down on your fats.

High-fat diets contribute to many chronic health problems, including high blood pressure, heart disease, stroke, diabetes and certain cancers. Also, since fats are rich in calories (270 calories per ounce as compared to 120 calories per ounce for carbohydrates or proteins), they promote overweight, and overweight contributes to poor health.

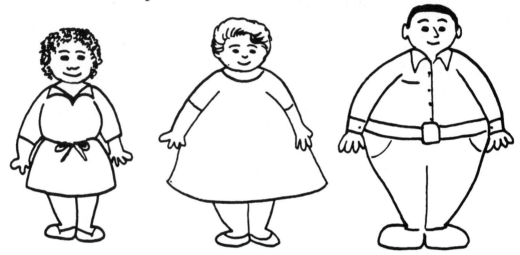

Here's another reason why high fat animal products are bad for you: Chemical toxins, including DDT and other insecticide residues, are concentrated and stored in the fat tissue of animals. So when you eat bacon, steak, pork chops or chicken (with the skin on it), you're taking in more chemical toxins.

A Special Word on "Bad Fats"

These fats that have sneaked into the foods you're eating every day are coconut, palm and palm kernel oils. They are more saturated than either butter or lard. Until recently many manufacturers used them in their processed foods to prolong shelf life. Beginning in 1985, an Omaha private citizen, Phil Sokolof, spent over a million dollars in a publicity blitz, highlighted by eye-grabbing newspaper ads which said, "Saturated fats in tropical oils make them poisonous."

Since that time, this concerned private citizen has continued

Saturated fats in tropical oils make them poisonous.

Sources of Pesticide Residues in the U.S. Diet

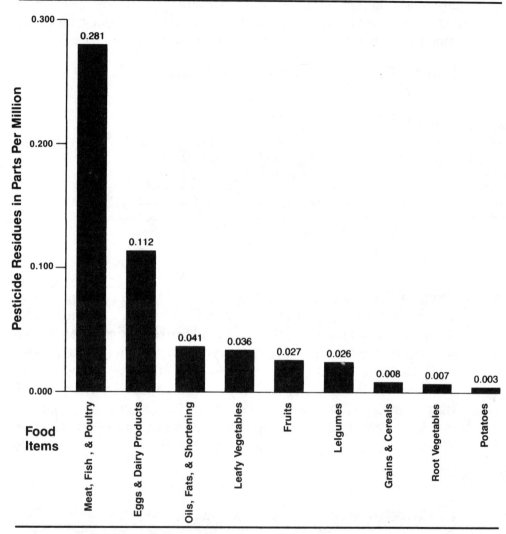

Source: Modified from data in G. Q. LIpscomb and R. E. Duggan, "Dietary Intake of Pesticide Chemicals in the U.S.," *Pesticides Monitoring Journal* 2 (1969): 162–69; and P. E. Cornelliussen, "Pesticide Residues in Total Diet Samples," *Pesticides Monitoring Journal* 2: (1969) 140–52, 5: (1872) 313–30.

his crusade. He has focused not only on tropical oils, but also on high-fat foods of all kinds. And because of his influence, major food manufacturers have removed tropical oils from many of their products. Moreover, McDonald's and other fast-food "eateries" have reduced the fat content in many of their foods. So have many food manufacturers and processors. And they're advertising these changes on TV and in magazines and newspapers every day. What's more, Kellogg's Corn Flakes, a food that never contained fat now comes in new boxes that say, "FAT FREE."

Complex Carbohydrates Are Good for You

Complex carbohydrates provide you with an even flow of energy.

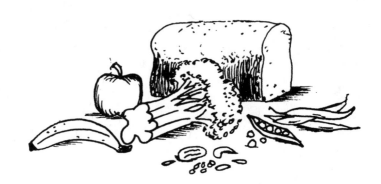

Vegetables, fruits and whole grains (and the grain alternatives amaranth, quinoa, buckwheat and teff) promote good health for many different reasons. Like the simple carbohydrates, they contain glucose, which provides energy. However, the glucose molecules in these foods—especially in vegetables and grains—are tied together in long chains. They are metabolized slowly, providing you with a more even flow of energy and a more pleasant disposition. Moreover, glucose in these foods is combined with fiber, vitamins and minerals, which are essential for their proper utilization.

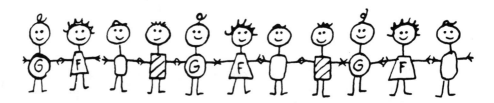

The good carbohydrates—especially vegetables and whole grains—promote friendly intestinal bacteria that counteract candida overgrowth. And the fiber contained in them promotes normal elimination, lessening the chances that you'll absorb food allergens and other toxins.

184

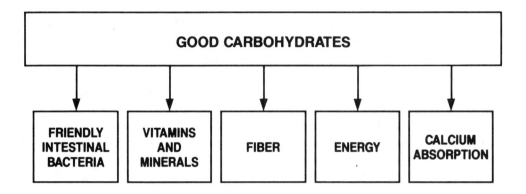

GOOD CARBOHYDRATES

| FRIENDLY INTESTINAL BACTERIA | VITAMINS AND MINERALS | FIBER | ENERGY | CALCIUM ABSORPTION |

The New Four Food Groups

On April 8, 1991, the Physician's Committee for Responsible Medicine, headed by Neal D. Barnard, M.D., unveiled a proposal to replace the four basic food groups which have been a part of U.S. Government recommendations since 1956. According to Barnard, diets which feature these foods are largely responsible for epidemics of heart disease, cancer, stroke and other serious illnesses in the country.

The old four food groups were meat, dairy, grains and fruits/vegetables. The New Four Food Groups are grains, legumes, vegetables and fruits.

The whole grain group includes breads, pastas, rice, corn, and all the other grains. Note the emphasis on whole grains, rather than refined grains.

The legume group includes anything in a pod. Beans, peas and lentils.

The vegetable group and the fruit group are no longer a single group as in the old four food groups.

The net effect of centering the diet on these groups is a reduction in fat and cholesterol intake and an increase in fiber, complex carbohydrates, beta carotene, and other important nutrients.

In commenting on the new diet recommendations in the *PCRM Update* newsletter May-June 1991, PCRM president Neal D. Barnard, M.D., said,

"The New Four Food Groups plan does not exclude all other foods from the diet. It simply prescribes the center of the diet. The New Four Food Groups are in line with Thomas Jefferson's statement . . . 'I have lived temperately, eating little animal food, and not as an aliment, so much as a condiment, for the vegetables which constitute my principal diet'.

"Two issues frequently arise in discussion of plant-centered diet: protein and calcium. Quantity of protein in a varied diet centered on plant foods is more than adequate, but is not excessive.

"Overly high protein intakes are common in meat-centered diets and are known to increase calcium losses in urine and to increase the work load of the kidneys. Diets which are more modest in protein are to be preferred.

"Calcium intake has been a selling point for the dairy industry. However, greens and legumes are also rich in calcium. In addition, there is substantial evidence that a lower protein intake actually reduces one's calcium requirement . . . In the New Four Food Groups, dairy products lose their status as an 'essential' food group.

> *I have lived temperately, eating little animal food . . . vegetables constitute my principal diet.*
> *Thomas Jefferson*

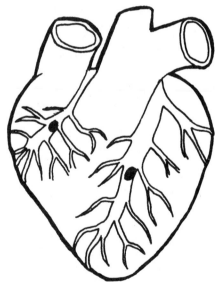

"If this new prescription is followed, the benefits will be profound. Heart attacks and strokes will become more rare, cancer risks will diminish, young women will have less risk of breast cancer and diabetes will diminish. It has even been hypothesized that sexual potency will remain unimpeded among men who age without the arterial damage of atherosclerosis. It may be that those who have no interest in protecting their coronary arteries have given other body parts a greater psychic presence!"

In his book *Power of the Plate*, in discussing osteoporosis, Dr. Barnard commented,

"To prevent osteoporosis we must use our bones. Weight bearing exercise helps build strong bones. In addition, we need to beware that alcohol and tobacco aggravate bone loss. And keeping our protein intake to more modest levels is important.

"The dairy industry, of course, is using osteoporosis as a marketing tool. They would like us to believe that the body's careful regulation of calcium absorption and bone structure can be tricked by simply ingesting a large amount of milk."

Drinking a lot of milk does not prevent osteoporosis.

In his continuing discussion Barnard cites the comments of the British physician, Denis Burkitt, who has for many years emphasized the importance of fiber in the diet. Burkitt also stated that people who take a lot of fiber-containing complex carbohydrates and a "quite low calcium intake get infinitely less osteoporosis" than people who drink a large amount of milk. Barnard also discussed the observations of Dr. John McDougall, who adds another reason to avoid dairy products,

"Dairy products are the most common cause of food allergies. Look at all the allergic reactions to dairy products that have been noted in the scientific literature: canker sores, digestive problems, skin conditions, respiratory reactions and so on . . . . People don't know until they get away from them for a while and then try them again. And they say, 'Oh, that's why I had a stuffy nose all the time' or 'That's why I have post nasal drip.'"

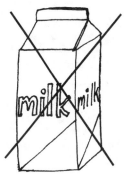

I share McDougall's thoughts about milk sensitivity. And during my many years of pediatric and allergy practice, I helped many children—and some adults—with complaints like fatigue, headache, abdominal pain, bedwetting, irritability, nasal congestion and hyperactivity by removing milk from their diet. In addition, my own nasal congestion and long lasting sinus trouble which wasn't helped by a submucous resection and the use of radium in my nose, improved dramatically when I stopped drinking milk.

187

McDougall, like Pritikin, Cheraskin, Brody, Blume, Burkitt, Barnard, Ornish and an increasing number of other professionals and nonprofessionals, is saying, *"The traditional American diet—rich in meat, milk and eggs—is hazardous to your health."*

McDougall has described his recommendations in a 1991 book, *Twelve Days to Dynamic Health*, and Ornish has outlined similar recommendations in his 1991 book, *Dr. Dean Ornish's Program for Reversing Heart Disease.*

A Good Diet *Is* a Good Diet *Is* a Good Diet

Will more complex carbohydrates and less meat and other proteins and less fat (especially the hydrogenated fats) help people with CFS? In my opinion, the answer is "Yes" and in discussing diet I like to quote comments by Emanuel Cheraskin, M.D., D.M.D., who served as Chairman of the Department of Oral Medicine, University of Alabama, for over 25 years. In responding to questions from a Jackson, Tennessee, audience in the late 1970's about the best diet for persons with diabetes, high blood pressure, overweight, underweight, fatigue or depression, he said in effect:

> "A good diet *is* a good diet *is* a good diet for anyone and everyone. And it should feature more complex carbohydrates and should avoid or sharply limit sugar, white flour, white shortening and other high fat foods."

In commenting about the concerns about the premenopausal woman who is concerned about obtaining enough iron and zinc on a diet low in protein and free of red meat, Bonnie Liebman* had this to say,

> "If you're still concerned, why not take a multi-vitamin-and-mineral supplement that provides 100% of the USRDA (15 mg. for zinc and 18 mg. for iron). Just make sure it has copper and that you're not at risk for hemochromatosis. 'I know it's against most others in my profession, but I don't see anything wrong with a supplement of RDA levels as a margin of safety' says nutritionist Jeanne Freelan-Graves' (University of Texas at Austin). One thing is certain. Taking a supplement is healthier than loading up on red meat."

A good diet should feature complex carbohydrates and should sharply limit sugar, white flour and high fat foods. Emanuel Cheraskin, M.D., D.M.D.

---

*B. Liebman, "What, Meat Worry?," *Nutrition Action Healthletter*, June 1991. CSPI, 1875 Connecticut Ave., N.W., Washington, DC 20009-5728.

Chemical Pollutants

Do chemicals play a part in causing CFS? In my opinion, and that of other clinicians and researchers, the answer is "yes." Here are some of the symptoms that may be caused by or aggravated by chemical exposures, including those you come in contact with in your home or in your work place:

- coughing and wheezing
- fatigue
- nasal congestion
- muscle aches
- burning eyes
- irritability
- burning, tingling and flushing of the skin
- headache
- drowsiness
- incoordination
- mental confusion
- short attention span

But in spite of growing evidence that our "chemical load" is increasing every year and that chemicals play a role in causing many health problems, you may have heard other voices saying, "Chemicals are a normal part of our life today. To maintain a high standard of living in our modern industrialized society we must use chemicals. Although a rare person may be bothered by them, the average person doesn't need to worry."

In my opinion, people who make such remarks resemble ostriches with their heads in the sand. Although I agree that chemicals (in certain ways) may promote better living, they play a part in causing many health problems.

Building Related Illnesses (BRI) and the Sick Building Syndrome (SBS)

In a recent article "Do Buildings Make You Sick?" (*Executive Health's Good Health Report*), Michael J. Hodgson, M.D., M.P.H., Director, Occupational and Environmental Medicine, University of Pittsburgh School of Medicine, discussed outdoor pollution from billowing smokestacks, exhaust fumes from cars and buses, and pollutants from oil refineries. He said,

"Just as insidious, although less apparent, is the threat posed by indoor air pollution. Apartment complexes, office buildings, hotels, even houses can present serious risks to our health.

"Since the mid-1960's, secretaries, executives, computer operators, maintenance workers and others have complained of symptoms and diseases that have been traced back to the workplace. We now group these illnesses under the headings of *building-related illnesses* (BRI) and *sick-building syndrome (SBS)*. Every year people miss up to 500,000 work days because of these illnesses."

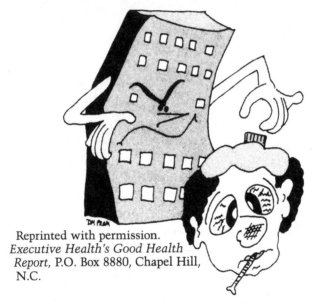

Reprinted with permission.
Executive Health's Good Health Report, P.O. Box 8880, Chapel Hill, N.C.

In discussing BRI, Dr. Hodgson pointed out that dust, mold spores, tobacco smoke, office products, microbial growth in ventilation systems, perfumes, dry-cleaned suits, volatile organic compounds, and other substances may pollute the indoor air. And he concluded,

Chemicals from seemingly innocuous office equipment can threaten both productivity and health.

"The battle against 'air pollution' must be waged on two fronts. Just as the smog which hovers over our major cities threatens urban dwellers, so too does the atmosphere inside the buildings we work and live in pose a threat.

"Inadequate filtration systems, poor ventilation, and the off-gassing of a variety of chemicals from seemingly innocuous office equipment can threaten both productivity and health.

"More attention from management, maintenance supervisors and individual employees must be given to the interdependent sys-

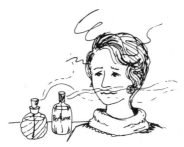

tems that make for either a healthy or threatening work environment."

Multiple Chemical Sensitivity (MCS)

More and more people seem to be bothered by perfumes, tobacco smoke, formaldehyde, carpet odors and other chemicals. People who develop these symptoms are said to have Multiple Chemical Sensitivity, or MCS. Yet, MCS, like CFS and the yeast connection, has stirred up a hornet's nest of controversy.

On one side, you'll find medical organizations like the American Academy of Allergy and Immunology, American College of Allergy and Immunology and the American College of Physicians who say in effect, "People who claim they're sensitive to all of these chemicals are hypochondriacs and their symptoms are psychoneurotic in origin." By contrast, members of the American Academy of Environmental Medicine (AAEM)* and other professional and lay organizations say these problems occur commonly.

In a comprehensive 17-page report in the *Chemical and Engineering News*, Bette Hileman included a 1987 report by Mark A. Cullen, Professor of Medicine Epidemiology at Yale University. In a book which he edited, titled *Workers with Multiple Chemical Sensitivities*, Cullen described a patient with the most debilitating and striking form of multiple chemical sensitivity (MCS).

This patient was a middle-aged man who developed pneumonia following a chemical spill on the job. Even though his X-ray cleared, he continued to have symptoms. Here are excerpts from Dr. Cullen's report:

"Particularly striking was the history that exposure to chemical odors would markedly exacerbate baseline dyspnea (difficult

*Formerly the Society for Clinical Ecology.

191

breathing) and chest pain. Upon return to work he 'passed out' on several occasions after a whiff of fume. Increasingly, even common household products and environmental contaminants induced debilitating respiratory and constitutional symptoms, reducing his formerly vigorous life to a pitiful existence at home."

In spite of extensive diagnostic investigations and clinical tests and treatment of various sorts, very little was accomplished. In his continuing comments, Dr. Cullen stated,

"Many of our colleagues practicing occupational medicine around the country began reporting similar cases. They too were stymied by them. Thus we became aware of how widespread the problem is and how incredibly expensive the costs are for medical care and disability in each case."

Hileman listed a number of milestones in the evolution of multiple chemical sensitivity, including a discussion of the work of MCS pioneers Theron Randolph and William Rea and their colleagues in the American Academy of Environmental Medicine (AAEM). She also stated that the Social Security Administration had added a section on MCS to the agency's program operations manual for disability determinations. And in briefly summarizing her report, she said,

"This enigmatic syndrome has no generally accepted definition or proved physiological mechanism. Yet it is increasingly being recognized in government regulations and the courts."

The New Ashford/Miller Book

In a 1991 book *Chemical Exposures—Low Levels and High Stakes,** Nicholas A. Ashford, Ph.D., M.D., and Claudia S. Miller,

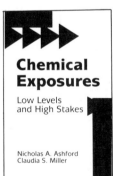

**Chemical
Exposures**

Low Levels
and High Stakes

Nicholas A. Ashford
Claudia S. Miller

---

*Nicholas A. Ashford, Ph.D., J.D., Associate Professor of Technology and Policy at the Massachusetts Institute of Technology. Former Chairman of the National Advisory Committee on Occupational Safety and Health, Fellow of the American Association for Advancement of Science and currently Chairman of the Committee on Technology Innovation and Economics of the EPA National Advisory Council for Environmental Policy and Technology.

Claudia S. Miller, M.D., M.S., Clinical Assistant Professor in Allergy and Immunology, University of Texas Health Science Center, San Antonio. Dr. Miller is Board Certified in internal medicine and holds a Masters Degree in Environmental Health from the School of Public Health at the University of California, Berkeley. She has served on the National Advisory Committee on Occupational Safety and Health. Before entering medicine she was an industrial hygienist for the University of California, San Francisco.

M.D., M.S., discussed the role that chemical pollutants play in causing a wide variety of symptoms including, in certain cases, fatigue. In their book these professionals identified four major groups of people with hypersensitivities to low levels of chemicals: Occupants of tight buildings; industrial workers who handle chemicals; residents of communities exposed to toxic chemicals; individuals with random and unique exposure to various chemicals.

Features of the book which provide invaluable information to professionals, lay persons, government officials and others interested in the "chemical problem" include:

- Clear, concise explanations of technical material on low level chemical exposure
- An extensive technical bibliography
- Table of contrasting medical approaches to chemical sensitivity
- Descriptions of recent research and proposed mechanisms
- An annotated bibliographical appendix highlighting illnesses that have been linked to environmental exposure
- Policy recommendations for federal and state government

In preparing their landmark work, Ashford and Miller interviewed key figures in the field and reviewed the relevant literature of the last 40 years. In a review of this book in the October 2, 1991, issue of the *Journal of the American Medical Association*, James E. Cone, M.D., M.P.H., San Francisco General Hospital, University of California-SF, commented,

"Clinicians and policy makers would do well to read and heed the advice of this book, for many of us are faced with the problems of how to best evaluate patients affected by this disorder, currently without adequate guidance about the best means of diagnosis, treatment, and, most important, prevention. Ashford and Miller do not give us any easy answers but do point the way out of the current quagmire of opinion and empiricism, which has hindered progress towards solving this challenge."

Clinicians and policy makers would do well to read and heed the advice of this book. James E. Cone, M.D., M.P.H.

Allergies

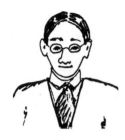

Unusual reactions to substances in a person's diet or environment have been recognized for thousands of years. Yet, it wasn't until 1906 that the term "allergy" was coined by the Austrian pediatrician Clemens von Pirquet. He put together two Greek words *allos*—meaning "other" and *ergon*—meaning "action." To von Pirquet *allergy* meant altered reactivity.

Today, most doctors feel that allergy means "hypersensitivity to a specific substance, which in a similar quantity doesn't bother other people." Incidentally, that's the definition you'll find in Websters New World Dictionary. However, if you moved from one city to another, you may run into different ideas about allergy—how it is defined, how it is diagnosed and how it should be treated.

Some doctors feel the term "allergy" should be limited to those conditions in which an immunological mechanism can be demonstrated using allergy skin tests or more sophisticated laboratory tests. But other conscientious physicians feel that the allergic and hypersensitivity diseases are much broader in scope. For example, the late Frederic Speer, M.D., of the University of Kansas said, "While immunological mechanisms are undoubtedly important in explaining allergic diseases, they don't tell the whole story."

> *Immunological mechanisms are important but don't tell the whole story. Frederic Speer, M.D.*

Types of Allergies

When you develop an allergy to something you breathe, such as grass, pollen, animal danders or house dust mites, the cause of your symptoms can be suspected from your history and identified through the use of the simple allergy scratch test. In carrying out such a test, a physician scratches or pricks your skin and applies a small amount of an allergy extract.

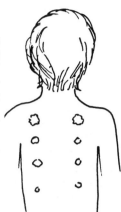

If you're allergic to the test substance in the abstract, as for example Bermuda grass, ragweed or cat dander, within a few minutes an itching bump or welt that looks like a mosquito bite will pop up on your skin.

Skin testing will usually produce similar welts if you're allergic to foods such as eggs, peanuts or strawberries. However, if you're obviously sensitive to these foods, skin tests aren't needed to identify them. Moreover, skin testing of foods that have caused severe reactions can be dangerous.

There are other types of food allergies and sensitivities you need to know about. Such allergies have been called "hidden," "masked," "variable," or "delayed-onset" food allergies. *Allergies or sensitivities of this type are caused by foods you eat every day.* You'll probably be surprised to learn that you're apt to be sensitive to some of your favorite foods, especially wheat, corn, milk, yeast, chocolate, citrus and coffee.

You're apt to be sensitive to some of your favorite foods.

Moreover, you may be "addicted" to foods that are making you tired or develop headaches, muscle aches or nasal congestion. Like the cigarette or narcotic addict, you may feel temporarily better after you've eaten some of the foods to which you're allergic.

Controversy over Allergy

Many subjects are controversial, including religion, politics, education, abortion and many others. What's more, if you read *USA Today,* you'll see opposing opinions on different issues expressed on the editorial page every day. Food allergy is another such controversial subject.

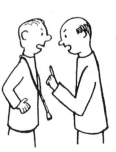

Early in 1987 a comprehensive new book by Jonathan Brostoff and Stephen Challacombe appeared on the medical scene. Its title: *Food Allergy and Intolerance* (London, Balliere Tindall, 1987). Eighty-three physicians and other scientists contributed to this book, which was favorably reviewed in the *Journal of the American Medical Association.*

Here are comments from the preface of *Food Allergy and Intolerance:*

Food allergy is an exciting, challenging, exasperating subject. J. Brostoff and S. Challacombe.

"As all who deal in the field will know, food allergy is an exciting, challenging, exasperating and sometimes controversial subject. Its study should be a clinical science with diagnosis based on a combination of clinical observations and scientific investigations . . . .

"The field of food allergy has generally been considered to be a clinical art rather than a laboratory science.

"There is more than an element of truth in this since clinical observations often have not been supported by reliable diagnostic tests or even laboratory data. This has led to skepticism of some of the clinical associations, especially when the mechanisms of any proposed food allergies are not understood . . . .

"There has been a strong tendency for the conventional physician to say that if the mechanism is not understood then food allergy does not exist . . . . This is of course unacceptable . . . . To make a diagnosis (of food allergy) certainly requires clinical skill, but does not necessarily need a complete understanding of a mechanism underlying the disease process or an exact understanding of the etiology. . . .

The cornerstone of diagnosis of food intolerance is the removal of that food from the patient's diet, with concomitant improvement (or not) of the patient's symptoms and their reappearance on adding that food back.

"A thread running through (this book) . . . is that the cornerstone of diagnosis of food intolerance is the removal of that food from the patient's diet, with concomitant improvement (or not) of the patient's symptoms and their reappearance on adding that food back."

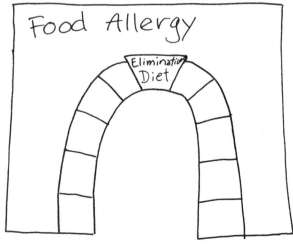

A discussion of food allergy from a different point of view was published in the November 27, 1987, issue of the *Journal of the American Medical Association*. In describing the clinical features of food allergy, Hugh A. Sampson, M.D., Rebecca Hatcher Buckley, M.D., and Dean D. Metcalf, M.D., emphasized immunologically mediated reaction to foods.

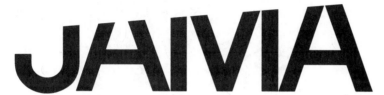

The Journal of the American Medical Association

They pointed out that such reactions are "expressed clinically by diversity of signs and symptoms that cause a diverse group of symptoms ranging from abdominal pain to generalized anaphylaxis." They also noted that, in addition to the GI system, food allergy can also affect other parts of the body, especially the skin, and less frequently the respiratory tract. Yet they expressed skepticism over the relationship of food allergy to systemic and nervous system symptoms, including fatigue and depression.

Although these allergy specialists suggested the use of double-blind or single-blind placebo-controlled oral challenges with suspected food, they also recommended the use of elimination diets. In discussing such diets, these physicians stated,

> "This approach has been used as an outpatient diagnostic aid for many years. The principle is somewhat the same, i.e., if the offending food is removed from the diet of the affected individual, the food-induced illness will be resolved . . . . Initiation of a severely limited diet is warranted if the removal of one or several foods from the diet is not successful in elimination symptoms or if multiple food sensitivities are suspected . . . . Continuation of symptoms following restricted diets indicates that symptoms are not due to foods or other avoided substances."

If the offending food is removed from the diet of the affected individual, the food-induced illness will be resolved.

197

Food Allergies Come Into The Allergy Mainstream

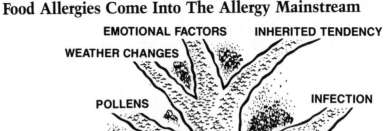

EMOTIONAL FACTORS   INHERITED TENDENCY

WEATHER CHANGES

POLLENS   INFECTION

HOUSE DUST AND MOLDS   FOOD

Allergies and Hypersensitivities

In a recent report "Food and Additive Sensitivity Presents Diagnostic Dilemma" (*Consult*—A Forum for Physicians, Cleveland Clinic Foundation, Vol. 7, No. 3, April 1988, pages 8-9) the tension-fatigue syndrome in children and headache were listed as occasional manifestations of food allergy according to that interview with Sami L. Bahna, M.D., then Chairman of the Foundation's Department of Allergy and Immunology 1987-1990.*

In a continuing discussion of the subject, the article stated,

The elimination challenge diet is the "Gold Standard" for diagnosis of food allergy. Sami L. Bahna, M.D.

"The majority of food sensitive patients cannot be diagnosed through routine tests. Dr. Bahna considers the elimination/challenge test the 'Gold Standard' for diagnosis . . . . When conducted properly, it is the definitive procedure for verifying a cause-and-effect relationship between exposure to a particular food and the occurrence of given symptoms. We apply it to every food suspected of causing or exacerbating symptoms.

"Once the offending food or additive is identified, management is usually straightforward and successful. Treatment consists primarily of dietary avoidance."

*Dr. Bahna is now Professor of Pediatrics and Medicine and Chief of the Division of Pediatric, Allergy and Immunology at East Tennessee State University, Johnson City, TN.

Still more support for the frequency and importance of food sensitivities came from health columnist Jane Brody. In the subtitle of her article in the July/August 1990 edition of *The Saturday Evening Post*, "Food Sensitivity: The Mystery Ailment*" Brody said,

THE SATURDAY EVENING POST

"Millions of Americans get sick when they eat certain foods. Some have known allergies but the majority of cases remain unexplained."

Brody briefly summarized the reactions of seven individuals who experienced food-related symptoms. One of these she said was . . . "Yours truly (who) suffered periodic attacks of abdominal pain that would last for days until dietary sleuthing revealed foods made with soybeans or dried peas as the likely cause."

In her continuing discussion, Brody said, "The seven of us are among the estimated 30 million Americans who experience adverse reactions to foods, reactions that most non-medical people call food allergies."

An estimated 30 million Americans experience adverse reactions to foods.

In discussing the controversy among physicians, Brody said,

"In researching this article I initially believed that most of the claims attacking this food or that as the cause of everything from hair loss to athlete's foot were elaborate hokum. But after looking at the medical research and learning about various people's experiences, I now wonder whether the rigid thinking of some doctors is not ill advised. Indeed, in dismissing symptoms that don't involve the immune system, these doctors might be doing a disservice to the health and well being of millions of Americans.

"Perhaps a food doesn't have to affect the immune system in order to ignite a yeast infection, cause the sinuses to fill, aggravate arthritis or bring on irritable bowel syndrome. Certainly foods might make some people feel tired or mentally foggy . . . or send some children into an orbit of hyperactivity."

Certain foods might make some people feel tired or mentally foggy. Jane Brody

---

*Reprinted from the *New York Times*, April 29, 1990.

Why People May Develop Adverse Food Reactions

In the August 24, 1991, issue of *The Lancet* (Vol. 338, pages 495-96), Dr. J. O. Hunter, FRCP, Addenbrooke's Hospital, Hills Road, Cambridge, CB2 2QQ, UK, presented a hypothesis to explain the mechanisms that take place in many people who experience adverse food reactions. Here are excerpts from his commentary:

> "Specific food intolerance has been implicated in many conditions. In controlled trials, exclusion diets are effective in migraine, irritable bowel syndrome, Crohn's disease, eczema, hyperactivity and rheumatoid arthritis."

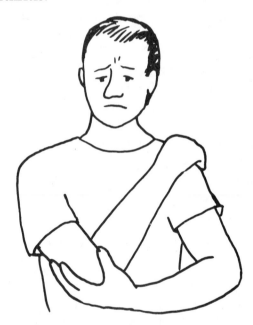

Yet, Hunter pointed out, because no evidence of the classical Type I allergic reaction can be found in most patients with food sensitivities, many investigators conclude that those who say, "I'm bothered by food allergies," are merely neurotic. In his discussion, he suggests that patients with food intolerance have an abnormal gut flora even though pathogens are not present.

In his concluding paragraph he stated,

> "Much further work, especially studies of gastrointestinal enzyme concentrations and of the colonic flora, is required to substantiate

this hypothesis. However, if food allergy is not an immunologic disease, but a disorder of bacterial fermentation in the colon, it might be more appropriately named an 'enterometabolic disorder.' This is of more than mere terminological importance: modern microbiology has opened the way to the manipulation of bacterial flora to allow the correction of food intolerances and thus the control of disease."

Food allergy may be a disorder of bacterial fermentation in the colon.

Another European researcher and clinician, Gruia Ionescu, Ph.D.,* shares Hunter's views about the relationship of gut flora to food sensitivities. Here are excerpts of Dr. Ionescu's interview with Marjorie Hurt Jones, R.N., Editor, *Mastering Food Allergies:***

"We have found approximately half of our allergics have a problem with candida overgrowth in their gut. And many people diagnosed with candida infections exhibit intolerances to foods also . . . . In our clinic in West Germany we focus our attention on improving the health of the gut . . . especially its lining, the intestinal mucosa. Here's an overview of our rationale:

"When the gut contains an overgrowth of candida the lining becomes very inflamed—and less efficient at handling food. Because the walls become more permeable, they start to leak . . . . We've found that the best diet in the world will not give the patient adequate nourishment if he has abnormal bowel flora. In healthy people, beneficial bacteria predominate in the delicate balance of organisms. They prevent the pathogenic bacteria, yeast, fungi or mold from running rampant."

Many people diagnosed with candida infections exhibit intolerances to foods.

Still other investigators, including Leo Galland, M.D.*** and W. Allan Walker, M.D., Professor of Pediatrics, Harvard Medical School, have also been studying the gut. Some of Walker's research studies have focused on the role of the mucosal barrier in handling allergens. In a recent comprehensive review of antigen handling by the gut, he commented,****

---

*G. Ionescu, Spezialklinik Neukirchen, Krankenhausstr 9, 8497, Neukirchen, West Germany.
**To obtain the entire four-page interview with Dr. Ionescu, send a SASE and $2.50 to *Mastering Food Allergies*, 2615 N. 4th St. #616, Coeur d' Alene, ID 83814.
***You'll find a detailed description of Dr. Galland's observations in Section VIII. (Intestinal Microbes and Systemic Immunity)
**** W. A. Walker, in Brostoff and Challacombe, *Food Allergy and Intolerance*, London, Balliere Tindal, and Philadelphia, W. B. Saunders, 1987, pages 209-22.

"There's increasing experimental and clinical evidence to suggest that large antigenically active molecules can penetrate the intestinal surface not in sufficient quantities to be of nutritional importance, but in quantities that may be of immunological importance.

"This observation could mean that the intestinal tract represents a potential site for the absorption of bacterial breakdown products such as endotoxins and enterotoxins, proteolytic and hydrolytic enzymes or other ingested food antigens that normally exist in the intestinal lumen."

"The intestinal tract represents a potential site for the absorption of . . . ingested food antigens that normally exist in the intestinal lumen."
W. Allan Walker, M.D.

Although neither Hunter nor Walker mentions the possible role that candida overgrowth contributes to abnormal gut flora, the observations of Ionescu and the favorable response of the person with food sensitivities to special diets and the administration of antifungal medications provide further support for the yeast connection to food allergies and in turn to CFS.

Other Comments About Food Sensitivity and Chronic Fatigue

At the Cambridge Symposium on Myalgic Encephalomyelitis, Robert Loblay, M.B., Ph.D., gave a presentation entitled "Clinical Immunology: Assessment and Treatment of Food and Chemical Sensitivity." Here's an excerpt of a summary of his presentation from the Spring/Summer 1990 issue of the *CFIDS Chronicle*. In discussing food intolerances, Dr. Loblay said,

One-third of CFIDS patients showed marked improvement on an elimination diet.

"Unlike true IgE-mediated food allergy, food intolerances can be difficult to recognize since they are delayed and accumulative, and occur with a large number of commonly eaten foods and drinks . . . . *After treatment with a very strict elimination diet, 1/3 of CFIDS patients showed marked improvement on an elimination diet.*" [emphasis added]

Foods incriminated by Dr. Loblay included naturally occurring salicylates (strawberries, orange juice, honey), amines (cheese, red wine) and glutamine (cheese, tomatoes, mushrooms). He noted that these dietary ingredients "may produce urticaria angioedema, migraines, irritable bowel syndrome and a variety of nonspecific symptoms, in CFIDS."

I agree with Dr. Loblay that the food groups and foods he listed often cause problems. Yet, I've found that commonly ingested foods, including milk, wheat, corn, chocolate, egg, coffee and tea or other of a person's favorite foods may cause food intolerances and/or other adverse reactions.

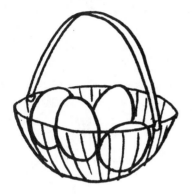 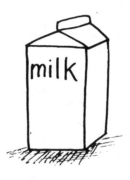

Here's more: In an article "Are We Really What We Eat?—Food and Our Moods—Food and Our Bodies,"* Dr. Richard M. Carlton, a New York psychiatrist in private practice, said,

"In my years as a psychiatrist, I've witnessed countless instances in which a simple change of diet led to a rapid recovery of mental health. It is now clear to me that what we eat has a profound effect on what we think and how we feel . . . .

"Different foods affect people differently. And any food can cause problems. But I've found coffee, chocolate, milk, sugar and wheat to be the most common culprits. In many cases my patients have been especially fond of the food that was causing them the trouble."

My patients have been especially fond of the food that was causing them the trouble.

In his article, Dr. Carlton discussed several "remarkable recoveries," including a nurse in her twenties whose anxiety disappeared when she stopped drinking milk; a young film maker whose depression and abdominal pain disappeared when he stopped drinking milk; a middle-aged business woman whose foggy thinking and chronic fatigue was caused by chocolate. Here's the story of one of the more fascinating patients described by Dr. Carlton:

*Bottom Line, Vol. 12, No. 15, August 15, 1991.

"A lawyer in his 30's was plagued by mid-afternoon sleepiness. So overwhelming that he would often fall dead asleep at inopportune times—even in the middle of conversations.

"Once while visiting my home, he fell asleep in my living room. When he woke up, I asked about his eating habits and discovered he had been eating lots of bread (wheat) at fancy lunches with clients. When he gave up the bread his afternoon sleepiness disappeared."

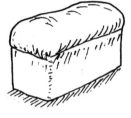

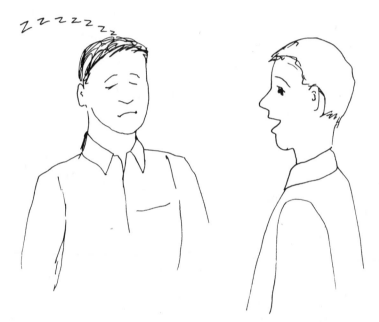

In a conversation with me in October 1991, Dr. Carlton pointed out that while food sensitivities are important, they're only one of many causes of mental and emotional symptoms in his patients.

Another New York physician, Morton Teich, M.D., in discussing CFS patients he's seen in his practice, commented,

"Food sensitivities occur commonly in these patients, and they often respond to dietary changes. Yet, most require other treatment measures, including avoidance of chemicals and molds in the home and workplace, antiyeast medication and psychological support."

Elimination Diets

In my medical practice during the past 35 years I've seen thousands of children and adults with fatigue, headaches, muscle aches, nasal congestion, irritability and other symptoms. Using trial elimination diets I've found that sensitivity reactions to foods my patients were eating every day were the main cause of their symptoms.

Then in the 1980s, I worked with and treated patients with yeast-connected health problems, I learned that *almost without exception, every person with a yeast-connected health problem was bothered by food sensitivities.* Moreover, my observations and experiences were confirmed by other physicians, including John Crayton, M.D.,* Robert Dockhorn, M.D., Leo Galland, M.D., and Sherry Rogers, M.D. and other professionals who made presentations at the September 1988 Candida Update Conference.

To identify the foods that contribute to your symptoms you must carefully plan and properly execute a trial elimination/ challenge diet. Here's an edited transcript of a tape-recorded visit with one of my patients:

Q: I've been tired ever since I had "mono" three years ago. I've also been bothered by headaches, muscle aches, poor memory, abdominal pain and a year-round stuffy nose. I'm wondering if my symptoms are food-related and I'd like to try an elimination diet. Please explain.

> *Almost without exception, every person with a yeast-connected health problem was bothered by food sensitivities.*

---

*You'll find a summary of Dr. Crayton's presentation in Section III.

205

A: On such a diet you eliminate many or all of your favorite foods. To make things easier for you I have prepared two diets. The first of these—a less restrictive diet—I call Diet A. Then there's a much tougher Diet B, which I call the "Caveman Diet."

Q: I believe I'd like to try Diet A first. What foods can I eat on this diet?

A: You can eat any meats but bacon, sausage, hot dogs or luncheon meats; any vegetables but corn; any fruits but citrus. You can also eat rice, rice crackers, plain oatmeal and the grain alternatives amaranth and quinoa (obtainable from health food store).

Foods you can eat include most meats, vegetables and fruits. Also rice, oats and the grain alternatives.

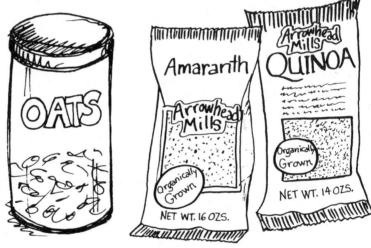

Q: Anything else?
A: Yes. Nuts in shell or unprocessed nuts of any kind.

Q: That doesn't sound too difficult, although it'll take careful planning to carry out the diet. What can I drink?
A: Water. I especially recommend bottled or filtered water.

Q: What foods do I need to eliminate?
A: Many of your favorite foods. Here's why: *The more of a food you eat, the greater your chances of developing an allergy to that food.* Here's a list of foods you must avoid on the diet: Milk, and all dairy products; wheat; corn, corn syrup and corn sweeteners; yeast; cane and beet sugar; orange and other citrus fruits; chocolate.

This diet also eliminates food coloring, additives and flavorings which are found in many packaged and processed foods.

If you are sensitive to foods you're eating every day, chances are you may also be sensitive to tobacco, insecticides and environmental chemicals. To gain maximum benefit from your diet detective work, do not smoke in the house or use perfumes, fumigants or other odorous chemicals.

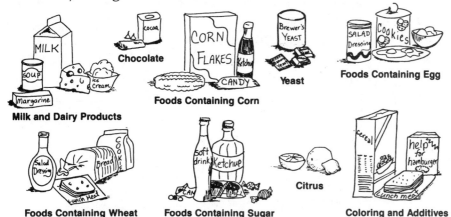

Milk and Dairy Products

Chocolate

Foods Containing Corn

Yeast

Foods Containing Egg

Foods Containing Wheat

Foods Containing Sugar

Citrus

Coloring and Additives

Getting started on your diet—what you do first.

Q: How do I get started on a diet? What do I do first?

A: Prepare menus and purchase foods you'll eat while on the diet. This requires careful planning. When you go shopping, avoid commercially prepared or processed foods. Here's why: Such foods usually contain sugar, wheat, milk, corn, yeast, food coloring and other hidden ingredients that may be causing some of your symptoms.

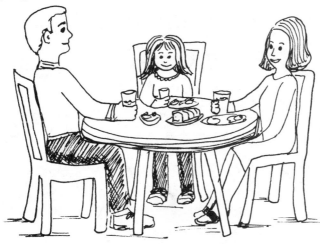

Discuss the diet with other family members. When you're planning your diet you'll feel less deprived if you think about the many foods you *can* eat rather than feeling frustrated because of the foods you must avoid.

Q: Tell me more about the diet.
A: The diet is divided into two parts: First you'll eliminate a number of your usual foods to see if your symptoms improve or disappear. Then, after five to ten days, when your symptoms show convincing improvement, eat the eliminated foods again—one at a time—and see which foods cause the symptoms to return.

An elimination diet is divided into two parts.

Q: How will I know the diet is really making a difference?
A: By keeping a record of your symptoms:
a. for three days (or more) before beginning the diet
b. while you're following the elimination part of the diet (five to ten days—occasionally longer)
c. while you're eating the eliminated foods again one food per day

You'll need, of course, to keep a detailed record of all foods you eat.

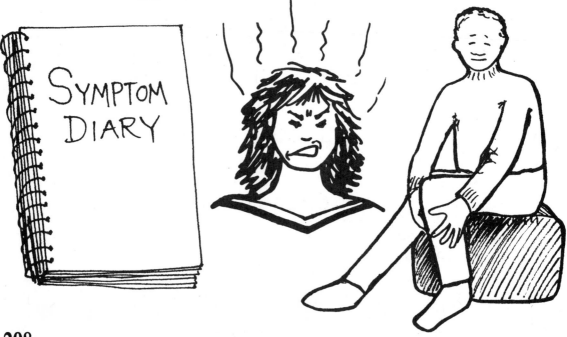

Q: How will I feel on the diet?

A: During the first two to four days of the diet, you're apt to feel irritable and hungry and you may not feel satisfied even though you fill up on the permitted foods. You may feel restless and fidgety or tired and droopy. You may also develop a headache or leg cramps.

You may be "mad" at the world because you aren't getting the foods you crave, especially sweets. You may act like a two-pack-a-day smoker who quit smoking "cold turkey." Here's why: People who suffer from hidden food allergies are often "addicted" to the foods causing their problems.*

Here's some good news. If the foods you've avoided are causing your symptoms, you'll usually feel better by the fourth, fifth or sixth day of the diet. Almost always, you'll improve by the tenth day. Occasionally, though, it'll take two or three weeks before your symptoms go away completely.

If the foods you've avoided are causing your symptoms you'll usually feel better by the fourth to sixth day of your diet.

Q: If I improve on the diet, what do I do then? When and how will I return the foods to my diet?

A: After you're certain that you feel better and your improvement has lasted for at least two days, begin adding foods back to your diet—one at a time. If you're allergic to one or more of the eliminated foods you'll usually develop symptoms when you eat the foods again.

Q: What symptoms should I look for?

A: Usually, but not always, your main symptoms will reappear. In your case you're apt to feel more tired and depressed; and you'll probably develop a headache or your nose will feel stopped up. However, sometimes you'll notice other symptoms, including some that had not bothered you previously—such as itching, coughing or urinary frequency.

Q: How soon will these symptoms appear after I eat a food that I'm sensitive to?

A: The symptoms will usually reappear within a few minutes to a few hours. However, sometimes you may not notice a symp-

---

*Dr. Elmer Cranton comments: "If you subsitute a nonallergic food of equal nutritional value for a frequently eaten food and feel cravings, you confirm the diagnosis of allergic addiction to that food. No matter how much you feel you need the formerly eaten food, you'll probably feel better long-term, without it!"

tom until the next day. *Nearly always, if you avoid an allergy-causing food for a short period-five to seven days—you'll develop symptoms promptly when you eat the food again.* By contrast, if you avoid the food for three or more weeks, your symptoms won't return until you eat the food two or three days in a row.

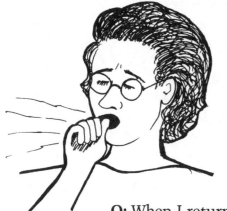 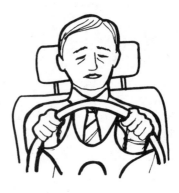 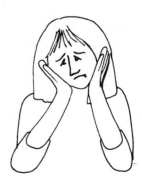

Q: When I return a food to my diet does it make any difference what form the food is in?

A: Yes! Yes! Yes! Add the food in pure form. For example, when you eat wheat, use pure whole wheat (obtainable from a health food store), rather than bread, since bread contains milk and other ingredients. If you're testing milk, use whole milk rather than ice cream, since ice cream contains sugar, corn syrup and other ingredients.

Here are suggestions for returning foods to your diet:

When you return a food to your diet, add it in pure form.

Egg: Eat a soft- or hard-boiled egg (or eggs scrambled in pure safflower or sunflower oil).

Citrus: Peel an orange and eat it. You can also drink fresh-squeezed orange juice (do not use frozen or canned orange juice).

Milk: Use whole milk.

Wheat: Get 100% whole wheat from the health food store. Add water and cook for 20 to 25 minutes. Add sea salt if you wish. Eat it straight or add sliced bananas or strawberries. If you want to "wet the cereal," you can put the fruit in a blender with a little water and pour in on the cereal like milk or cream.

> *To test wheat, get 100% whole wheat from the health food store.*

If you don't like hot cereals, you can use shredded wheat. However, shredded wheat contains the additive BHT, which may cause symptoms. So a pure wheat product without additives is better.

Food coloring: Buy a set of McCormick's or French's dyes and colors. Put a half teaspoon of several colors in a glass. Add a teaspoon of mixture to a glass of water and sip on it. If you show a reaction, you'll later need to test the various food dyes separately. Red seems to be the most common offender.

Chocolate: Use Baker's cooking chocolate or Hershey's cocoa powder. You can sweeten it with a little liquid saccharin (Sweeta or Fasweet). Eat the powder with a spoon or add it to water and make a chocolate-flavored drink.

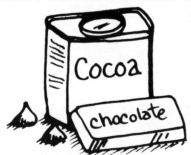

Corn: Use fresh corn on the cob, pure corn syrup, grits or hominy. Eat plain popcorn. Don't use microwave popcorn because it contains other ingredients.

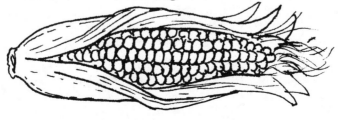

Sugar: Get plain cane sugar. Perhaps the easiest way to do this is to eat some sugar lumps or add the sugar to a glass of water. Do the same with beet sugar.

Q: I think I understand what you want me to do. However, a few points aren't clear. Please go over them again.

A: Okay, here they are:

1. Carefully review all your instructions. Plan ahead. Don't start your diet the week before Christmas, Thanksgiving or some other holiday—and don't start it when you're traveling or visiting friends or relatives. Ask—even beg—other family members to help you and to cooperate. Study your instructions and purchase the foods you'll need. Keep a diary of your symptoms for at least three days before you begin your diet.

   Remain on the diet until you're absolutely certain your symptoms have improved. Remember that your symptoms are apt to worsen the first 48 to 72 hours on the diet.

   Usually, you'll feel better by the fourth or fifth day although some people won't notice a significant change until they've followed the diet for seven to ten days—occasionally longer. Still other individuals with a hidden food allergy won't show a lot of improvement until they've avoided an offending food for two or three weeks. However, such people are the exception.

2. If you don't feel significantly better in 10 to 14 days,* start eating your usual foods—even pig out. If your symptoms worsen (including your headache, fatigue, irritability or stuffiness), chances are they're food related and you'll have to do further detective work to identify the troublemakers.

3. If you improve on the diet, return the eliminated foods one at a time and see if you develop symptoms. Here's how you go about it.

Don't start your diet the week before Christmas, Thanksgiving or some other holiday—or when you're visiting friends or relatives.

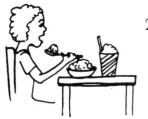

---

*Your failure to improve substantially on an elimination diet may be related to other offending substances in your living and work environment (exhaust fumes, paint fumes, insecticides sprays, carpet odors, etc.). Accordingly, before beginning your diet, clean up your environment.

A: Add the foods you least suspect first. Save the foods you think are causing your problems until last. Remember, you're apt to be allergic to your favorite foods.

B. If you have no idea what foods are causing your symptoms, here's a suggested order to returning foods to your diet.

1. Eggs
2. Citrus
3. Yeast
4. Wheat
5. Food coloring
6. Chocolate
7. Corn
8. Sugar
9. Milk

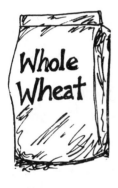
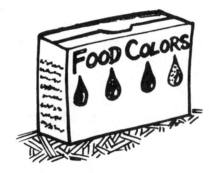

4. Eat a small portion of the eliminated food for breakfast. If you show no reaction, eat more of the food for lunch and for supper and between meals too.*

5. Keep the rest of your diet the same while you're carrying out the challenges. Here's an example: Suppose you eat wheat on the first day of your diet and show no reaction. Does this mean you can continue to eat wheat? No. Eat wheat only on the day of the challenge and don't eat it again until you've tested all the foods and the diet has been completed.

6. If you show no symptoms after adding a food the first day, add another food the second day, eating all you want—unless you show a reaction.

---

*If a person suffers from severe asthma, hives, or swelling, the food challenges should be supervised by a physician and carried out in his office or clinic.

7. If you think you develop symptoms when you add a food but aren't certain, eat more of the food until your symptoms are obvious. But don't make yourself sick.

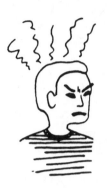 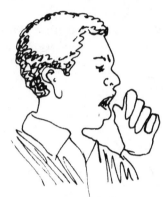

If you show an obvious reaction after eating a food, such as stuffiness, cough, irritability, nervousness, drowsiness, headache, stomach ache, flushing or wheezing, don't eat more of that food.

If you show an obvious reaction after eating a food, don't eat more of that food.

Wait until the reaction subsides (usually 24 to 48 hours) before you add another food.

If a food really bothers you, shorten the reaction by taking a teaspoon of "soda mixture" (two parts baking soda and one part potassium bicarbonate—your pharmacist can fix up this mixture for you). Or dissolve two tablets of Alka Seltzer Gold* in a glass of water and drink it. A saline cathartic such as Epsom salts will also shorten your reaction by eliminating the offending foods from your digestive tract rapidly.

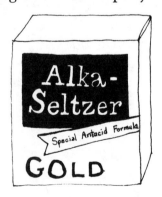

*Alka Seltzer Gold contains no asprin.

Q: Thank you for those explanations. They make sense. But while we're discussing diets, let's go ahead and talk about Diet B.

A: I call Diet B the "Rare Food" or "Cave Man" Diet. On this diet you'll eliminate all the foods listed on Diet A. In addition, you must avoid beef, chicken, pork, white potato, tomato, rice, oats, coffee, tea and any food or beverage you consume more than once a week.

For example, if you eat bananas and apples daily or several times a week, add them to the list of the foods you eliminate. If you snack on pecans, avoid them. But if you rarely eat a food, you need not leave it out of your diet.

Q: I can see that this is a truly comprehensive diet. Would I be able to get enough to eat?

A: Yes. Although early on you'd probably suffer food cravings, which we've already discussed. But you can eat as much as you want of the allowed foods. So you get plenty of nutrition. My purpose in prescribing the Cave Man Diet is to avoid foods you usually eat. But to repeat—as difficult as this diet seems to be, it provides you with a variety of wholesome foods. Do you think you'll be able to carry out this Diet B?

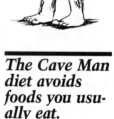

The Cave Man diet avoids foods you usually eat.

Q: Yes—I can do anything I have to do. But let me repeat your instructions so I can be certain I understand them.

If I feel Diet A hasn't given me the answers I'm looking for, you're suggesting I try Diet B. On this diet, I eliminate all the foods on Diet A plus pork, beef, chicken, potato, rice, oats and any food I eat more than once a week. So I'll have to eliminate twenty or more foods?

A: That's right.

Q: How about returning these foods to my diet? Do I add one food a day?

A: That's one way to do it. However, it would take you three or four weeks to complete the diet.

Q: That's a long time. And it would be hard for me to hold the line and keep from cheating. Is there another way to do Diet B in less time?

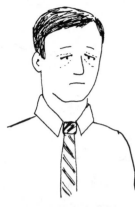

A: Yes. Carry out the elimination phase of the diet until your symptoms improve, just as we've already discussed. However, if you improve promptly (as, for example, in four or five days), you can begin returning the foods to your diet sooner. You can also shorten the period you'll have to stay on the diet by adding the foods you've eliminated four times a day.

Q: How would I do this? Please explain.

A: After your improvement is convincing and you've continued to feel better for at least 48 hours, add a single food—such as orange—for breakfast. But before you add the food, take a few minutes to make an inventory of your symptoms.*

Before you add the food, make an inventory of your symptoms.

Think about how you feel. Does your head hurt? Are you tired? Is your nose stopped up? Do you have a burning in your stomach or aching in your legs? It's important for you to "tune in" to symptoms that are present before eating the food. If you fail to do this, you're apt to blame symptoms that are already present on the food you're testing.

After you've finished your symptom inventory, eat the orange. If no new symptoms develop, wait 15 minutes and eat another orange, and then a third. If no symptoms develop, oranges aren't causing your problems.

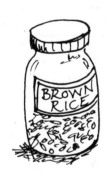

Wait four hours, then introduce a second food (such as rice). Follow the same procedure that you followed in testing the orange. If this food causes no reaction, in another four hours, try a third food (such as baked chicken). Then eat a fourth food an hour before bedtime.

So each day you'll be eating four foods. By doing this you'll reduce the "adding back" phase of your diet from three weeks to seven to ten days.

Q: Would that work as well?

A: Perhaps. Such a rapid addition of foods would have several advantages. One of these would be completing Diet B in less time—two weeks rather than three more weeks. Another advantage relates to the peculiarities of a "hidden" food allergy.

---

*Counting your pulse before and after you eat a food may also help you determine a food reaction. A pulse acceleration of six to eight beats following a food challenge is usually significant.

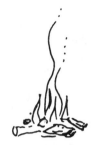

Q: Could you explain.

A: I'll try. If you avoid a food you're allergic to for a week and then eat it again, it'll nearly always cause a reaction. But if you avoid it for four to six weeks, like a fire that dies down, your sensitivity to that food will decrease. And you may show a little reaction when you eat it again, especially if you consume only a small amount.

Q: From what you've told me, I believe it'll be best for me to add one food four times a day. Will that be okay?

A: Yes. I feel that's the best way.

Q: Okay, now that's settled. I'd like your suggestions for getting my family to cooperate.

A: Plan the diet carefully. Discuss it with other family members ahead of time. Where possible, feature foods all the family members will eat (although they may want other foods to keep them satisfied and happy). Don't worry if your diet is limited. Even if you lose several pounds it won't hurt you and you'll soon regain them.

Plan the diet carefully. Discuss it with other family members ahead of time.

Q: Can I follow the diet at work?

A: Yes, if you "brown bag" it. If you're invited out to dinner, tell your host or hostess what you're doing and eat before you go or decline the invitation and ask for a raincheck.

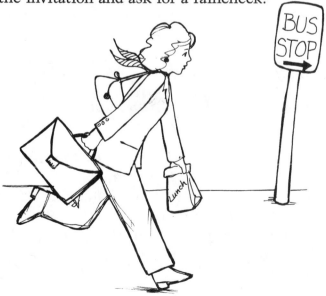

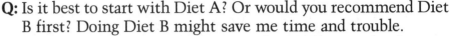

Q: Is it best to start with Diet A? Or would you recommend Diet B first? Doing Diet B might save me time and trouble.

A: Sometimes I recommend Diet A for my patients and sometimes I recommend Diet B. It depends on how the patient feels about it and how severe and long lasting his symptoms are. However, in most patients I recommend Diet A.

Here's why: Most food-sensitive people improve on Diet A and Diet A is easier to follow than Diet B. It eliminates many of the major food troublemakers. Yet, it allows a person to eat pork, chicken, potatoes, apples and other foods which he likes but which he doesn't eat every day. And the rest of your family can eat the same diet. This makes things easier.

Q: When, why and under what circumstances should I try Diet B?

A: As I've already indicated, it depends on many different things. For example, although I've found that milk, wheat, corn, yeast, sugar, egg, chocolate and food additives are the most common troublemakers, any food can cause a reaction.

So even if you improve when you remove these foods from your diet, you may continue to show symptoms because beef, pork, chicken, apple, potato tomato, banana, oats or other foods may be causing some of your symptoms. The only way you can tell if these foods bother you is to eliminate them from your diet and see if your symptoms improve. Then you can eat the foods again and see if your symptoms return.

Sometimes I recommend Diet A for my patients and sometimes I recommend Diet B.

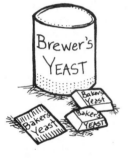

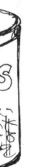

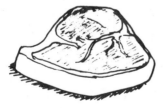

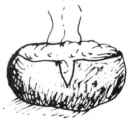

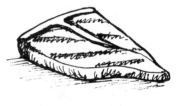

Q: I think I understand. But to make sure, let me repeat your instructions. You want me to do Elimination Diet A for seven to ten days, keeping a record of my symptoms for three days before I start the diet. I continue to record my symptoms for the seven- to ten-day elimination phase of the diet. Then after I'm sure my symptoms have improved, I eat the foods again, one at a time, to see which foods bother me and which foods do not. I continue my records.

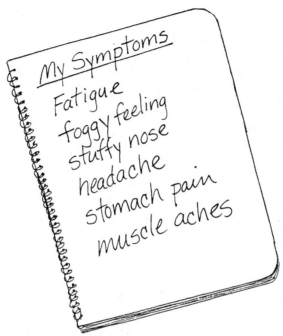

A: That's right.

Q: Suppose I complete the diet and note obvious reactions to a couple of foods, yet, there are other foods I'm not sure about—what do I do then?

A: Keep the foods that cause reactions out of your diet indefinitely. Retest the foods you're uncertain about. Here's one way you can do this. Eat the suspected food several days in a row, as for example, Friday, Saturday, Sunday, Monday and Tuesday. Eliminate the food on Wednesday, Thursday, Friday, Saturday and Sunday and then load up on the food you've eliminated the following Monday. If you're allergic to it, you should develop symptoms. If you show no symptoms, chances are you aren't allergic to that food.

Keep the foods that cause reactions out of your diet indefinitely. Retest the foods you're uncertain about.

Mon.	Tue.	Wed.	Thu.	Fri.
1	2	3	4	5

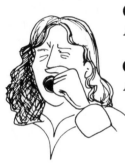

Q: I think I understand, but suppose I show a reaction when I eat wheat or egg or when I drink milk. Does this mean I'll always be allergic to these foods?

A: Yes, to some degree. Your symptoms will nearly always return if you consume as much of a food as you did before you began your diet. However, if you avoid a food you're allergic to for several months, you'll usually regain some tolerance to it. And you may not develop symptoms unless you eat it several days in a row.

If you avoid a food you're allergic to for several months, you'll usually regain some tolerance to it.

Q: How do I find out?

A: By trial and error.

Q: I'm not sure I understand—please explain.

A: I'll do my best. When you avoid a food you're allergic to for several months, you'll generally lose some of your allergy to the food (like a fire that dies down).

For example, if you're bothered by a stuffed-up nose, headache and fatigue while drinking a quart of milk a day, you may be able to eat yogurt or cheese occasionally after you've eliminated milk from your diet for several months. However, suppose you eat milk-containing foods after you've avoided them for several months and show no reaction. In such a situation you may say to yourself, "The yogurt and cheese didn't bother me so maybe milk allergy isn't one of my problems. But if you start drinking milk or eating dairy products every day, within a few days or weeks some of your symptoms will return. Before you know it, you'll develop the same health problems you had before you eliminated milk.

Sometimes, though, it takes even longer for your symptoms to recur and you may not connect them to the food.

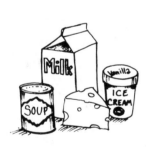

Q: I think this point is clear but why does a food bother me on some occasions and not on others. For example, I've heard of people who became congested when they drank milk in the winter but who could drink it in the summer without showing any symptoms.

A: It has to do with the "allergic load" or concomitant allergies. Along with other physicians interested in food allergy, I have found that allergic individuals may tolerate foods in the summer which they can't eat in the winter.

Part of the problem relates to chilling. Also, wintertime furnaces which stir up dust and dry out the respiratory membranes may lessen a person's resistance and make him more susceptible to wintertime infections and allergies.

In addition, during the wintertime, you spend more time indoors. Windows and doors are usually closed so there is less ventilation. Accordingly, disease-producing germs are more prevalent. Other factors include the household and office indoor air pollutants (tobacco smoke, perfumes, janitorial supplies and other odorous chemicals).

Cold weather, dust, cold germs and chemicals, plus food allergies, cause many wintertime health problems.

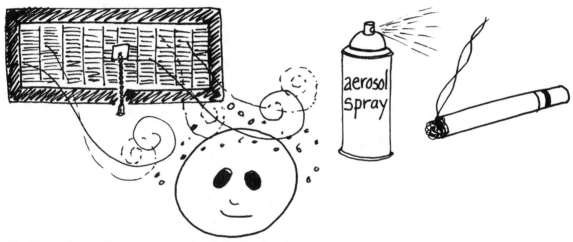

Q: Do other allergies such as hay fever due to grass or bronchitis due to house dust mites or cat dander have anything to do with the amount of an allergy-causing food I can eat?

A: Yes. The more allergy troublemakers you're exposed to, the greater are your chances of developing an allergic illness. For example, let's suppose you're allergic to milk, corn, chocolate, spring grass and house dust mites. Yet, you aren't severely allergic to any one of these substances.

Accordingly, you may play golf in the spring without being bothered by hay fever and you may be able to eat an occasional piece of cornbread or chocolate without symptoms. But if you eat a sack of popcorn, a candy bar and drink a chocolate milk

The more allergy trouble makers you're exposed to, the greater are your chances of developing an allergic illness.

shake on the same day (after cutting the grass), you may become irritable and nervous and develop nasal congestion or bronchitis.

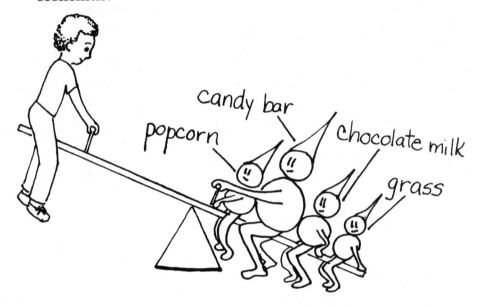

Q: I'm beginning to understand more about hidden food allergies. But suppose I'm allergic to egg and I avoid egg for three months. Then I eat an egg for breakfast and it doesn't bother me. How will I know how much and how often I can eat egg in the future?

S	M	T	W	T	F	S
1	2	**3**	4	5	6	7
8	9	**10**	11	12	13	14
15	16	**17**	18	19	20	21
22	23	**24**	25	26	27	28
29	30	**31**				

⌐ EGG DAY

A: I'm glad you asked. It'll give me a chance to talk about a rotated diet. Along with many physicians interested in hidden food allergies. I've found that my allergic patients who rotate their diets usually get along well and develop fewer new food allergies.

Rotating a diet means eating a food only once every four to seven days. For example, if you're allergic to egg and after avoiding it for several months you eat an egg and it doesn't bother you, you can try eating an egg once a week and see if you tolerate it. You can do the same with other foods.

Rotating a diet means eating a food only once every four to seven days.

Q: Aren't some foods "kin" to each other—like chicken and egg, wheat and corn or milk and beef? Is a person who is allergic to one food more apt to become sensitive to foods in the same "family?"

A: The answer to both of your questions is yes. Foods are "kin" to each other. Familiar food families include the grain family, citrus family and the legume family (peas, peanuts, beans and soybeans). While there are many exceptions, people who are sensitive to one food in a family are more apt to be sensitive—or become sensitive—to another food in the family, especially if they eat a lot of it.

People who are sensitive to one food in a family are more apt to be sensitive to another food in the family.

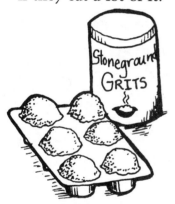
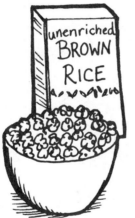
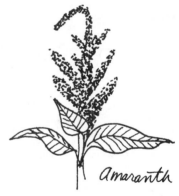

amaranth

I've found that wheat-sensitive patients are apt to become sensitive to all other grains—especially if they eat them repeatedly or in quantity. Although I permit rice and oats on Diet A, if you find you're allergic to wheat or corn, experiment further with your diet to see if other grains cause reactions.

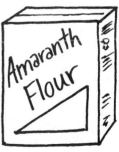

If you're allergic to grains, here's another suggestion: Go to your health food store and get some quinoa, amaranth and buckwheat. You can make bread and other grainlike products from these grain alternatives. Yet, they aren't "kin" to the grains.

223

Now for a word on milk and beef. Most milk-sensitive individuals seem to be able to eat steak and hamburger without a reaction. However, because cow's milk and beef come from the same animal, if you're allergic to milk, avoid beef for a week, then add it back and see what happens. If you're allergic to egg, limit your intake of chicken to a serving every four to seven days.

Is there anything else you'd like to know—anything at all?

Q: Nothing I can think of at the moment—my head is spinning. Do you have further suggestions?

A: Read, review and study all the instructions I've given you. When you've finished, you'll find that detecting your hidden food allergies won't be as hard as you thought it would be.

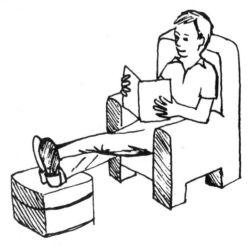

Prescription Yeast-Control Medications

Three prescription medications, nystatin, Nizoral (ketoconazole) and Diflucan (fluconazole) are now being used by physicians in North America to eradicate or control *Candida albicans* and/ or other yeasts and molds. A fourth antifungal medication, amphotericin B* (Fungizone, Squibb) is used commonly in Europe. Still another antifungal medication, itraconazole (Janssen) is undergoing testing in the United States and may become available in 1992 or 1993.

Nystatin**

If your CFS is yeast connected, you'll be hearing about the antiyeast medication nystatin. So I think you'll be interested in knowing how it was discovered and where it got its name.

You'll be especially interested if you're a woman. Here's why: Two brilliant women scientists collaborated in discovering this remarkable antifungal substance over 40 years ago. In the late 1940s, mold researcher Elizabeth Hazen and organic chemist Rachel Brown began looking for agents in the soil which might be useful in controlling fungus disease. And while working at the Albany laboratory of the New York State Health Department, they found many antifungal substances. However, most of them were toxic, not only to yeasts, but also to laboratory animals.

How nystatin was discovered and where it got its name.

*This antifungal medication is closely related to nystatin and given orally it is extremely well tolerated and is virtually non-toxic. You'll find further information on pages 281-285 of the third edition of *The Yeast Connection*.
**Brand names include Mycostatin (Squibb) and Nilstat (Lederle). Generic preparations of nystatin are also available.

Then, while vacationing with friends on a farm in Warrenton, Virginia, Elizabeth Hazen dug a soil sample and took it back to her laboratory. Cultures of this soil revealed a mold that kept other molds (including *Candida albicans*) from growing. Moreover, tests showed that this mold did not harm the animals. These scientists named their discovery after New York State, nystatin (NY-Stat-In).

In 1951, Hazen and Brown signed an agreement with E. R. Squibb and Sons to study the drug, patent it and produce it. In their agreement with Squibb, royalties were put in a special scientific and educational fund. Neither of these women asked for or received personal financial gain from their discovery.

Nystatin was marketed exclusively by Squibb until 1974 and since that time has been manufactured and marketed by other companies. During the decades after its discovery it was used mainly in suppositories to treat vaginal yeast infections. And not until the reports of C. Orian Truss in the late 1970s was it used to discourage yeast growth in the intestinal tract.

Then, during the decade of the '80s, physicians began using oral forms of this medication along with a sugar-free special diet in treating patients with fatigue, headache, depression, PMS and other symptoms.*

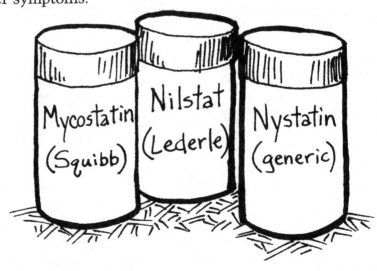

---

*The research studies of Mary L. Miles, M.D. published in the *Journal of the American Medical Association* document the importance of intestinal yeast in women with recurrent beginal yeast infections. (Se Section III.)

Dosage forms for oral use: Tablet, capsules, liquid solutions and powder.* Although the tablets are convenient and easy to obtain on prescription, I usually recommend the nystatin powder. Here's why:

1. Yeasts live in your digestive tract from your mouth to your anus. Accordingly, the powder helps you get rid of yeasts in your mouth, esophagus and stomach, as well as in your intestines.

2. The powder contains no food coloring, chemicals, dye or other similar ingredients that may cause reactions in chemically sensitive patients.

3. The powder is more economical.

I like nystatin for a number of reasons. Here's one of them. It is perhaps safer than any medication a physician can prescribe for his or her patients. According to the *Physician's Desk Reference* (which gives information on over 2,500 prescription drugs), "Nystatin is virtually nontoxic and nonsensitizing, is well tolerated by all age groups, even on prolonged administration."

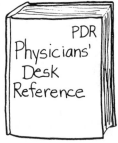

Here's a major reason for the safety of nystatin—*Very little is absorbed from the intestinal tract. Accordingly, it helps a person with yeast-connected CFS by controlling candida growth in the intestinal tract.*

Nystatin is unusually safe because very little is absorbed from the intestinal tract.

The usual starting dose is 500,000 to 1 million units, four times a day. (Each tablet equals 500,000 units; 1/8 teaspoon of powder equals 500,000 units.) For a further discussion of nystatin, see pages 45-49 and 349-53 of the third (paperback) edition of *The Yeast Connection.*

If your pharmacy does not stock powdered nystatin you can fill your prescription from the following pharmacies: Wellness Health and Pharmaceuticals (800-227-2627), Bio-Tech (800-345-1199), N.E.E.D.S. (800-634-1380), Freeda Pharmaceuticals (800-777-3737), Medical Tower Pharmacy (205-933-7381) and Willner Chemists (212-685-0441).

A special word to physicians about nystatin powder: If you are prescribing nystatin for many of your patients, ask your pharmacist to order it in bulk. They can obtain it by calling 1-800-LEDERLE. It comes in one billion and five billion unit containers.

---

*If your physician prescribes the powder, make sure it is the powder for oral administration and not the foot powder.

Nizoral*

A broad spectrum antifungal agent introduced in the United States in 1981. It is preferred by some physicians. For example, Francis Waickman, an Akron, Ohio, physician who has treated hundreds of patients with Nizoral commented,

> "I put all of my patients with severe candida-related problems on Nizoral, 200 mgs. a day for two weeks. Ninety percent of them show significant improvement. It is remarkable! I then switch them over to nystatin.
>
> "In my opinion, the much greater improvement on Nizoral takes place because hyphal forms of candida burrow into the deeper tissues of a person's body and nystatin simply doesn't get to them."

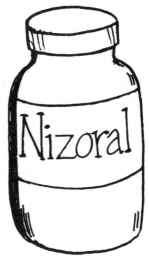

I've used Nizoral in over 200 of my patients, especially those with persistent or long-standing candida-related health problems and I've never run into a significant toxic reaction. I've also been impressed by the success Dr. Carol Jessop experienced in treating 1,100 of her patients with the Chronic Fatigue Syndrome using Nizoral, 200 mgs. (1 tablet) a day and a special sugar-free diet.**

---

*Nizoral is the trade name for ketoconazole. It is produced and marketed by Janssen Pharmaceuticals.

**See also Dr. Jessop's comments at the April 1989 CFS Conference in San Francisco and the November 1990 CFIDS Conference in Charlotte. During her question and answer session at the latter conference in discussing medication, Dr. Jessop said that in patients with a yeast overgrowth "my treatment of choice is 3 weeks of fluconazole (Diflucan, 100 mg. daily.)

Serious side effects may occur in one person out of 10,000 who take this medication. Accordingly, a blood test to check liver function is recommended every two to four weeks for people who take this medication for one month or longer. See also pages 49-52 of *The Yeast Connection*, third edition and Dr. Carol Jessop's comments at the San Francisco CFS Conference (which are described in Section III).

People who take Nizoral for a month or longer should have a blood test.

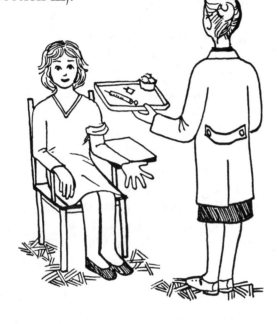

Diflucan*

This broad spectrum antifungal agent is a "cousin" of Nizoral and has been used in England and other foreign countries for several years. In informal discussions at the Candida Update Conference, Memphis, Tennessee, in September 1988,* Dr. Stephen Davies and Dr. Jean Monro of London reported favorable experiences using this medication in treating patients with the Candida-Related Complex.

In September 1989, I obtained two 25-page brochures from the British branch of Pfizer Pharmaceuticals and I was impressed by what I read. *For example, one study cited in this literature showed that a single Diflucan tablet (150 mgs.) taken by mouth*

A single oral Diflucan tablet was more effective than five days of vaginal suppositories.

*Diflucan is the trade name for fluconazole. It is produced and marketed by Pfizer-Roerig Pharmaceuticals.
**This conference was organized and conducted by the International Health Foundation, Inc., P.O. Box 3494, Jackson, TN 38303

was more effective in treating vaginal yeast infections than five days of vaginal suppositories and/or five days of Nizoral therapy.

Diflucan is less apt to cause toxic effects in the liver or disturbances of the endocrine system.

A number of research studies have shown that although Diflucan was kin to Nizoral, it was less apt to cause toxic effects in the liver or disturbances of the endocrine system. Diflucan was introduced for use in the United States by the Roerig Division of Pfizer, Inc., in February 1990. Initially, the company has advertised it mainly for the treatment of candida infections in individuals suffering from marked immunosuppression.

During 1990 and 1991, I received reports from clinicians throughout the United States who used Diflucan in treating their patients with the Candida-Related Complex (CRC) and the Chronic Fatigue Syndrome (CFS). Dosages have ranged from 200 mgs. to start, followed by 100 mgs. two to three times a week, on up to 200 mgs. (occasionally more) daily for 30 to 60 days. *The dose and duration of therapy has depended on the severity of the illness and the response of the patient.*

In the March 1991 *Physician's Forum* issue of the CFIDS *Chronicle*, Jay A. Goldstein, M.D., Director of the Chronic Fatigue Syndrome Institute, Anaheim, California, discussed treatment. And in a paragraph entitled "Battling Yeast" he said:

"I'm still unclear about the role of the candida hypersensitivity syndrome. Yet, I'm impressed with the sincerity of certain clinicians who believe in the entity, some of whom are conducting research about the effectiveness of its diagnosis and treatment. Although fluconazole (Diflucan) is quite expensive (one 200 mg. tablet costs about $10 to $12), it is also quite safe, and a quick trial of this agent may help make the diagnosis and establish a treatment.

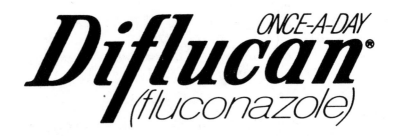

Compassionate ("free") supplies of Diflucan are available. The person requesting this medication must have clinical and/or laboratory confirmation of infection by *Candida albicans*; the patient must be uninsured; that is, not covered by private insurance, Medicaid, Medicare, the state AIDS Drug Assistance Program or any other third-party payer; the patient's annual income must be less than $25,000 if single with no dependents, $40,000 if married or with dependents.

Diflucan tablets must be prescribed; the IV dosage form is not available through this program. The drug must be taken in an outpatient setting. Inpatient use in an acute or chronic care setting is not recovered. To obtain more information, call Barbara Jenkins, information specialist, Roerig Division, Pfizer, Inc., 1-800-869-9979.

Free supplies of Diflucan are available for some persons with laboratory confirmed yeast infections.

Nonprescription Yeast-Control Medications

During the past decade a number of nonprescription agents have been used by professionals and nonprofessionals in helping patients curb yeast overgrowth in the digestive tract. Included among these substances are caprylic acid, citrus seed extracts, probiotics and garlic.*

Caprylic Acid

In the 1950s this short-chain, saturated fatty acid was studied by Dr. Irene Newhouser of the University of Illinois, who found it effective in treating persons with yeast overgrowth in the intestinal tract. Because it is a food substance, it is available without a prescription. It is marketed by a number of different companies under various brand names, including Mycopryl 680, Caprystatin, Caprycidin-A, Capricin, Capralin and Caprinex.

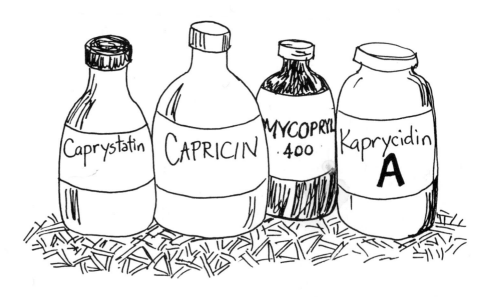

*You'll find a discussion of probiotics and garlic in Section VI.

These preparations appear to be safe and effective and I know of no serious side effects. However, as is the case with nystatin and other antifungal medications, some persons may experience a temporary accentuation of symptoms during the first week they take the medication. These symptoms have been called, "die-off" reactions. Here's the probable mechanism:

When you kill yeast germs in your intestinal tract, you absorb metabolic products, which temporarily worsen your symptoms. Although annoying, they're rarely serious and usually subside in a few days. In addition, other persons may experience digestive complaints. If you do not tolerate this yeast-control substance discontinue it and check with your physician.

Here are the comments of Ralph Golan, M.D., Seattle, Washington, who has been using Mycopryl 680 in treating many of his patients:

> "I begin my patients with yeast-related health problems on Mycopryl 680, 1 capsule daily. If it is well tolerated, in two or three days I add a second capsule. I continue to increase the dose of Mycopryl every two to three days until the patient is taking three capsules three times a day with meals.
>
> "In approximately 35–40% of my patients with yeast-related illness, no other antifungal agent is needed. I like to begin with Mycopryl because of its low toxicity, ease of use and relative effectiveness. If, in three to four weeks there has not been a sufficient response, I will often prescribe nystatin or another antifungal agent."

Citrus Seed Extracts

I first learned about this biologically active botanical from Dr. Leo Galland several years ago. It is produced and distributed by a number of different companies under various trade names, including ParaMicrocidin, Paracan 144, DF100, Citricidal™ and Seed-a-Sept-II™. Here are comments of two physicians who have been using citrus seed extracts.

Leo Galland, M.D., New York:

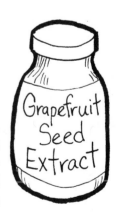

> "It will be hard for me to overestimate the value of ParaMicrocidin to my medical practice. It is a broad spectrum antimicrobial product derived from the extracts of tropical plants. It is not ab-

In the treatment of candiasis citrus seed extracts appear as effective as nystatin, caprylic acid and other non-absorbed intestinal antifungal agents.

sorbed from the intestinal tract and has no inherent toxicity except for a concentration-dependent local irritant effect.

"For the past year I've used the ParaMicrocidin formula in the treatment of intestinal parasitism and chronic candidiasis with excellent results. In the treatment of candidiasis it appears as effective as nystatin, caprylic acid and other non-absorbed intestinal antifungal agents . . . . The dose which I prescribe is 2 drops, twice daily. It must be diluted in at least 4 oz. of liquid and stirred in well because the straight preparation is irritating to the mucous membranes.

"ParaMicrocidin has a bitter taste which is quite noticeable in water but which is barely detectable in orange or grapefruit juice . . . . The duration of treatment will depend upon the individual. In giardiasis I maintain treatment for 8 weeks. In candidiasis treatment may continue for a longer time. I've have some immunosuppressed patients taking the preparation for over a year with no apparent development of side effects or drug resistance."

Charles Resseger, D.O., Norwalk, Ohio:

"I've found this medication to be extremely effective in my patients with the Candida Related Complex. Now that I've been using it, I rarely use nystatin. A word of caution: The liquid preparation must be diluted or it will cause burning of the mucous membranes of the mouth. Also even when diluted and taken by mouth I've had some female patients complain of vaginal burning."

Tanalbit™

This internal intestinal antiseptic consists of natural tannins, combined with zinc. It has been found to be effective in the management of yeast overgrowth in the intestine, acute and chronic diarrhea, colitis, constipation and spastic colon.

Here are the comments of physicians who have used this product.*

James Brodsky, M.D., Chevy Chase, Maryland:

"I've found that Tanalbit™ has helped a number of my patients, who aren't responding to nystatin as well as I think they should or

---

*Further information about Tanalbit can be obtained from Scientific Consulting Service, 466n Whitney, San Leandro, CA 94577 (415) 632-2370.

those who cannot tolerate nystatin. The usual dose is 3 capsules, 3 times a day. I've experienced few if any side effects . . . especially when it is taken with meals."

Gus J. Prosch, Jr., M.D., Birmingham, Alabama:

"About two years ago I began using Tanalbit . . . I've been so impressed with the results I see in treating candida patients that I routinely start all my patients on Tanalbit. I'm convinced that it is superior to other antifungal agents in the treatment of candida infections. My usual dose is two capsules, three times a day. I give it along with a special diet, probiotics and nutritional supplements."

You can usually obtain these and other products from your health food store or from:

Bio-Tech, Box 1992, Fayetteville, AR 72702. 1-800-345-1199.
Freeda Vitamins, 36 E. 41st St., New York, NY 10017. 1-800-777-3737.
National CFIDS Buyers Catalog, 1187 Coast Village Rd., #1-280, Santa Barbara, CA 93108. 1-800-366-6056.
N.E.E.D.S., 527 Charles Ave., 12-A, Syracuse, NY 13209. 1-800-634-1380.
Wellness & Health Pharmaceuticals, 2800 S. 19th St., Birmingham, AL 35209. 1-800-227-2627.
Willner Chemist, 330 Lexington Ave., New York, NY 10016. (212) 685-0448.

Psychological Support

I disagree strongly with professionals who say, "CFS is caused by depression." Such critics usually ignore the role of viral infections, food allergies, chemical sensitivities and other organic causes of CFS. And they're especially skeptical of the "yeast connection." Yet, psychological factors are important in every illness, whether it's heart disease, arthritis or asthma. And they can play a role in weakening the immune system.

Psychological factors are important in every illness and can play a role in weakening the immune system.

Several years ago, the late Phyllis Saifer, M.D., of Berkeley, California, commented, "In dealing with patients with a yeast connected health problem, and environmental sensitivities, I'm impressed by the number of patients—especially women—who give a history of having been physically or sexually abused during childhood or adolescence. And I've found that attention to my patient's psychological needs is an important part of a comprehensive treatment program."

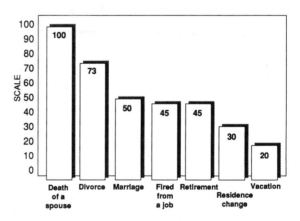

Here's more. Over 20 years ago, two University of Washington researchers, Thomas Holmes and Richard Rahe,[*] devised a scoring system to measure lifetime events according to their degree of stressfulness. They included both positive and negative experiences since both can produce stress.

---

[*]T. H. Holmes and R. H. Rahe, *Psychosom. Med.* 11 (2) 2:213-18, 1967.

Here are other examples. A study I read in a medical journal showed that T-lymphocytes (the cells which protect people from viral and other infections), were reduced to a significant degree following the death of a spouse or child. And in a recent report, the rates of both respiratory infections and clinical colds increased in a dose-response manner with increases in the degree of psychological stress.*

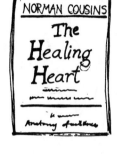

On a more favorable note, the observations of Norman Cousins (published in his books *Anatomy of an Illness* and *The Healing Heart*) show that the immune system can be strengthened and recovery from many illnesses accelerated by laughter and other psychological nutrients.

In the mid-80s I visited Mr. Cousins in his office at UCLA. During our conversation he told me of his work with groups of people with arthritis, cancer and other chronic, disabling and painful illnesses. And he said, "I always tell them jokes. And after about the third joke I have them laughing so hard they have to hold their sides. Then when my session with them is completed, I ask 'How many of you are still hurting as much as you were when you walked into this room?' And no hands are raised."

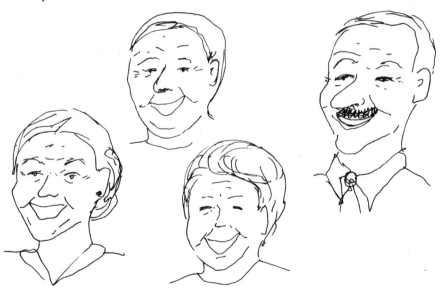

*S. Cohen, D.A.J. Tyrrell and A.P. Smith, "Psychological Stress and Susceptibility to the Common Cold," *The New England Journal of Medicine*, 325:606-12, 1991.

Surgeon, writer and lecturer Bernie Siegel in his book *Love, Medicine and Miracles*, eloquently explores the link between mind and body and tells people with cancer and other chronic illnesses how they can become a survivor. And he said, "We must learn to give fun a high priority in life . . . . Each of us must take time to find humorous books and movies, play the games we enjoy, tell jokes to friends, doodle or have fun with coloring books, whatever the choice is of the child inside you."

In his book *Maximum Immunity*, Michael A. Weiner, Ph.D., (Houghton-Mifflin, 1986) described a study carried out on cadets at West Point to see how psychological factors influenced their susceptibility to infectious mononucleosis.

. . . cadets who became sick with infectious mononucleosis had experienced greater pressure than those who remained well.

"Cadets were selected at the beginning of the study who were free of the antibody for the Epstein-Barr Virus, . . . During their stay at the academy, some of the young men developed the Epstein-Barr Virus antibody; but only some of these actually developed mononucleosis. The others remained symptom free, indicating that they had better resistance. The cadets who became sick with infectious mononucleosis were generally found to have experienced greater academic pressure and to have shown poorer academic performance than the resistant group of cadets."

Weiner cited another study of a group of students in which "it was found that failure, social isolation and unresolved role crisis was often associated with respiratory infections. The more serious the sickness, the more likely it was that stressful situations had occurred during the preceding year."

Psychological vitamins can help you get well.

What do these observations mean? *Psychological stress can play a part in making you more susceptible to illnesses of many types and psychological support can help you get well.* In talking to my patients about such support, I like to use the term "psychological vitamins." Here are some of them:

- You need caring, empathetic people to encourage you, work with you and help you. Included, of course, would be your spouse or companion who lives with you, or a relative or best friend. It could also include a professional who understands your illness and works to help you. Support groups consisting of people who are experiencing similar problems can also help.

- *You need to be noticed, praised and encouraged.* You need smiles, touching, holding, patting and petting. Physical contact stimulates the release of endorphins, a chemical which lessens anxiety and pain.

In his book *Touching*, Ashley Montagu told of scientific studies with rats: "The more handling and petting the rats received, the better they did in laboratory situations."

- In spite of your illness, you need to have a feeling of accomplishment. You need to do something, however small, that makes you feel useful—tasks that you can complete successfully. It could be something as simple as knitting a sweater, if you like to knit, painting a picture if you like to paint or cooking one of your favorite recipes.

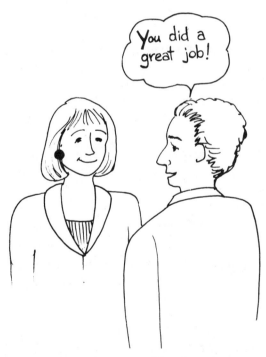

To summarize. CFS isn't caused by depression or psychological stress. Yet, psychological factors can play a part in weakening your immune system and contributing to your health problems. Conversely, love, laughter, praise, touching and other psychological nutrients can hasten your recovery.

Nutritional Supplements

Will nutritional supplements help my CFS? In my opinion, the answer is yes. Yet some physicians and other professionals may disagree with me. In a report, "Vitamin Preparations and Dietary Supplements as Therapeutic Agents" published in the April 10, 1987, *Journal of the American Medical Association*, the Council on Scientific Affairs commented,

"Application of sound dietary practices should eliminate any need for supplemental vitamins after infancy . . . In situations when an individual is unable or unwilling to eat an adequate diet—the physician must decide whether vitamin supplementation is necessary. All health practitioners should repeatedly emphasize a properly selected diet as the primary basis for good nutrition."

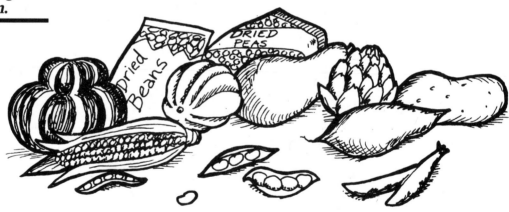

If a person is healthy—really healthy—

- and eats a truly "good" diet with lots of vegetables, whole grain, fruits, beans, nuts and seeds, and occasional fish, lean meats, skim milk and yogurt—
- and if the foods are grown organically on nutritionally rich soil—
- and if he avoids or sharply limits the "junk foods" (refined and processed foods that contain hydrogenated or partially

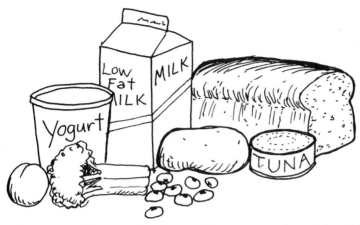

hydrogenated fats and oils) and beverages loaded with sugar, phosphates, food coloring and additives—

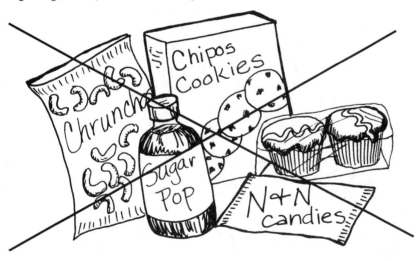

- and isn't exposed to environmental chemicals including traffic fumes, tobacco, insecticides and other home chemicals, then—he doesn't need nutritional supplements.

I recommend nutritional supplements in addition to a truly good diet.

BUT, persons with CFS do not fulfill these requirements.

Accordingly, I recommend nutritional supplements in addition to a truly good diet.

A number of authorities also support the use of supplements in providing "nutritional insurance" and fortifying the body's immune system. Several years ago, Robert A. Good, M.D., Ph.D., of the University of South Florida, Tampa, said,

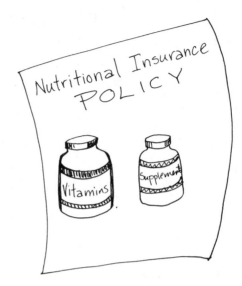

The proper combination of nutrients—will help fortify the body's immune system and aid in fighting disease. Robert A. Good, M.D., Ph.D.

"An explosion of new information shows that the proper combination of nutrients fortified with the reduction of caloric intake will help fortify the body's immune system and aid in fighting disease."

Recently a scientific study supporting the use of nutritional supplements in children was published in *The Lancet*.* In this article, researchers reported that children who took a multivitamin mineral supplement every day for eight months showed a significant increase in nonverbal intelligence.

Stephen S. Schoenthaler, Ph.D.**, Department of Sociology and Criminal Justice (California State University, Stanislaus), commented,

"Collectively the data from our studies show that selected individuals with behavioral, psychological and mood problems are likely to be marginally malnourished and/or suffering from chemical or food sensitivities. The pragmatic solution is straightforward:

"Individuals who suffer from behavioral, psychological and mood problems would be well advised to eat balanced diets containing adequate fruits, vegetables and whole grain products each day, backed up with a good multivitamin mineral supplement, as an insurance policy of adequate nutrition."

*D. Benton, G. Roberts, "Effective Vitamin Mineral Supplementation on Intelligence of a Sample of School Children," *The Lancet*, 1988; i:140-43.
**For reprints or additional information contact S. Schoenthaler, Ph.D, California State University, Stanislaus, Turlock, CA 95380.

In a recent article* nutritonal biochemist Jeffrey S. Bland, Ph.D. said that to obtain "optimal health" we may have to consume more than the RDA (recommended daily allowances) of various vitamins and minerals throughout our lives. And Bland cited research studies published in the *New England Journal of Medicine* (Vol. 314, No. 3, 1986, p. 157) and the *American Journal of Clinical Nutrition* (Vol. 52, pp. 93-102, 1990) to support his point of view.

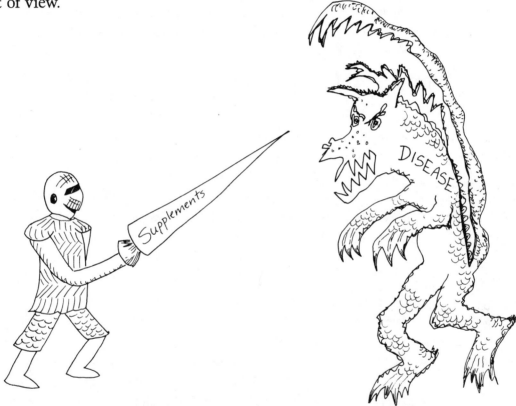

Do these reports indicate that the person with CFS can take nutritional supplements and continue to eat sweetened, refined, processed and fabricated nutritionally deficient foods? No, absolutely not.

In discussing the importance of nutrition with me recently, Donald R. Davis, Ph.D. (a long-time associate of the late Roger J. Williams, Ph.D.), Clayton Foundation Biochemical Institute, University of Texas, Austin 78712 said,

*J.S. Bland, "Vitamin Supplements—Why Take Them?", *Delicious*, Vol. 7, October 1991, pp. 30-32, 36. New Hope Communications, 1301 Spruce St., Boulder, CO 80203.

"We do not eat enough whole tissues of plants and animals. Instead, ⅔ of the calories we consume come from 'dismembered' or 'partitioned' foods which lack the vital nutrients found in whole foods.

"Our most fundamental goal should be to reduce the consumption of purified sugars, separated fats,* alcohol and milled grains. We need to refocus nutrition education on the benefits of whole food and the little known pitfalls of dismembered foods. Although I recommend a broad spectrum nutritional supplement, supplements are just supplements, and not a practical substitute for good nutrition."

In a utopian world you'd be consuming a wide variety of nutritious foods grown organically on nonchemically polluted soil. You'd also be breathing clean air at home and in your community and you would not be exposed to tobacco smoke, lawn chemicals, diesel fumes and other toxic substances.

BUT, in the real world of the 1990s, I recommend insurance vitamins, minerals and other nutritional supplements. Those I recommend for my adult patients with yeast-connected health problems and/or CFS contain:

Vitamin A	5,000-10,000 IU	Calcium	500 mgs.
Beta-carotene	15,000 IU	Magnesium	500 mgs.
Vitamin B1	25-100 mgs. daily	Inositol	100 mgs.
Vitamin B2	25-50 mgs. daily	Citrus bioflavinoids	100 mgs.
Niacinamide	100-150 mgs. daily	PABA	50 mgs.
Pantothenic acid	100-500 mgs. daily	Zinc	15-30 mgs.
Vitamin B6	25-100 mgs. daily	Copper	1-2 mgs.
Folic acid	200-800 mcg.	Iron**	15-20 mgs.
Vitamin B12	100 mcg.	Manganese	20 mgs.
Biotin	300 mcg.	Selenium	100-200 mcg.
Choline(Bitartrate)	100 mgs.	Chromium	200 mcg.
Vitamin C***	1000-10,000 mgs.	Molybdenum	100 mcgs.
Vitamin D	100-400 IU	Vanadium	25 mcgs.
Vitamin E	400-600 IU	Boron	1 mg.

---

*A separated fat means separated from original food source, i.e. butter separated from milk, lard from pig, oil from corn, soybeans, olive, etc.
**Iron supplements are given only to individuals who are anemic or who are losing blood.
***Vitamin C dosage is determined by the bowel tolerance test. You'll find further information on Vitamin C in Section VI.

When supplements are prescribed by a knowledgeable professional, the amounts may vary considerably from those I've outlined, and his or her experience, expertise and clinical judgment will override my recommendations. Although the use of vitamin/mineral supplements continues to be "controversial," there appears to be increasing interest and support for their use.

SECTION **VI**

Other Therapies

Magnesium

If you're like most folks, you've been reading and hearing about the importance of calcium for many years. And many people, especially women, have been taking calcium supplements in the hope of preventing the development of osteoporosis and other disorders. Calcium is important, but so is magnesium.

During my pediatric residency training many years ago, we used injections of magnesium sulfate to control elevated blood pressure in children with acute kidney disease. Magnesium was also used as a laxative. Yet, it wasn't until the mid-60s, after reading several papers by Mildred Seelig, M.D., that I began to learn about the importance of magnesium.

Then, in September 1977 I read an article in *Executive Health,* "On the Dangers of Not Getting Enough Magnesium in the Foods You Eat." Although emphasis was placed on the abnormalities of the heart and blood vessels, observations were cited that showed that many patients who sought help for insomnia, tension and anxiety were magnesium deficient.

Many patients who sought help for insomnia, tension and anxiety were magnesium deficient.

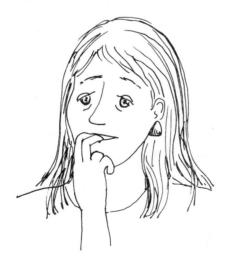

In a study of more than 200 patients, Dr. W. S. Davis, University of Pretoria used magnesium chloride tablets as a possible means of combating insomnia. *They reported that sleep was induced rapidly, was uninterrupted and waking tiredness disappeared in 99% of the patients.*

In addition, anxiety and tension diminished during the day. And no ill effects were noted in a group of patients in a long-term study in which before retiring they took eight tablets of 250 mgs. each of magnesium chloride over a 12-month period. (W.H. Davis and F. Ziady, "The Role of Magnesium in Sleep," Montreal Symposium, 1976.)

The *Executive Health* article also cited the observations of Dr. Edmund B. Flink, West Virginia University School of Medicine in Morgantown. In his address at the international meeting, this magnesium researcher stated that:

- Magnesium deficiency not only exists but is common.
- Although it is common, it is often undetected.
- Chronic* deficiency can produce long-term damage and can be fatal.
- The manifestations of the deficiency are many and varied.

Comments by Baker, Galland and Gaby

In spite of these reports, I didn't emphasize the use of this important mineral in managing my pediatric and allergy patients. Then in the early 80s, after learning about candida-related disorders, I consulted Sidney M. Baker, M.D., a former member of the Clinical Faculty at Yale University. I said, "Sid, tell me about magnesium." Here are his comments:

"Magnesium deficiency is widespread. The average daily need for magnesium for an adult is between 500 mg. and 1000 mg. and a lot of people simply aren't taking in that much. For my patients, I recommend oral magnesium chloride.

"The pharmacist can make it up in a 25% solution. The usual dose is 1-2 teaspoons a day. However, it should be diluted in water or another liquid so as to make it palatable and non-irritating. After people have been taking the magnesium solution for a while and obtain a good clinical response, I sometimes switch them to SLOW-MAG (Searle), the pill form of magnesium chloride."

*Acute magnesium deficiency may also occur following several weeks of diuretics, cisplatin or amino glycoside use. (Personal communication Edmund B. Flink, September 1991.)

Sleep was induced rapidly, was uninterrupted and waking tiredness disappeared in 99% of the patients.

Magnesium deficiency is widespread. The average daily need for magnesium is between 500 mg. and 1000 mg.

A year or two later, as I was working to update and expand *The Yeast Connection*, I learned more about magnesium from Leo Galland, M.D., a former associate of Dr. Baker's.

Galland, like Baker, pointed out that magnesium deficiency occurs more often than generally recognized. In discussing the food sources of magnesium, he said,

"The richest sources of magnesium are also the richest sources of essential fatty acids. . . . Seed foods (including whole grains, nuts and beans). Other foods which are relatively rich in magnesium include buckwheat, baking chocolate, cottonseed, tea, whole wheat and leafy green vegetables including collard greens and parsley. The mineral is also plentiful in seafood, meats, nuts and fruit. What's more, you can protect your magnesium stores by avoiding the magnesium wasters: saturated fats and soft drinks, especially those containing caffeine."

You can protect your magnesium stores by avoiding saturated fats and soft drinks. Leo Galland, M.D.

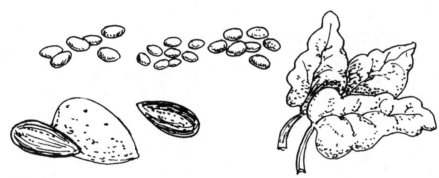

Here's more: In discussing magnesium in an editorial in the *Journal of Advancement in Medicine*, (Vol. 1, No. 4, Winter 1988, pages 179-181) Alan R. Gaby, M.D., said,

"*Properly administered magnesium is entirely free of adverse side affects. Equally important, its cost is negligible.*" [emphasis added]

"The neglect of magnesium as a safe, effective and exceptionally inexpensive treatment for cardiovascular disease parallels a similar neglect of other inexpensive and less toxic therapies in the treatment of virtually all major categories of disease. Broad scale adoption of those medically sound alternatives most of which are not under patent by pharmaceutical companies could save countless lives and save billions of dollars each year."

Properly administered magnesium is entirely free of adverse side affects. Equally important, its cost is negligible.

251

Reading about the effectiveness of magnesium and other non-prescription remedies (including the essential fatty acids) makes me wonder about the need for some of the expensive and potentially toxic drugs that are sometimes used to control symptoms in people with CFS.

Intramuscular Magnesium in CFS

In a recent study carried out in the United Kingdom, investigators described the efficacy of intramuscular magnesium in people with CFS (I.M. Cox, M.J. Campbell and D. Dowson*, "Red Blood Cell Magnesium And Chronic Fatigue Syndrome," *The Lancet*, 1991; 337:757-60).

THE LANCET

Twenty patients with CFS had lower red cell magnesium concentrations than did twenty healthy control subjects.

In a randomized, double-blind, placebo-controlled trial, 20 patients with CFS had lower red cell magnesium levels than did 20 healthy control subjects matched for age, sex and social class.

Responding to questions by Dr. Barry Shurlock, reporting for *The Medical Post*, Dr. Dowson stated that intramuscular magnesium is safe to use in all patients who do not have impaired renal function. In discussing CFS and magnesium therapy, he commented:

> "This is a devastating illness that affects young people and ruins their lives—and orthodox (drug) treatment has nothing to offer. Because the (magnesium sulfate) treatment is so safe and the disorder so devastating, and the response is so quick, I wouldn't hesitate in using it even if I couldn't check magnesium levels beforehand. We have found it effective in 80% of individuals."

In the concluding paragraph of their article in *The Lancet*, the authors stated,

---

*In a September 3, 1991, letter to me Dr. Dowson said, "I've recently found that patients who take selenium in a dose of 100 micrograms a day require less magnesium supplementation. Early research would indicate that this may be due to the fact that selenium is an essential of glutathione peroxidase, which 'locks' the magnesium in the cell. This may also explain why plasma magnesium levels are not a ready indicator of magnesium status."

"We've shown that patients with CFS have slightly lower magnesium levels than healthy controls and that treatment with magnesium seems to benefit patients, especially with respect to their energy and emotional status. However, we realize that our trial was small and that follow-up was only six weeks; therefore the results should be viewed with caution. There are some unresolved questions. Would the benefit that we have recorded be maintained and for how long? Should magnesium be given by injection, or taken orally? We hope that our findings will stimulate more GPs to take an interest in the disease."

More About Magnesium

Comments by Dr. Carol Jessop at the November 1990 CFIDS Conference (Charlotte, North Carolina):

"Low magnesium levels are common and can only be found using a test whereby you collect a 24-hour urine sample to test for magnesium. You then load the patient with 400 to 500 mgs. of magnesium a day for three days. You take another magnesium urine test on the third day to see how much the body retains. If they retained greater than 50%, it is significant because magnesium is very important in muscle relaxation. Many of my fibromyalgia patients improved with the addition of magnesium to the diet.

Many fibromyalgia patients improved with the addition of magnesium to the diet.

"Low zinc levels are also common although only 32% of patients show this on the blood tests. Blood tests are not as accurate as sweat tests which are hard to do in the office. But many patients either have poor wound healing or leukonychia (white spots on the fingernails) which are signs of zinc deficiency. Both of these trace minerals are absorbed in the gut and, I think, are being malabsorbed by our patients."

Comments by Dr. Stephen Davies, editor of the *Journal of Nutrition in Medicine*.
In a conversation with me in August 1991, Dr. Davies said,

CFS patients are nearly always deficient in magnesium and frequently deficient in zinc and copper.

"CFS patients are nearly always deficient in magnesium. Our research studies show that they're frequently deficient in zinc and copper too."

To summarize, magnesium appears to be safe, inexpensive and effective in helping patients with a variety of health problems including CFS. And, even in the absence of laboratory studies, magnesium sulfate or magnesium chloride should be a part of the treatment of the person with CFS.

Comments by Dr. Sherry Rogers:*

Magnesium deficiency is under-appreciated and under-diagnosed . . . it can be responsible for a vast array of seemingly un-related symptoms.

"It is becoming increasingly apparent that magnesium deficiency (MD) is underappreciated and underdiagnosed. At the same time it can be responsible for a vast array of seemingly unrelated symptoms. . . . To compound the problem, medications that are usually prescribed for these symptoms have the side effects of further lowering the magnesium. Since there is no reliable blood test for MD, we devised a magnesium loading test (MLT) with a before and after 24 hour urine magnesium. . . . 51% of patients had marked relief in over 40 different symptoms. 10% of the patients reported marked reduction in chemical sensitivity."

A Word of Caution

Like all medications of any type, magnesium may occasionally cause adverse side effects. In discussing the use of magnesium in CFS, in August 1991, Dr. Edmund B. Flink commented,

"Chronic renal failure causes chronic fatigue so it could be dangerous to give magnesium chronically to such individuals. It is also important to know that patients with chronic renal failure may actually be magnesium deficient. Such patients need to be monitored carefully during treatment."

Commenting on magnesium load testing, Dr. Flink said,

"An intravenous test is more reliable because of variable GI absorption."

---

*S. A. Rogers, M.D., "Unrecognized Magnesium Deficiency Masquerades as Diverse Symptoms: Evaluation of an Oral Magnesium Challenge Test," 2800 West Genesee Street, Syracuse, NY 13219. *International Clinical Nutrition Review*, Vol. 11, No. 3, 117-29, July 1991.

Essential Fatty Acids

Just about everybody knows that most people in the Western world are eating too much fat. And, in the United States, when you turn on your TV set, you're apt to hear somebody say, "If you want to enjoy better health, cut down on the fats in your diet." That's good advice.

You should not avoid all fats because there are good fats as well as bad ones. The good ones are called *Essential Fatty Acids* (EFAs). You need them to enjoy good health. EFAs are found in plants and their seeds, including flaxseed (linseed), walnut, sunflower, safflower, corn, canola and evening primrose. They're also found in the fat of cold water fish, including salmon, mackerel, sardines, tuna and herring. Like vitamins, EFAs cannot be manufactured in the body and so must be supplied in the diet.

You should not avoid all fats because there are good fats as well as bad ones.

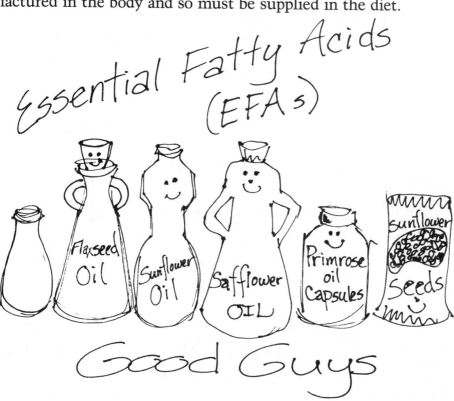

255

EFAs have many essential functions in the body. Here are a few of them. They store energy and furnish raw materials for making prostaglandins and other "short-lived" substances required for the second-by-second regulation of almost all of the tissues of the body. Equally important, they are required for the structure of all cells and all other membranes of the body. Because of these many diverse functions, they are important in preventing health problems of many types, including eczema and other skin disorders, arthritis, heart disease, PMS and malignant diseases.

EFAs are required for the structure of all cells and all other membranes of the body.

There are two general classes of EFAs. One group are called the Omega 3 fatty acids and the other group are Omega 6 fatty acids. Here's how they get their names. Each long chain of fatty acids begins with a carbon atom that has three hydrogens hitched on to it. This is called the CH_3 end of the molecule. Omega 3 fatty acids have the first double bond on the third carbon atom from the CH_3 end of the molecule and the Omega 6 fatty acids have the first double bond on the sixth carbon.

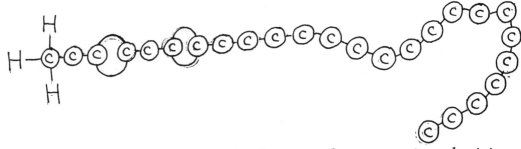

During the past decade, almost without exception, physicians treating patients with yeast-connected health problems have used EFA supplements as an essential part of their treatment program. The usual recommendations include flax oil, one or two tablespoons daily, and evening primrose oil, one or two capsules three times a day. Along with these supplements, patients are instructed to eat more vegetables and to avoid sugar, alcohol and the bad fats (hydrogenated vegetable oils and saturated fats).

Dr. C. Orian Truss found that patients with yeast-connected health problems showed significant abnormalities.

EFAs and CFS

In the summer of 1990, I appeared on a television program in Toronto* which dealt with the CFS/M.E. Other program partici-

---

*Dr. Peter Behan also participated in the program by transatlantic telephone.

pants included both physicians and patients. While waiting in the "green room" for the program to start, I met an enthusiastic young man, Paul Beatty, who told me this story: "I was severely disabled by M.E. until I started taking essential fatty acids. They worked like a miracle in helping me turn my life around."

Paul gave me mimeographed copies of reprints and commentaries from the medical literature, including a chapter he'd copied out of a 1990 book, *Omega-6 Essential Fatty Acids—Pathophysiology and Roles In Clinical Medicine*, editor D. F. Horrobin. The article was written by Peter O. Behan and Wilhelmina M. H. Behan, Departments of Neurology and Pathology, Glasgow University, Glasgow G12 Scotland.

These researchers used a special EFA preparation, Efamol Marine,* in treating patients with the Post-Viral Fatigue Syndrome. Patients receiving the EFAs improved significantly as compared to a control group of patients who received placebo capsules containing only olive oil. *The symptoms that showed improvement included dizziness, vertigo, depression, memory loss, exhaustion, musle weakness, aches and pains, and lack of concentration.*

Here are excerpts from a paper entitled "Effect of high doses of essential fatty acids on the post-viral fatigue syndrome" by P.O.

> *Patients receiving the EFAs improved significantly as compared to a control group of patients who received placebo capsules.*

> *I was severely disabled by ME until I started taking essential fatty acids.*

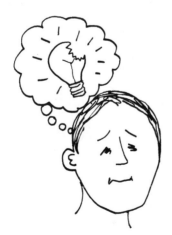

---

*This product is produced by Scotia Pharmaceuticals Ltd., Woodbridge Meadows, Guildford, Surrey GU1 1BA, England. (Tel. 0483 574949) (Fax: 0483 506682) It is generally available in Europe and at this time is not available in the U.S. or Canada. The equivalent would be 3 to 4 g. of Efamol coupled with about 1 g. of fish oil or 3 to 4 g. of flaxseed oil.

Behan, W.M.H. Behan and D. Horrobin,* Departments of Neurology and Pathology, University of Glasgow, Scotland (Behan & Behan), and Scotia Pharmaceuticals, Guildford, Surrey, England (Horrobin):

> *Sixty-three adults with . . . postviral-fatigue syndrome were enrolled in a double-blind, placebo-controlled study.*

"Sixty-three adults with the diagnosis of the post-viral fatigue syndrome were enrolled in a double-blind, placebo-controlled study of essential fatty acid therapy. The patients had been ill for from one to three years after an apparently viral infection, suffering from severe fatigue, myalgia and a variety of psychiatric symptoms. . . .

"At 1 month, 74% of the patients on active treatment and 23% of those on placebo assessed themselves as improved over the baseline with the improvement being much greater in the former. At 3 months, the corresponding figures were 85% and 17% (p0.0001) since the placebo group had reverted toward the baseline state while those in the active group showed continued improvement. The essential fatty acids were abnormal at the baseline and corrected by the active treatment. There were no adverse events. *We conclude that essential fatty acids provide a rational, safe and effective treatment for patients with the post-viral fatigue syndrome.*" [emphasis added]

> *Essential fatty acids provide a rational, safe and effective treatment for patients with post-viral fatigue.*

In a second article entitled "Essential Fatty Acids, Immunity and Viral Infections" (D.F. Horrobin, *Journal of Nutritional Medicine*, 1990, 145-151), Horrobin stated, "There is evidence of a close interrelationship between essential fatty acid (EFA) metabolism and the ability to respond to viral infections." In this article, he also discussed the importance of a whole series of "cofactors" (including magnesium, biotin, pyridoxine, nicotinic acid, iron, zinc and ascorbic acid) which are required for the normal metabolism of linoleic acid. And he said, "All these nutrients must be present in adequate amounts if EFAs are going to have their expected effects."

EFAs and Yeast-Related Illness

In 1984, C. Orian Truss** described a number of metabolic abnormalities in patients with yeast-related illness. Included

---

*Acta. Neurol. Scand. 1990: 82:209-16
**C.O. Truss, "Metabolic Abnormalities in Patients with Chronic Candidiasis," *Journal of Orthomolecular Medicine*, 13: 66-92, 1984.

were disturbances in proteins, carbohydrates and essential fatty acids.

Twenty-four patients with symptoms typical of mold sensitivity and yeast susceptibility were studied. Fat metabolism was evaluated by measuring fatty acids in plasma and in red blood cell membranes. Abnormalities in these patients were noted especially in the 20 and 22 carbon highly unsaturated fatty acids. Following treatment with a sugar-free special diet and nystatin, fatty acid measurements improved.

Following treatment with a sugar-free special diet and nystatin, fatty acid measurements improved.

I've found the clinical observations of Behan, Behan, Horrobin and Truss exciting. They show that EFAs help many people with chronic symptoms, including individuals with CFS and/or chronic candidiasis. In commenting on the treatment of patients with these and other chronic health disorders, Sidney M. Baker, M.D. said in effect, "For the sick person to regain his health he has to play with a full deck. And the EFAs are an essential card."

Sources of EFAs

You can usually find flax oil, evening primrose oil and other essential fatty acids in your health food store or you can obtain them from the following:

Allergy Resources, P.O. Box 888, Palmer Lake, CO. 80133. 1-800-USE-FLAX.

Freeda Vitamins, 36 E. 41st St., New York, NY 10017. 1-800-777-3737.

National CFIDS Buyers Catalog, 1187 Coast Village Rd., #1-280, Santa Barbara, CA 93108. 1-800-366-6056.

N.E.E.D.S., 527 Charles Ave., 12A, Syracuse, NY 13209. 1-800-634-1380.

Wellness and Health Pharmaceuticals, 2800 S. 19th St., Birmingham, AL 35209. 1-800-227-2627.

Willner Chemist, 33 Lexington Ave., New York, NY 10016. (212) 685-0448.

Probiotics

Probiotics are a group of friendly bacteria that help us stay well. They include *Lactobacillus acidophilus and Lactobacillus bifidus* and other bifidobacteria. These bacteria, which are found in yogurt, were first identified about 100 years ago. And in 1908, Metchkinoff, a Bulgarian, recommended the daily consumption of yogurt because he felt it promoted good health and prolonged life.

During the years since that time, preparations of these friendly bacteria have been used by both physicians and nonphysicians to treat complaints ranging from constipation and diarrhea to skin problems.

Lactobacillus acidophilus and *Lactobacillus bifidus* (and other bifidobacteria*) are perhaps the best-known probiotics and preparations of these organisms can be found in health food stores and pharmacies. A third friendly bacterium, *Streptococcus faecium*, has also been found to be effective in curbing the growth of harmful bacteria in the digestive tract.

During the last seven or eight years, many professionals and nonprofessionals have described the effectiveness of probiotics in helping control their yeast-connected health problems. One woman reported, "I've tried various remedies for my bloating, constipation, abdominal pain and recurrent vaginitis. Finally I found that by taking probiotics regularly, I'm better than I've been in years. Of course, I also have sharply reduced my intake of sugar."

> **Probiotics helped persons with yeast-connected health problems.**

During the past decade, several conferences have been held on the candida/human interaction. And almost without exception both professionals and nonprofessionals described their use of probiotic products for persons with yeast-related health problems.

---

*For a further discussion, see pages 257-60 of *The Yeast Connection*.

Bifidobacteria were discussed in a recent article by Tomotari Mitsuoka, Department of Biological Science, Faculty of Agriculture, University of Tokyo, Japan, *Journal of Industrial Microbiology*, 6 (1990) 263-68:

"There is a growing consensus on the beneficial effects of bifidobacteria in human health. It is now clear that bifidobacteria that exist in the large intestine are helpful for maintenance of human health and are far more important than *Lactobacillus acidophilus* as beneficial intestinal bacteria throughout human life. Oral administration of bifidobacteria may be effective for the improvement of intestinal flora and intestinal environment . . . (and) for stimulation of the immune system."

In researching probiotics I read reports from many different sources. One of the best of these was a discussion in the book *Childhood Ear Infections*** by Dr. Michael A. Schmidt. In a section entitled "The Importance of Intestinal Bacteria," he listed 15 beneficial functions performed by *Lactobacillus acidophilus* and bifidobacteria in the intestinal tract. Here are a few of them: Contribute to "germ-eating" activity of some of the body's immune cells; produce organic acids and hydrogen peroxide, which kill invading microbes; synthesize important B vitamins; allow for better utilization of nutrients from foods; prevent the fungus *Candida albicans* from forming invasive germ tubes; inhibit the growth of *Candida albicans* in the digestive tract and vagina.

Lactobacillus acidophilus and bifidobacteria in the intestinal tract contribute to "germ eating" activity of some of the body's immune cells.

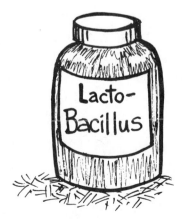

---

*M.A., Schmidt, *Childhood Ear Infections*, North Atlantic Books, 2800 Woolsey St., Berkeley, CA 94705.

In discussing probiotics with nutrition researcher Jeffrey Bland, Ph.D., I asked, "Do you use plain *Lactobacillus acidophilus* or a combination product?" He responded,

> "I think we all recognize that the most important criteria for activity of probiotic substances is that there must be an adequate number of live organisms, they must be reasonably resistant to oxgall (bile) and they must be able to adhere to the gastrointestinal epithelium. If any one of these three criteria is not present, then the activity of the product is limited.
>
> "At our center we start patients on preparations of *Lactobacillus acidophilus*. If we don't get a response we go with bifidobacteria as well. So they get them both. I don't think there's any harm in giving these products in combination form because they're combined in the intestinal tract at all times."

I recommend probiotics for my patients—especially those who are taking or have taken broad spectrum antibiotic drugs.

You can find a number of probiotic products in your health food store. I recommend them as a nutritional supplement for my patients—especially those who are taking or have taken broad spectrum antibiotic drugs.

Garlic

According to a report by the *New York Times* columnist Jane Brody (Tuesday, September 4, 1990), "After 4000 years of folklore extolling garlic as a preserver and restorer of health and youth, modern scientists have begun to define the complex condiment's medically important effects and substantiate several of its reputed benefits."

Brody attended the First World Congress on the Health Significance of Garlic and Garlic Constituents. Other participants included people from all over the world, and more especially from China and Japan, where garlic preparations have been a mainstay of traditional medicine for many centuries. According to Brody,

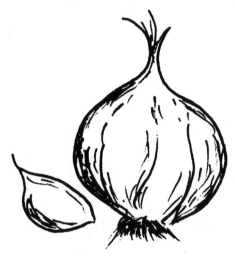

"Only a few facts about the use of garlic are clear. Garlic does not have to be consumed raw to be effective; in fact, raw garlic is more likely than cooked or processed forms to cause adverse reactions. Furthermore, the characteristic odor of garlic or its freshness are not critical to its health benefits; aged, deodorized forms seem to work as well or better than pure unadulterated fresh garlic."

In summarizing reports at the conference, Brody said, "The scientists reported in humans as well as laboratory animals garlic, or one or more of its active ingredients, can do these things:

- Suppress cholesterol synthesis.
- Lower levels of triglycerides.
- Reduce the tendency of blood to clot.
- Stimulate various immunological factors that may help the body combat cancer as well as stubborn fungal infections like *Candida albicans*, a yeast that plagues millions.
- Protects cells against damage by oxidizing agents and heavy metals that are widespread in modern industrial environments."

In the concluding paragraph of her article, Brody said,

Garlic can stimulate the body to combat stubborn fungal infections like Candida albicans.

> "While scientists continue to sort out the benefits and risks of garlic and its constituents, Dr. Lin and other researchers suggested that those who can tolerate garlic would be wise to eat it at least every other day in cooked form. An alternative for those wishing to avoid garlic breath is regular use of aged garlic extract, a deodorized supplement sold in health food stores under the trade name Kyolic."

In another report of this conference, Joy Ashchenbach, in an article in the April 20, 1991, *Rocky Mountain News* quoted Herbert Pierson, head of the National Cancer Institute's "designer foods program," who said, "Chopping, steaming and food processing does marvelous things to garlic."

Ashchenbach also quoted Eric Block of the State University of New York at Albany, an authority on garlic's chemistry who said, "Undisturbed, the garlic bulb has limited medicinally active compounds. . . . Cutting triggers the formation of a cascade of compounds that are quite reactive and participate in a complex sequence of chemical reactions. Ultimately an amazing collection of chemical compounds is produced."

An amazing collection of chemical compounds is produced by garlic.

Here's more. Recently Dr. Benjamin H. Lau, M.D., Ph.D.,* et al., Loma Linda University, Loma Linda, California, reported the effectiveness of aged garlic extract against *Candida albicans* in-

---

*P. P. Tadi, R.W. Teel and B.H.S. Lau, "Anticandidal and Anticarginogenic Potentials of Garlic," *International Clinical Nutrition Review,* 10:4, 1990; *Nutrition and Cancer,* 15:87-85, 1991.5; *Molecular Biotheraphy,* 3:103-107. 1991

fection in mice. After candida exposure, one group was treated with aged garlic extract while the other group was given a garlic-free control. The treatment with aged garlic extract hastened the clearance of candida cells from the blood and reduced their growth in the kidney.

The treatment with aged garlic extract hastened the clearance of candida cells from the blood.

In addition, germ killing activity of macrophages was observed in the mice treated with aged garlic extract. According to Dr. Lau, this study suggests that the control of *Candida albicans* may be mediated through enhancement of phagocytic ("germ-eating") function by garlic extract.

To obtain more information about the value of garlic in helping people with chronic health problems of various sorts, I interviewed Jeffrey Bland, Ph.D. Here are some of his comments:

"Garlic is one of those really interesting phyto-pharmaceutical substances that has a whole host of different therapeutic potential applications due to the fact that it is almost a chemical storehouse of many different pharmacologically active substances. Some of those can prevent platelets from sticking together and therefore are natural blood thinners.

"Others of those are antibacterial or bacteriostatic due to the effect that they have on the immune system. Others may be actually anticarcinogenic and help prevent cell transformation and enhance the surveillance system activity."

Which garlic products are best? During the past five years, many claims have been made about the efficacy of various garlic products. In *The Yeast Connection* I quoted a garlic researcher who said,

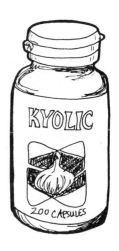

"The major chemical constituent of whole garlic which is responsible for its therapeutic qualities is allicin. Allicin is also responsible for most of the strong odor it gives to your breath."

During the past several years I've received information of a different sort. For example, Osamu Imada, Ph.D., visiting scientist, University of Texas, M. D. Anderson Cancer Center, Houston, Texas, in reviewing the proceedings of the First World Congress on the Health Significance of Garlic and Garlic Constituents commented,*

More than 50 scientists from 15 countries presented their recent research finding on garlic at the Congress.

"More than 50 scientists from 15 countries presented their recent research findings on garlic at the Congress. The beneficial effects of aged garlic extract have become the center of the presentations at the Congress. Fourteen of the 46 presentations were related to the efficacy of aged garlic extract (Kyolic)."

Dr. Imada reviewed a number of the beneficial effects of aged garlic extract, including lowering of cholesterol levels, inhibition of clot formation, inhibiting of free radicals and peroxide formation, protection against radium toxicity and anti-cancer activity. He also reviewed his own studies, which showed that aged garlic extract has no undesirable effects, even when taken in large doses. And he cited the comments of Dr. Robert I-San Lin, the Congress Chairman, who stated,

"Allicin is a transient and highly unstable compound and there's no evidence showing that allicin is the active compound in the body. The studies presented at this Congress demonstrated that many thioallyl compounds and their derivatives contribute to garlic's various nutritional/pharmacological properties. Thus the claim that allicin is the only active principle of garlic is unfounded; rather, it has little direct contribution to garlic's nutritional/pharmacological properties. Excessive consumption of allicin may cause toxicity."

You'll find whole garlic in your supermarket and garlic products of many types in your health food stores. If you have CFS, whether yeast connected or not, based on the reports I've cited, garlic and/or aged garlic extract may help you regain your health.

*Townsend Letter for Doctors, February/March, 1991, page 194.

Coenzyme Q_{10}

In 1986 and 1987 I received a number of anecdotal reports by phone and by mail about a substance I'd never heard of . . . CoQ_{10}. People who wrote and called said, "You should read about CoQ_{10}. It helps the immune system."

Then one day, in late 1987, I picked up a book in a health food store entitled *The Miracle Nutrient, Coenzyme Q_{10}*, by Emile G. Bliznakov, M.D. (President and Scientific Director of the Lupus Research Institute), and Gerald L. Hunt. I read the book almost from cover to cover and I was impressed. Here are some of the things I learned:

CoQ_{10}, also known as ubiquinone, is a nutrient that was first extracted from beef heart mitochondria by scientist F. L. Crane and his group in the United States in 1957. A great deal of the work on this substance has been carried out since that time by Dr. Carl Folkers and research colleagues at the University of Texas, Austin. It has also been researched and used extensively in Japan, where 252 commercial preparations of CoQ_{10} are supplied by over 80 pharmaceutical companies. According to the authors of *The Miracle Nutrient, Coenzyme Q_{10},*

"On April 14, 1986, Carl Folkers was honored with the Priestley Medal, the highest award bestowed by the American Chemical Society in recognition of superior accomplishments in chemistry and medicine. It was presented to Dr. Folkers in recognition of his work with Coenzyme Q_{10}, vitamin B_6 and B_{12}."

The book reviews many reports that describe the value of Coenzyme Q_{10} in people with congestive heart failure and other types of heart disease. It also discusses its effectiveness in reversing gum disease and in strengthening the immune system. Mice experiments were cited to show that CoQ_{10} boosts the performance of immune system cells, not by stimulating the production of more cells, but by inducing more energy and thus increasing the immunocompetence in the existing ones."

Research studies show that CoQ_{10} can produce a profoundly beneficial effect on the immune system.

Although so far research into CoQ_{10} and the immune system has received less emphasis and publicity than its role in treating heart disease, the authors of the book concluded, *"Our research with animal models and the studies of other scientists have proved conclusively that CoQ_{10} can produce a profoundly beneficial effect on the immune system* [emphasis added] . . . no toxic effects whatsoever . . . clinical studies under the auspices of the FDA show that CoQ_{10} is much safer than many drugs presently on the market."

However, in the "disclaimer" in front of the book appears the following statement:

"The authors must stress the importance of consulting with your family physician before making any nutritional changes to your regular diet. Although Coenzyme Q_{10} has been found to have no side effects during extensive toxicological studies, we point out that it is important that you do not self medicate. . . . CoQ_{10} is regarded as a dietary factor and as a food supplement and should be looked upon strictly as such."

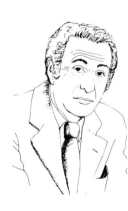

I agree that people with health problems should stay in touch with their family physicians and be guided by his or her advice. At the same time, I'd like to point out that most physicians have been given relatively little training in nutrition and preventive medicine. Moreover, at a conference in Florida almost 20 years ago, Emanuel Cheraskin, M.D., D.M.D., who was then chairman of the Department of Oral Medicine at the University of Alabama, made this comment, which I have repeated many times,

"The average physician knows as much about nutrition as his secretary, unless his secretary belongs to Weight Watchers—then he doesn't know half as much."

The average physician knows as much about nutrition as his secretary.

Resistance to CoQ$_{10}$

In spite of the research studies of Dr. Carl Folkers (and other scientists) which provide evidence for the safety and effectiveness of CoQ$_{10}$ in helping persons with various health problems, this substance has recently received some verbal rotten tomatoes. For example, I was talking to a reputable distributor of nutritional supplements, including probiotics and vitamin/mineral perparations. During our conversation I asked her about Coenzyme Q$_{10}$. She said, "Based on research studies, we feel CoQ$_{10}$ is a valuable nutritional supplement. However, we haven't added it to our product line because efforts are being made in some quarters to ban its distribution and use."

Support for CoQ$_{10}$

I recommend CoQ$_{10}$. During the past 3½ years, I've used CoQ$_{10}$ in doses of 25mg, 1 to 4 times daily, as one part of a comprehensive program in treating my chronically ill patients with chronic fatigue, headache, PMS and other disorders. I take it myself, give it to my wife and daughters and I've also recommended it to friends. Although I can't claim that it is a magical cure which is "good for everything," here are a couple of anecdotal reports:

A 46-year-old woman with recurrent asthma, sinusitis, rhinitis, fatigue, headache and other symptoms had failed to improve on repeated courses of antibiotic drugs and bronchial dilators. She had also taken allergy extract injections for 10 years. On a comprehensive treatment program which included an improved diet, vitamin-mineral supplements, small doses of nystatin for a short period of time and CoQ$_{10}$, she showed remarkable improvement in her health status. And in an August 1991 letter to me she said,

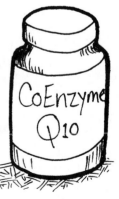

"I'm enjoying very good health, better than I can remember in my life. I've never gone this long without a bronchial infection since I was 12 years old. I believe CoQ$_{10}$ has certainly contributed to my being able to stay well. I took 75 mgs. a day for quite a while, but

269

now I'm doing great on 50 mgs. daily. I'm also taking the vitamin/mineral preparation Basic Preventive. Also, my mother and stepfather have been taking CoQ_{10} for over a year and have had no colds since they started taking it."

A 70-year-old professional enjoyed reasonably good health. However, he was subject to colds followed by sinusitis several times a year. Moreover, he would always "catch a cold" whenever his wife had a cold . . . even though his diet was a good one and he took extra vitamin C and other nutritional supplements.

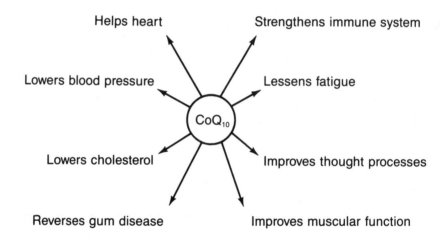

In late 1987 he began taking CoQ_{10} regularly, 25mg twice daily. Since that time he has experienced no respiratory infections, even though his wife has had several bad colds. And he didn't develop a cold after sitting next to a woman who coughed and sneezed repeatedly during a 12-hour plane trip from New Zealand.

Here's more. According to a report in the August 1991 issue of *Capsulations,* Thorne Research, Inc. (800-228-1966), Coenzyme Q_{10} protects against exercise-induced muscle injury. Here are excerpts from this report:

"The effect of Coenzyme Q_{10} administration on exercise induced muscle injury was examined in rats. . . . After exercise . . . serum creatine kinase lactate dehydrogenase activity was elevated in the control rats, but not in the Coenzyme Q treated rats... These results suggest that the Coenzyme Q_{10} treatment protects skeletal muscle against injury caused during exercise." (Shimomuray, et al., Protective Effect of Coenzyme Q$_{10}$ on Exercised Induced Muscular Injury, *Bio-Chem Biophys*, Res. Commun., 1991; 176:349-55)*

Here's still more. In their *Chronic Fatigue Syndrome Self-Care Manual*, February 1991, Charles W. Lapp, M.D. and Paul R. Cheney, M.D., Ph.D., outlined their recommendations. These included lifestyle, exercise, diet and nutrition, vitamins and optional supplements. In discussing CoQ$_{10}$ they said,

> "This enzyme (metabolic catalyst) is thought to be involved in 95% of a cell's metabolic reactions. It has additional benefits of lowering cholesterol and blood pressure and stabilizing heart conditions. Particularly useful for improving fatigue, thought processes, muscular function and cardiac complaints. A threshold effect occurs and it may take 5 to 6 weeks for full benefit. We recommend 90-200mg daily (one dose or divided), for a 5 to 6 week trial. Expensive, so we discontinue if no benefit is noted in 6 weeks. We use sublingual form to increase its bioavailability."

We recommend CoQ$_{10}$, 90 to 200 mgs. daily for a five to six weeks trial. Charles W. Lapp, M.D. and Paul R. Cheney, M.D., Ph.D.

In the *National CFIDS Buyer's Catalog*, 1187 Coast Village Road, #1-280, Santa Barbara, California 93108, under the heading, "Why CoQ$_{10}$?" appeared a comment by Alan Goldberg, Charlotte, North Carolina, which had been published in the Summer/Fall 1989 issue of the *CFIDS Chronicle*. And here's an excerpt of Goldberg's comment:

> "I am among a group of CFIDS patients in Charlotte who have been taking the product for a few months. I cautiously state, that, for the most part, those of us in the Charlotte CoQ$_{10}$ network feel better, have more energy and enjoy an amelioration of some of our bizarre symptoms. I am cautious in what I say because my superstitious nature inhibits me from mentioning good news."

---

*A number of other reports have been published in the peer-reviewed literature which provide evidence of the effectiveness of CoQ$_{10}$ in cardiac and other conditions. Langsjoen, A.U., et al, *American Journal of Cardiology*, 65:521, 1990. Mortensen, S.A., *Int. J. Tissue-React.*, 12:155, 1990.

Vitamin B$_{12}$

Although I've rarely used vitamin B$_{12}$ injections in treating my patients, I've received anecdotal reports from others, including professionals and nonprofessionals who say, "Vitamin B$_{12}$ really helps." Here are excerpts of a letter from Linda A., a 28-year-old third grade teacher:

I've been receiving B$_{12}$ shots for several years. . . . I find I have much more energy and stamina.

"I've been receiving B$_{12}$ shots for several years to combat the Allergic Tension-Fatigue Syndrome. When I take the shots, I find I have much more energy and stamina to make it through a long day. The effects seem to wear off gradually within 8 to 10 days so I try to get a shot once a week. The B$_{12}$ shots are only one part of my health regimen, but when I miss a shot, I definitely begin to feel draggy. The shots may not work for everyone, but I would certainly recommend them to my fellow sufferers."

In discussing treatment measures that help patients with CFS, Dr. Paul Cheney* said,

"After sleep disturbance the most important symptom to attempt to treat is fatigue itself. Since fatigue is at the heart of chronic fatigue syndrome, it is difficult to treat that symptom apart from the disease process as a whole. Despite this, I think there are agents and drugs that seem to improve the fatigued state.

"The primary ones that we usually include are B$_{12}$, given as a self injection, two times to three times per week, high dose sublingual Coenzyme Q$_{10}$ and Prozac.

Vitamin B$_{12}$ injections help many persons with fatigue.

"Many patients will have a dramatic response to B$_{12}$ although there appears to be a threshold effect, usually at 2000 mcg. We therefore recommend a trial dose of 3000 mcg., two times to three times per week. If there is no response by the end of two weeks, I will then only consider giving B$_{12}$ as a monthly or bi-monthly shot.

---

*From the *CFIDS Chronicle* "Physician's Forum," Vol. 1 Issue 1, March 1991, pages 4 and 5.

B$_{12}$ appears to work for only a few days and therefore it needs to be given relatively frequently. If patients feel like B$_{12}$ might be helping but are not quite sure, it can be stopped and then restarted and the efficacy determined.

"We do not understand at this time why B$_{12}$ works in Chronic Fatigue Syndrome. Typically, once the B$_{12}$ receptors have been saturated the excess B$_{12}$ will be rapidly excreted in the urine over several hours. Why we see effects lasting several days is really quite peculiar and does not fit within the normal pharmacokinetics of B$_{12}$ utilization. We feel that high dose B$_{12}$ must trigger some other effect that lasts longer than the B$_{12}$ itself as it is rapidly excreted."

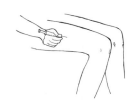

Here's more. For over 20 years, H.L. Newbold, M.D , * 115 E. 34th St., New York, NY 10016 has been writing and talking about the beneficial effects of vitamin B$_{12}$ orally and by injection in the treatment of many types of illness, including tension, fatigue, backache, depression and poor memory. Moreover he noted "often, even seriously ill patients with normal vitamin B$_{12}$ levels and a variety of diagnoses showed great improvement. Moreover, these same patients failed to respond favorably to placebo injection (water)."

Beginning in 1971 he started giving larger amounts of B$_{12}$ to patients who failed to improve on 1000 mcgs. And he found that for best results some patients need to repeat the injection from twice a week to twice a day. A few patients required 6000 to 9000 mcg. daily and he cited the story of one patient who could not function well enough to work unless he took 26,000 mcg. daily.

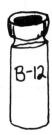

I found more support for the efficacy of vitamin B$_{12}$ in treating patients with fatigue, depression, confusion and memory defects in a recent edition of the *Journal of Nutritional Medicine*.** One brief report by Damien Downing reviewed a 1956 article in the *British Medical Journal* (2:1394-1398) by J. MacDonald Holmes which showed that severe psychological symptoms could be caused by Vitamin B$_{12}$ deficiency in the absence of pernicious anemia.

---

*H.L. Newbold: *Dr. Newbold's Type A/Type B Weight Loss Book*, Keats Publishing Company, New Canaan, CT 1991
**The Journal of Nutritional Medicine*, P.O. Box 3AP, London, W1A 3AP.

A second commentary in the *Journal of Nutritional Medicine* was a review of an article in the *New England Journal of Medicine* (318:1720-1728, 1988) by Jay Lindenbaum et al. entitled "Neuropsychiatric disorders caused by cobalamin (Vitamin B_{12}) deficiency in the absence of anaemia or macrocytosis." In his review of this paper, editor Stephen Davies commented:

A double-blind trial showed vitamin B_{12} to be more effective than placebo in the treatment of tiredness.

"It is interesting that fatigue was common in the absence of anaemia but this cleared on cobalamin therapy; this observation is reminiscent of the report by Ellis et al (*Brj. Nutr.* 1973; 30:277-283) who conducted *a double blind trial of cobalamin administration showing it to be more effective than placebo in the treatment of 'tiredness' for which no other physical cause could be found.* [emphasis added] In Ellis' study, no subject was included in the trial whose initial serum B_{12} values were not in the normal range."

Vitamin C

If you're like most North Americans, you've read and heard about Nobel Prize winner Linus Pauling, Ph.D., a strong advocate of large doses of vitamin C. In his book *How to Live Longer and Feel Better,** Pauling talked about scurvy, which commonly affected sailors and soldiers on long voyages and campaigns. According to Pauling,

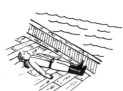

> "The idea that scurvy could be prevented by proper diet developed only slowly. In 1536, the French explorer, Jacques Cartier, discovered the St. Lawrence river and sailed upstream to the present site of the city of Quebec where he and his men spent the winter.
>
> "Twenty-five of the men died of scurvy and many others were very sick. A friendly Indian advised them to drink tea made of leaves and bark of the *Arbor Vitae* tree. The treatment was beneficial. The leaves of this tree were later shown to contain 50 mgs. of vitamin C per 100 grams."

Then, just before the middle of the 18th century, James Lind, a physician in the British navy found that limes (and other fresh fruits) kept sailors from developing scurvy. Yet, because Lind's superiors didn't believe him, they ignored his observations and recommendations. And British sailors on long ocean voyages continued to suffer and die from this disease.

But in 1795, the lime juice story spread and limes (and other fresh fruits) were made a part of the ration on all British ships. That's how the British sailors got the name "limeys." Soon afterward, the scurvy "epidemic" disappeared. Yet, it wasn't until 1933 that the Hungarian researcher Albert Szent-Gyorgi learned why lime juice worked. It contained vitamin C. Gyorgi received the Nobel Prize for his discoveries.

People in North America began to read and hear about taking larger doses of vitamin C following the publication of Dr. Paul-

*New York, W. H. Freeman, 1986.

ing's 1970 book, *Vitamin C and the Common Cold*. Pauling's interest in vitamin C continued, and in a report in the January 1977 issue of *Executive Health*, "On Vitamin C and Cancer," he pointed out that a number of studies showed that vitamin C helped extend the life of patients with advanced cancer. He also suggested it could help people in the early stages of the disease.

In his article, he referred to the observations of Dr. Ewan Cameron, a Scottish physician who gave 100 patients with advanced cancer 10 grams of vitamin C a day. The results of Cameron's study showed that those receiving the large doses of vitamin C lived on an average four times longer than matched controls.

Cancer patients who received large doses of vitamin C lived four times longer.

In spite of these observations, until relatively recently, most people in the medical establishment said, "Forty-five mgs. of vitamin C is all a person needs." But support for larger doses of vitamin C increased in the 1980s. A leading proponent, Robert F. Cathcart, M.D., an orthopedic surgeon, became interested in vitamin C in 1969 because it helped his own respiratory symptoms.

During the '70s and '80s, Cathcart began to use "mega" doses of vitamin C in individuals with suppressed immune systems. Included were patients with cancer, AIDS and Chronic Fatigue Syndrome. In comments in a number of professional publications he told of his remarkable success in treating severely ill patients with oral and intravenous vitamin C. He also described his experiences on *The Donahue Show*.

Cathcart and Pauling found that persons with viral infections could take 10, 20, 100 or more grams of vitamin C during a viral illness, whereas, at other times, more than 5 or 10 grams would usually cause diarrhea or other types of digestive upset. And Cathcart used the term "bowel tolerance test" to determine the appropriate dose of vitamin C.

In a 1985 report* he described his experiences in giving "mega" doses of ascorbic acid to people with various illnesses using bowel tolerance as a method of gauging the correct dose. And he stated, "A person—might be able to tolerate 30 to 60 grams (of vitamin C) for 24 hours if he has a mild cold, 100 grams with a severe cold, 150 grams with influenza and 200 grams with mononucleosis or viral pneumonia."

Persons with viral infections can tolerate "mega" doses of Vitamin C.

*R.F. Cathcart, "Vitamin C: The non-toxic, nonrate-limited, antioxidant free radical scavenger." *Medical Hypotheses* 18: 61-77, 1985.

In an October 15, 1991, letter to me, Dr. Cathcart commented on intravenous vitamin C and pointed out that fatigue is one of the manifestations of free radicals. And he said that large doses of intravenous vitamin C can neutralize these free radicals and play a significant role in relieving a person's fatigue.

Large doses of intravenous vitamin C can neutralize free radicals and play a significant role in relieving a person's fatigue.

More on Intravenous Vitamin C

During the past five years I've talked to a number of other practitioners who have used (and are using) large doses of intravenous vitamin C in treating their patients with severe immune system disorders. One physician commented, "I'm certain—absolutely certain—that IV vitamin C helps my patients. And I've experienced no adverse reactions. One problem, however, insurance doesn't cover costs."

Jay A. Goldstein, M.D., also commented on the frustrating problems faced by both patients and physicians since insurance companies usually do not cover the cost of treatment which hasn't been proved by multiple double-blind studies. And he said,*

"The use of intravenous vitamin C for CFIDS treatment provides a good example of these problems. I've had many patients tell me that they had received the treatment from other physicians and it had helped them. If a treatment is safe and has a scientific rationale, I like to try it in selected patients. *I use IV vitamin C and have found it to be effective according to the patients' self reports.*

"Insurance companies initially reimbursed me for it and I continued to infuse it in patients who did not respond to H2 blockers and anti-depressants. Then they began to withhold payments pending medical review. I did not feel I could stop treating patients who were improved and continued to do so.

"The bills of some patients receiving IV vitamin C got very large and many were ultimately not reimbursed. The patient often could not pay for the total cost of their treatment. I began to be bombarded by requests for information from insurers and ultimately decided to discontinue the use of IV vitamin C.

---

*The CFIDS Chronicle, Physician's Forum, Vol. 1, Issue 1, March 1991, page 13.

"I still believe IV vitamin C to be an effective treatment for some patients with CFIDS, but shall not resume it until I, or someone else, does a double-blind experiment, which is very costly for an individual practitioner to perform."

The problems Dr. Goldstein described with vitamin C administration resemble those many practicing physicians faced (and continue to face) in treating their patients with food and chemical sensitivities and with yeast-related health problems. Although double-blind placebo controlled studies have a place in medicine, the clinical experience of the skilled, conscientious, caring physician is of even greater importance. Support for this point of view can be found in an editoral by Gene H. Stollerman, M.D., "The Gold Standard."*

> *Clinical experience is the Gold Standard on which patient care should be based.*

"As the insights of medical science and technology increase our medical powers, I find renewed strength in my clinical skills. . . . *Clinical experience is the gold standard on which patient care should be based.*"

Vitamin C and Fatigue

For many years Emanuel Cheraskin, M.D., D.M.D, of the University of Alabama, has carried out research studies on the relationship of diet to health problems that affect many people. Studies have included research on vitamin C. Here's an excerpt from one of his reports:

> "It has long been known, actually since about 1750, that sailors on long voyages frequently suffered with inordinate fatigue. For this and other reasons, 411 dental practitioners were queried by a simple seven point questionnaire regarding tiredness. Additionally, vitamin C consumption by means of a simple food frequency questionnaire was ascertained. It was discovered that the 81 subjects who consumed less than 100 milligrams of vitamin C per day recorded a fatigability score approximately twice that of 330 subjects who ingested more than 400 milligrams of vitamin C on a daily basis.**"

> *Dentists who took less than 100 milligrams of Vitamin C per day showed more fatigue.*

Taking Vitamin C

You'll find vitamin C combined in most multiple vitamin prep-

---

*Hospital Practice, January 30, 1985, page 9.
**As cited in E. Cheraskin, Health and Happiness, Bio Communications Press, 1989, p. 31.

arations and in tablets of ascorbic acid. Powdered forms of ascorbic acid and calcium ascorbate are available in most health food stores. A teaspoon of the powder usually contains 3000 to 4000 mg. of vitamin C.

In my own practice during the past two decades, vitamin C in doses of 2000 to 20,000 mg. (or more) daily, has seemed to help many of my patients with food and chemical sensitivities and with yeast-related health problems. In such patients I often recommended the bowel tolerance dose.

A New Form of Vitamin C

During the past decade, researchers in the United States and Scandinavia have studied a new patented form of vitamin C known as Ester-C.* In studies carried out in the Department of Pharmacology at the University of Mississippi, Marilyn J. Bush and Anthony J. Verlangieri** administered Ester-C and L-ascorbic acid (plain vitamin C) to two groups of rats. In analyzing their observations they concluded, "These results support the hypothesis that Ester-C is absorbed more readily and excreted less rapidly than L-ascorbic acid."

In a subsequent human clinical study comparing Ester-C and ascorbic acid, Jonathan V. Wright, M.D. and Raymond M. Suen, M.T., ASCP,*** carried out blood studies on 12 men, ages 27 to 45. Here's a brief summary of their findings: "Ester C produced higher WBC levels, was excreted less in the urine, and was associated with lower urinary oxalate output than L-ascorbic acid."

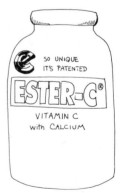

In another animal study, a Norwegian veterinarian, found that C-Flex (Ester-C labelled for animals), provided symptomatic relief of chronic joint problems while a group given a placebo preparation showed no improvement. In still another study in rats, Ester-C was found to be 4-5 times more potent or effective than ascorbic acid in preventing scurvy.****

---

*Information about Ester-C can be obtained from Inter-Cal Corp., 421 Miller Valley Rd., Prescott, AZ 86301. (602) 445-8063.
**M.J. Bush and A.J. Verlangieri, "An Acute Study on the Relative Gastrointestinal Absorption of a Novel Form of Calcium Ascorbate," Research Communications in Chemical Pathology and Pharmacology, Vol. 57, No. 1, July 1987.
***J.W. Wright and R.M. Suin, "A Human Clinical Study Ester-C vs. L-ascorbic Acid," International Clinical Nutrition Review, Vol. 10, No. 1, January 1990.
****A.J. Verlangierl et al., Life Sciences: 48, 2275-81, 1991.

Viral Vaccines

Observations of Joseph B. Miller, M.D.

Tiny doses of flu vaccine helped patients with fever blisters, shingles and other types of herpetic viral infections.

Beginning over 20 years ago, Joseph B. Miller, M.D., a Fellow of the American Academy of Allergy and Immunology, noted that tiny doses of flu vaccine helped patients with fever blisters, herpes simplex, shingles, herpes zoster and other types of herpetic viral infections. He reported his findings in the *Journal of the Alabama State Medical Association* (41:493, 1972) and subsequently in the *Annals of Allergy.** Here's an excerpt from Dr. Miller's report:

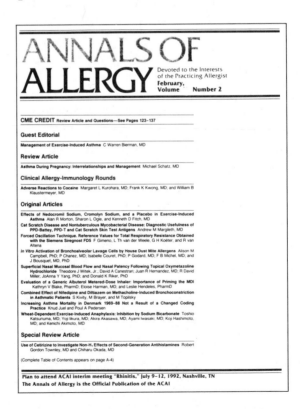

---

*J.B. Miller, "Treatment of Active Herpes Virus Infections with Influenza Virus Vaccine", *Annals of Allergy*, 42:295-305, 1979.)

"This system for treating active virus infections with very small precisely determined doses of specific killed-virus vaccine could be termed 'immunologic antibiosis.' They apparently operate through enhancement of some facet of the body's own innate defense mechanism to eliminate or diminish the infectious process as well as its symptoms . . . and, most importantly, bring relief to many patients for whom no relief has been heretofore available."

Subsequently, Dr. Miller published further observations on his use of immunotherapy in a book entitled *Relief at Last* (Charles C. Thomas Publishers, Springfield, Ill. 1987.) Included in this book is a discussion of the treatment of a variety of health problems caused by food and chemical sensitivities and by viral infections, including acute attacks of influenza and herpes zoster. In a personal conversation with me in 1991, Dr. Miller said, "I have been able to help a number of people with CFS using tiny 'neutralizing' doses of flu vaccine."

Tiny doses of flu vaccine may help people with CFS.

Observations of Other Physicians

During a trip to New Zealand in March 1988, I visited Bruce Duncan, a Fellow of the Australian Academy of Otolaryngology and the American Academy of Otolaryngology. Based on the pioneer work of Dr. Miller, Dr. Duncan has tested and treated several hundred patients with M.E. (CFS) using the Miller technique.** Dr. Duncan has not only used flu vaccines, but other viral vaccines.

Here's an excerpt from Dr. Duncan's paper entitled "Post-Viral Syndrome—Serial Vaccination Therapy:"

"Post-viral syndrome with allergy and candidiasis was the clinical diagnosis of 185 patients. All initially were investigated for inhalant, mould, food allergies, food intolerances and *Candida albicans* and *Candida tropicalis* sensitivity. . . . Serial vaccinations with one or more virus solutions . . . relieved symptoms in patterns that loosely fitted each virus . . . No explanation is offered for this new approach to post-viral syndrome therapy. Responses suggest organ cell immune activity occurs, together with heightened immune response."

**Professionals can obtain additional information by writing to Joseph B. Miller, M.D., 5901 Airport Blvd., Mobile, AL 36608, or Dr. Bruce Duncan, 33 Churchill Ave., Palmerston, North NZ.

A further report of the successful use of viral vaccines in treating patients with CFS was published in a 1989 issue of, *Journal of Orthomolecular Medicine,* Vol. 4, No. 4, pages 185-92 (Publication office, 7375 Burnaby, British Columbia, Canada V3N 3B5.) In this article R. Radulescu, Ph. D. and J. Krop, M.D., stated that flu virus vaccine (Fluogen) controlled recurrent flu-like symptoms in 100% of 28 patients with chronic active Epstein-Barr virus (EBV) who were tested and treated.

In discussing their observations, Radulescu and Krop said,

> "Although we realize that it is not a cure, the therapy applied to the CEBVS patients as described (in their article) can provide people with a substantially improved physical state and with a better way of life. However, it would be simplistic to see only the EBV infection in so many patients suffering today from Chronic Fatigue Syndrome.
>
> "The causes are multiple and one has to look at the patient and the surrounding environment. . . . Water, food, air, homes and work places are contaminated. We must remember that we are dealing with a globally compromised immune system in the whole human species. Infections with bacteria, fungus, viruses and parasites are only an expression of our diminished defense against them. To better fight these infections, we must learn to live in harmony with our environment."

A number of other physicians, including Young Shin, M.D., Atlanta, Georgia, have found viral vaccines, as a part of a comprehensive treatment program, helpful in treating patients with CFS. In a letter to me in September 1991 Dr. Shin said,

The causes of CFS are multiple and include environmental contaminants, bacteria fungi, viruses and parasites.

> "We have found that multiple symptoms in most CFS patients are due to many different causes rather than a single isolated factor such as a viral infection.
>
> "In my practice, I use a combination of treatment modalities including proper diet, management of allergies, treatment of candidiasis, chemical sensitivities, auto-immune thyroid conditions, hypoglycemia and viral infections.
>
> "If the fatigue continues, I use influenzal viral vaccine in neutralizing doses. It has been very effective in increasing energy levels and improving alertness in some patients. The response to this vaccine has often been dramatic."

Testing and Treatment

To carry out this testing and treatment program, serial dilutions of flu vaccine are made in saline. Each dilution is 1/5 as strong as the prior dilution. The 1 to 5 dilution is labeled #1; the 1 to 25 dilution is labeled #2; the 1 to 125 dilution is labeled #3, etc.

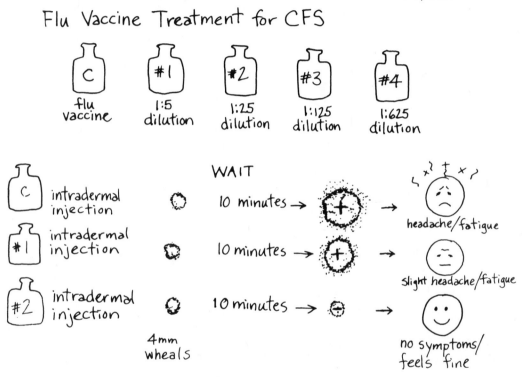

Flu Vaccine Treatment for CFS

According to Dr. Miller, testing is usually begun with the concentrate with the injection of 0.01 ml. If after 10 minutes this dilution causes a "positive" wheal (a wheal which is hard, raised, blanched and increases in size by 2 mm or more) or if symptoms are produced, the patient is given an injection of the #1 dilution.

The patient and the wheal size are again observed. If this wheal increases in size and is judged to be positive and if the patient's symptoms continue, in another 10 minutes the patient is given 0.01 ml. of the #2 dilution. If after a 10 minute wait the examination the the wheal shows that is has not increased in size, (meaning it is "negative") and the patient's symptoms, which have been previously present, are relieved, this dose is the neutralizing or treatment dose.

The treatment dose of viral vaccine is determined by serial dilution testing.

283

Administration of this same neutralizing or treatment dose to the patient one to four times daily initially, then one to three times weekly, was effective in helping many of their patients with CFS.*

---

*In a report to me on October 21, 1991, Dr. Miller stated that 25% of the patients showed no reaction on testing with the concentrate (undiluted flu vaccine) and 0.01 cc of the concenterate is the treatment dose; in 50% of the patients the #1 dilution is the treatment dose; in 15% of the patients it is the #2 dilution; in 7% of the patient it is the #3 dilution; and the remaining 3% is the #4 dilution.

Prozac

Prozac* (fluoxetine hydrochloride) is one of a new generation of antidepressants. It is the nation's most prescribed antidepressant and was first made available in December 1987.

Prozac is related to Elavil, Tofranil, Nardil and Parnate and other antidepressants which have been used for the past 30 years. These medications appear to act through bolstering the action of *serotonin* and *norepinephrine*. (These substances that relay impulses through the nervous system are called "neurotransmitters.")

Although Prozac acts in a manner somewhat similar to other antidepressants, it appears to work exclusively on *serotonin*. Moreover, the dose is easy to regulate, and Prozac causes fewer unpleasant side effects.

As a general rule, Prozac becomes effective in about three weeks and a dose of one or two 20 mg. capsules is usually sufficient. Side effects, which occur in a limited number of patients, include headache, nausea, insomnia, jitteriness and weight loss.

In a comprehensive review article, in the March 26, 1990, issue of *Newsweek* appeared the following comments:

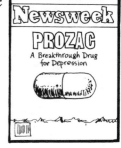

"In the light of Prozac's many virtues, its specificity, its low toxicity and the confidence with which doctors and patients can use it, the excitement it generates is not hard to fathom. But, as Lilly itself concedes, there are good reasons for handling Prozac with care. One concern is that therapists, not to mention family doc-

---

*This drug is produced and marketed by Dista Products Company, Division Eli Lilly and Co. In a September 24, 1991, letter to me, Charles M. Beasley, M.D., Clinical Research Physician, Eli Lilly and Co. commented, "I must point out that Prozac is not approved for the treatment of chronic fatigue syndrome. We are enclosing a copy of the current, approved package literature for Prozac and request any discussion of Prozac be consistent with the contents of this Prozac package literature." The package literature provides a description of Prozac, the clinical pharmacology, indications and usage, contraindications, warnings, precautions, including adverse reactions, dosage and recommendations. A copy of this information can be found in the *Physician's Desk Reference* or can be obtained by writing to Eli Lilly and Company, Indianapolis, IN 46285.

tors, may be giving the drug to people without fully diagnosing their problems."

One psychiatrist (who was quoted in the *Newsweek* report) pointed out that psychiatrists rarely hand these and related medications out without a complete physical and psychological examination. Such a workup may show that the depression stems from some hidden illness or from a job or marriage problem that no drug can possibly solve.

Because Prozac is perceived as safe, the temptation is to prescribe first and ask questions later.

A small minority of patients may not improve on Prozac, and others may develop worse symptoms. These include, in rare cases, manic, violent or suicidal behavior. In addition, the long-term side effects of this drug are unknown.

In my own pediatric and allergy practice, I've had no experience with Prozac. Yet, I've received phone reports from physicians and persons with yeast-connected health problems who have said, "Prozac really helps me." One such person (I'll call him Tom) had experienced headache, fatigue, respiratory allergies and other symptoms for many years.

Tom had sought help from many different physicians. He'd taken both nystatin and Nizoral. Both helped. He'd also taken vitamins, minerals and essential fatty acids. These nutritional supplements also helped. He had received a series of intravenous gamma globulin injections. Tom commented, "I didn't feel any different after having these injections and they were expensive."

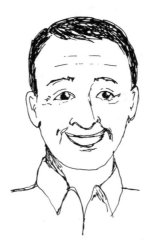

Then, about three years ago, blood tests carried out by the Mayo Clinic laboratory showed a zinc deficiency. So a consulting physician recommended zinc supplements. About the same time, another physician prescribed Prozac, which he began to take on a regular basis. Recently, I bumped into Tom and asked him how he was getting along. He replied,

"Absolutely fantastic. I don't know whether it's the zinc or the Prozac or the combination. But, since I've been taking both, my overall health status is 100% improved. The spaced out feeling and fatigue have gone. So has my depression. My energy level has increased and I have even taken on more volunteer work in addition to forming two new business companies.

"I now have the health and energy to keep up with my four kids and teach a Sunday School class of about 30 to 40 Junior High kids. In addition to my full time investment job, I own and run two other companies. This would have been impossible five years ago. Incidentally, I've been able to cut down my Prozac to one capsule every two or three days."

Further Support for Prozac*

In the March 1991 issue of the *CFIDS Chronicle*, the results of a patient survey were published. Persons with CFIDS were asked, "What treatment measures have helped you and which ones have not?" Prozac ranked high on the list (but almost as many who gave it a positive rating, reported that it did not help.)

A concluding comment: Because I've found that many people will respond to the comprehensive program described in this book (dietary changes, antifungal medication, nutritional supplements, avoidance of environmental pollutants and psychological support), I feel that such a program should be tried before prescribing Prozac. Yet, in spite of the possibility of adverse side effects from the medication, Prozac appears to be a valuable adjunct in the treatment of some individuals with CFS.

Prozac appears to be a valuable adjunct in the treatment of some individuals with CFS.

---

*See also the comments of Nancy Klimas, M.D., in Section VIII.

Ampligen

In searching for a therapy for persons with severe Chronic Fatigue Syndrome, researchers have been using Ampligen in a select group of patients. Here are excerpts from a presentation by Dr. Dan Peterson at the CFIDS Association Research Conference reported in the Spring 1991 issue of the *CFIDS Chronicle*.

Ampligen is a biological response modifier with anti-viral and immunomodulatory activity.

"Ampligen is mismatched double-stranded RNA. It is a known biological response modifier that has been proven in the past to have a broad spectrum of antiviral and immunomodulatory activity. The mismatched structure of the molecule . . . significantly decreases the toxicity without a significant loss of efficacy, making it quite useful. The mechanism of action of Ampligen is known to augment natural killer cell function and also influences the 2-5A synthetase pathway."

Peterson then describes the response of an extremely ill patient who began treatment with Ampligen in 1988. Prior to treatment she had been hospitalized on many occasions. Her response was dramatic, even spectacular. Her IQ increased 46 points, up to 134 and she had a dramatic increase in exercise tolerance.

Because of the response of this patient, treatment was started on 15 additional patients. In commenting on their response, Peterson said,

"Cytopathic changes in the cells markedly decreased in 13 of the 15 patients over the course of Ampligen therapy, which again confirmed the antiviral properties of this particular drug. . . . Statistical analysis of the clinical and laboratory findings suggest that Ampligen is a biologically active drug in CFS. Based on this analysis we had further justification to construct a double-blind, placebo-controlled study which was indeed designed and implemented.

"The first infusions began this summer (1990) and ultimately 120 patients will be enrolled at five different sites with five different investigators."

In his conference report on Ampligen, under the heading "CFS: What It's Not," Dr. Peterson discussed some of the difficult and often frustrating problems the researcher runs into. And he described several polysymptomatic patients with fatigue, arthralgia, cognitive dysfunction, sore throat and other symptoms who had diseases other than CFS. Included were patients with brain tumors, Hodgkin's lymphoma, Lyme disease, senile dementia, diabetes and multiple sclerosis.

In discussing Ampligen in The *CFIDS Chronicle*, Physician's Forum, (Vol. 1, Issue 1, March 1991) Dr. Paul Cheney said,

"Ampligen may be the ultimate in immune modulation and may shortly become the first scientific validated treatment for Chronic Fatigue Syndrome. Ampligen can down-regulate an anti-viral enzyme pathway, which is excessively turned on in most patients with Chronic Fatigue Syndrome. It also down-regulates the production of tumor-necrosis factor-alpha . . .

"Besides its immune modulating effects, Ampligen also has direct anti-viral effects. Ampligen, in our experience and in others, causes a significant improvement in cognitive dysfunction and a general lessening of all symptoms seen in Chronic Fatigue Syndrome."

According to an AP report by Daniel Q. Haney, October 2, 1991, Dr. William Carter of Hahnemann University (Philadelphia), co-inventor of Ampligen, presented new observations on this drug at the meeting of the American Society for Microbiology. Here are excerpts from the Haney report,

Anti-virus drug relieves chronic fatigue syndrome

By Daniel Q. Haney
Associated Press

An experimental anti-virus drug can dramatically relieve the extreme tiredness, memory loss and other debilitating miseries of people severely afflicted with <u>chronic fatigue syndrome</u>, researchers said Tuesday.

Doctors tested the medicine on people so gravely ill that they toms much worse.

In the latest study, doctors at four hospitals tested Ampligen on 92 people whose lives had been ruined by chronic fatigue syndrome. Half received Ampligen injections for up to six months; the rest got placebo shots.

"As a result of Ampligen therapy, the typical patient wa~ needing help mos~ needin~ ~ ~

In the study, doctors found th victims had elevated levels of i terleukin-1, an immune syst~ chemical that prompts the b~ make infection-figh~ bodies.

The re~~ the ~

"In the latest study, doctors at four hospitals tested Ampligen on 92 people whose lives had been ruined by Chronic Fatigue Syndrome. Half received Ampligen injections for up to six months; the rest got dummy shots of a medically inert substance.

"Before treatment, the patients needed custodial care. They could not cook, shop or realiably perform the simplest household tasks.

> *Routine activities of living completely turned around by the use of Ampligen.*

"'As a result of Ampligen therapy, the typical patient went from needing help most of the time to only needing help now and then for sustained tasks such as cutting the grass', Carter said. 'The routine activities of living completely turned around by the use of the drug.' Those in the comparison group were unchanged during the study period. . . .

"Dr. Anthony Komaroff of Brigham and Women's Hospital in Boston, an authority on the syndrome, cautioned that the study does not settle several important issues, such as whether benefits last when treatment is stopped and whether there are unwanted side affects of long term use of Ampligen. 'To me the most interesting aspect of the study is that whether this turns out to be a useful long-term treatment or not, by seeming to show an effect, it clearly implies that there is an immunological or viral cause to this illness', Komaroff said. 'There's no way this medicine is treating a psychological disorder.'"

Still More on Ampligen

In an article, "U.S. Declines to Expand Use of Chronic Fatigue Drug" (*Wall Street Journal*, October 8, 1991), staff reporter Ron Winslow said,

"The U.S. Food and Drug Administration, citing concerns about 'serious and potentially life-threatening' side effects, refused . . . at least for now . . . to permit wider use of an experimental drug for chronic fatigue syndrome.

"The decision was in response to a request by Hem Pharmaceuticals Corp., to make its drug Ampligen available under FDA regulations and tentatively provide desperately ill patients with promising experimental drugs before the drugs are fully licensed for marketing."

In his report Winslow pointed out that the Philadelphia company doesn't believe that Ampligen provokes life-threatening reactions and Dr. William Carter, president of the company, "told a meeting of the American Society of Microbiology that there wasn't any statistical difference in the incidence of adverse events among 45 patients who were treated with Ampligen compared with 47 who were treated with a dummy drug or placebo. No patient was taken off treatment or put on a reduced dose as a result of adverse reactions."

Patients treated with Ampligen had no more adverse events than those treated with placebo.

Kutapressin™

In the Spring/Summer 1990 issue of The *CFIDS Chronicle* and at the November 1990 CFIDS Conference in Charlotte, North Carolina, Thomas L. Steinbach, M.D., and William J. Hermann, Jr., M.D., Memorial City Medical Center, Houston, Texas, described their experiences in using Kutapressin ™,* a mixture of polypeptides derived from pig liver, on 270 patients with CFIDS.

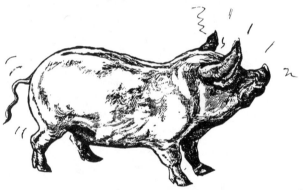

Kutapressin is given by injection for periods up to six months.

The initial therapeutic protocol involved the use of injectable Kutapressin ™ on a daily basis for 4 to 10 injections, followed by three injections a week until recovery for a period up to six months.

Patients were advised to follow a prudent diet, take one multi-vitamin tablet daily, abstain from all alcoholic beverages and get adequate rest. Thyroid and estrogen replacement therapy were allowed to continue with proper monitoring. Ninety-five percent of the patients had tried various therapies, including vitamins, acyclovir, gamma globulin, antidepressants, antihistamines and/or Tagamet. All patients indicated that these previous therapies had been unsuccessful.

The therapeutic outcome was rated as successful in the great majority of patients. In summarizing their observations, these physicians said,

*Produced by the Kremers Urban, Inc., Mequon, Wisconsin 53201.

"We describe a successful, concise and reasonable program for treatment of Chronic Fatigue Immune Dysfunction Syndrome. The large number of patients yield validity to the success of the drug Kutapressin.™ . . . The exact mechanism of Kutapressin™ action is not clear, however, these clinical findings certainly warrant basic research into the purified components of this apparently valuable drug."*

In the March 1991 Physician's Forum, *The CFIDS Chronicle*, Paul R. Cheney, Ph.D., and J. A. Goldstein, M.D., discussed Kutapressin.™ Here are Dr. Cheney's comments,

"Kutapressin™ is another immune system modulator useful in the treatment of Chronic Fatigue Syndrome. The dosage for Kutapressin™ has wide variability and ranges from maintenance doses of 2 cc. intramuscular, 2 times to 4 times per week, to accelerated uses of Kutapressin™ 2 to 4 cc. daily for several days up to 10 days for acute relapses. . . .

"Interestingly as far back as 1939 Kutapressin™ was used to treat a condition known as neuraesthenia, which might well be another name for Chronic Fatigue Syndrome. Kutapressin™ appears to improve fatigue and endurance and sometimes reduces myalgic and arthralgia pain. I have seen it also improve herpetiform blisters of the mouth and buccal mucosa, as well as shingles in the setting of Chronic Fatigue Syndrome. I have not found Kutapressin™ very helpful in treating cognitive impairment."

> *Kutapressin is an immune system modulator useful in treating CFS.*

Dr. Goldstein's comments were less positive:

"I have been rather disappointed in the results of Kutapressin, although I continue to try it when many other treatments have failed. I try to follow the methods outlined in *The Chronicle*. It has been occasionally effective in my patients although many of them will not want to try it for 6 months if it has not worked after 3 or 4 months. I wonder whether the physicians in Texas who popularized this treatment are seeing a different population than I am. A double blind study of this medication would be very helpful."

---

*For a more detailed report see pages 25-30 of the Spring/Summer 1990 issue of the *CFIDS Chronicle*, P.O. Box 220398, Charlotte, NC 28222-0398.

Further comments about Kutapressin

To obtain more information about Kutapressin I wrote to Dr. William J. Hermann, Jr. Here's a copy of his November 8, 1991 response:

Kutapressin is more effective when given by intramuscular injection.

"Thank you for the inquiry regarding Kutapressin in CFIDS. We continue to enjoy success at approximately the same rates as previously reported. No double blind study has been performed as we are waiting another formulation to proceed on that front. Enclosed is a copy of a brief synopsis we prepared for the North Carolina Group's hotline. Included in this transcript is our exact protocol.

"I would emphasize the greatest variable leading to lower success rates is the use of subcutaneous rather than, our specified, intramuscular injection. I cannot, with complete scientific validity, account for this observation but it does seem to influence the efficacy and the lower incidence of local side effects at the injection site. Thank you for your interest on behalf of myself and Thomas Steinbach, M.D."*

---

*To obtain a 2-page summary, The Diagnosis and Treatment of CFIDS with Kutapressin by Thomas L. Steinback, M.D. and William J. Hermann, Jr., M.D., and the transcript of their exact protocol, send a SASE to William J. Hermann, Jr., M.D., Director of Laboratories, Memorial City Medical Center, 920 Frostwood, Houston, TX 77024. (923-3000).

Recommendations of CFS Leaders

In Vol. 1, Issue 1, of the March 1991 *Physicians' Forum* issue of the CFIDS Chronicle, David S. Bell, M.D.; Paul R. Cheney, M.D., Ph.D.; Jay A. Goldstein, M.D.; and Charles W. Lapp, M.D. were asked—"Given the complexities and diversity of symptoms of CFIDS, how do you approach the treatment of CFIDS patients?"

In a letter introducing this dialogue, Marc M. Iverson, President and Publisher of *Physicians' Forum*, said,

> "In this premier issue we address the question that we most often hear . . . 'How can CFIDS be treated?' . . . And this topic is destined to be continually discussed: The fact that there is presently no scientifically validated treatment for CFIDS impedes, but cannot halt, the search for help conducted by PWCs (person's with CFIDS) and those who truly care for them."

Treatment is based on trial-and-error application of anecdotal evidence . . . I lack the strength to wait years for controlled studies. Thomas English, M.D.

> "Dr. Thomas English, (a surgeon with CFIDS and a *Chronicle* contributor, in an editorial published in *JAMA*, February 27, 1991, Vol. 265, No. 8, page 964) said, 'Treatment is palliative and based on trial-and-error application of anecdotal evidence, but it helps most patients. I enjoy passable existence, not a miasma of misery. I lack the strength to wait years for controlled studies; life is short, science is slow.'"

Each of the physicians who responded to Mark Iverson's question has been on the cutting edge of CFIDS research and each has treated hundreds of CFIDS patients.

David S. Bell, M.D.

This Cambridge, Massachusetts, pediatrician and author of the recent book *The Disease of a Thousand Names*, said,

"The question of treatment approaches in CFIDS is extremely dif-

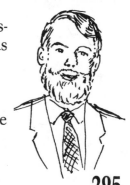

ficult because of numerous variations in the clinical course and prognosis seen with this condition."

Dr. Bell divided patients into three different groups: those with mild to moderate symptoms and a good prognosis; those with moderate symptoms and a prolonged course with less likelihood of recovery; those with severe symptoms and small chance of spontaneous recovery.

Included in the latter group were those who had been ill for five years or longer, and who have prominent neurologic symptoms and a gradual onset.

Dr. Bell recommended lifestyle adjustments, nutritonal support, stress reduction and symptomatic treatment.

In treating all groups of patients Dr. Bell recommended lifestyle adjustments, nutritional support, stress reduction and symptomatic treatment of specific symptoms. In the moderate group he said,

"I would consider the use of intramuscular gamma globulin, more aggressive use of anti-depressants and certain vitamin preparations to attempt to improve mitochondrial function . . . If the most debilitating symptom was fatigue, I would consider bupropion and/or amantadine, both of which require careful monitoring because of possible unpleasant side effects."

For those with severe symptoms, he said,

Dr. Cheney divides his treatment program into three parts: lifestyle issues, symptom relief and primary therapy.

"I would be more likely to move to treatment agents considered aggressive or experimental (including) intravenous gamma globulin, transfer factor and Ampligen."

Paul Cheney, M.D., Ph.D.

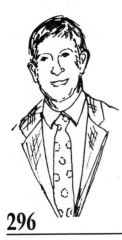

This Charlotte, North Carolina, clinician and researcher, has for a number of years been a vigorous advocate for persons with CFIDS. Dr. Cheney and Dr. Daniel Peterson first characterized the 1984-85 CFIDS epidemic in Incline Village, Nevada (on Lake Tahoe), which brought the disease to national attention.

During the past several years Dr. Cheney has conducted, coordinated and participated in dozens of CFIDS research projects and has seen over 2,000 CFIDS patients. He divides his treatment program into three parts: lifestyle issues, symptom relief and primary therapy. He emphasized stress reduction and appropriate exercise. (Not too little and not too much.) He also stated,

"The final lifestyle elements that require adjustment are nutrition and vitamins. . . . While food allergies do exist in some patients, I think that food sensitivities are far more common and are believed to significantly affect up to 1/3 of all patients with chronic fatigue syndrome. . . . Vitamins appear to be very important . . . we recommend that multi-vitamin therapy be employed in the treatment of chronic fatigue syndrome."

Food sensitivities significantly affect up to 1/3 of all patients with CFS. Paul Cheney, M.D.

" . . . Probably the single most important symptom to treat is the sleep disorder associated with chronic fatigue syndrome. . . . We have attempted to avoid sleeping pills. . . . We rely primarily on a combination of low dose Sinequan, plus Klonopin at low doses."

Dr. Cheney also said he uses vitamin B_{12} injections two to three times a week, high doses of sublingual Coenzyme Q_{10} and Prozac. In discussing this treatment of cognitive dysfunction Dr. Cheney stated that he used different kinds of Diamox as well as Nimodapine and Cardene and other therapies in some patients, especially those with pain. These have included Toradol, deep tissue massage, TENS unit therapy, physical therapy, biofeedback therapy, Tegretol, Elavil, Prozac and the calcium channel blockers such as Calan or Cardene.

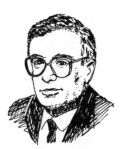

In his continuing discussion Dr. Cheney stated that the final issue of the treatment of Chronic Fatigue Syndrome is what I would describe as "primary therapy" which encompasses immunomodulation as its principal effect. Such therapy includes gamma globulin, Kutapressin and Ampligen, which has immune modulating effects and direct antiviral effects.

Jay A. Goldstein, M.D.

This Anaheim, California, physician has spent over five years researching and writing about CFIDS. He is also the author of a recently published book, *The Chronic Fatigue Syndrome: The Struggle for Health.* Dr. Goldstein said, "Contrary to popular view, there are a vast number of useful treatments for CFIDS although they have to be carefully and intelligently employed case-by-case . . . and 'experimental' methods are increasingly being limited."

Among the basic drug therapies he uses are the H2 blocker, ranitidine (which results in a beneficial response in 20% of CFIDS patients). Other medications he uses include Sinequan, Pamelor and Prozac and Wellbutrin. In discussing other agents, Dr. Goldstein said, "In my approach to CFIDS treatment it is important to have a good grounding in biological psychiatry because of the psychoneuroimmunologic nature of CFIDS."

A basic tenet of CFIDS treatment—the patient must get a good night's sleep. Jay A. Goldstein, M.D.

He pointed out that sleep disorders occur commonly and that a basic tenet of CFIDS treatment is still that the patient must get a good night's sleep. He then discussed several different medications, including the Desyrel, Klonopin, Doral and chloral hydrate.

For those with temporal lobe dysfunction he points out that Tegretol, Depakote and nimodipine (Namotop) and Cardene may be of help. He expresses support for the judicious use of gamma globulin "despite the astounding negative report recently published in the *American Journal of Medicine.*" He says, "I've been rather disappointed in the results of Kutapressin, although I continue to try it when many other treatments have failed. He also had only occasional success with acyclovir (Zovirax).

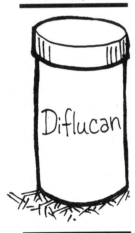

Goldstein also discussed the candida hypersensitivity syndrome and states that he had found the antiyeast medication Diflucan effective in a few of his patients. And even though this medication is expensive, he said that "It is also quite safe and a quick trial of this agent may help make the diagnosis and establish the treatment." And he stated that he had had success with this approach in patients who had been resistant to almost every other treatment. (See also Dr. Goldstein's comments entitled "Battling Yeast" in Section III.)

I've had success with Diflucan in a few patients who had been resistant to almost every other treatment. Jay A. Goldstein, M.D.

Goldstein stated he had not been able to document the role that giardia and other intestinal parasites may contribute to CFIDS but that new anti-giardia antibody studies may be helpful. He noted that an occasional patient responds to antibiotics, particularly Vibramycin. Yet, he pointed out that there are potential adverse drug reactions.

He then discussed herbal remedies and nutritional supplements of various kinds, including zinc, garlic, echinacea and the antioxidants such as vitamin C, vitamin A and selenium. Also Coenzyme Q_{10}. Although he said, "I'm still waiting for my first unambiguous response to this substance." He stated that immunomodulatory drugs such as Ampligen show great promise. In discussing diagnostic challenges he said,

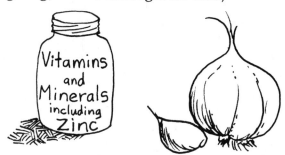

"Because CFIDS patients are tired of being told their problem is 'all in your head', they often rebel against any suggestion that the illness has a psychological component. It is, therefore, very important to stress that, increasingly emotional problems are being recognized as having a physiologic basis."

"As CFIDS is better understood, a rapprochement between the two camps (ie, psychiatrists and physiologists and immunologists) may occur with the elucidation of a common pathophysiology, even considering that CFIDS is a multifactorial disorder."

Finally, he discussed the problems of third party payment which continue to exist. And he said,

"The use of intravenous vitamin C for CFIDS treatment provides a good example of these problems. I had many patients tell me they had received the treatment from other physicians and it had helped them. If a scientific treatment is safe and has a scientific rationale, I like to use it in selective patients."

CFIDS in most cases is a quite treatable disorder. Jay A. Goldstein, M.D.

In his concluding remarks, Dr. Goldstein said,

"We must all come to our own terms with the rapidly changing medical scene in the United States when, in the absence of research funding, innovative decision-making must be tempered more and more with circumspection. Nevertheless, I believe the CFIDS is, in most cases, a quite treatable disorder and I anticipate that new discoveries will make it even more so."

In an article in the Fall 1991 issue of the *CFIDS Chronicle*, "CFS: Limbic Encephalopathy in a Dysfunctional Neuroimmune Network," Dr. Goldstein made these additional observations on CFS,

"Chronic Fatigue Syndrome can be viewed as a multicausal disorder of the neuroimmune network which occurs in genetically predisposed individuals. Infectious agents, probably viral, may activate the immune system and dysregulate the central nervous system, particularly the temporolimbic area.

"Many symptoms are neurologic and the fatigue appears to be central, not peripheral. Since the symptoms fluctuate and can be altered by neuropharmacological intervention, they may be mediated by neuroimmune transmitter substances. A latent infection or predisposition may be triggered by a number of possible stimuli. . . .

"If the neuroimmune system is viewed as a network, then it could possibly be disrupted by agents influencing the network in various locations. Thus, it would be possible to treat CFS with neuro-pharmacologic, immunomodulatory and anti-infective modalities, particularly since it increasingly appears that lymphocytes and neural cells share many receptor systems. Most of the symptoms of CFS can be explained on the basis of a limbic encephalopathy."

Charles W. Lapp, M.D.

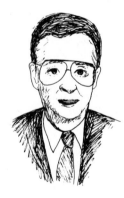

This board-certified internist and pediatrician and former medical director, Piedmont Associates, Raleigh, North Carolina, is now working with Dr. Paul Cheney in the treatment and management of CFIDS patients with particular attention toward children. In his comments, Dr. Lapp said,

"First, it must be made clear that there are no cures, no panaceas. We have not identified a cause for this disorder, so naturally we cannot specify an exact cure. . . . Perhaps the most important part of any 'treatment' is the inexpensive, drug free, low tech, high touch advice that we dispense. A whole drugstore full of medicine cannot accomplish what a little reassurance, a positive attitude and some self-care can accomplish."

Reasurance, a positive attitude accomplish more than medicine. Charles W. Lapp, M.D.

In collaboration with Dr. Paul Cheney, Dr. Lapp prepared a self-care manual in February 1991. Major divisions of this manual include:

1. Lifestyle changes. Included is appropriate rest and the management of stress.
2. Exercise. Carefully tailored to the individuals needs and abilities.

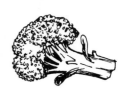

3. Diet and nutrition. Emphasized are complex carbohydrates and the avoidance of foods that cause sensitivity reactions, also "The Big Five," sugar, caffeine, nicotine, alcohol and Nutrasweet.

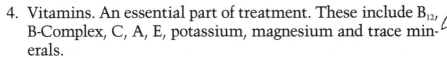

4. Vitamins. An essential part of treatment. These include B_{12}, B-Complex, C, A, E, potassium, magnesium and trace minerals.
5. Optional supplements (which are available over the counter). Those recommended included Coenzyme Q_{10} (ubiquinone) 90-200 mg daily for five to six weeks; Omega 6 fatty acids and Omega 3 fatty acids; L-Carnitene and L-Lysine.

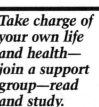

6. General recommendations. Keep a daily log, avoid sunshine, avoid corticosteroid drugs, do not take an annual flu shot. Take precautions to avoid the possible spread of infection.
7. Complete annual physical examination.

In his final words of advice, Dr. Lapp urged persons with CFS to take charge of their own lives and he said,

Take charge of your own life and health— join a support group—read and study.

"In many cases you will have to be your own medical advisor because few people—even doctors and counselors—will know as much about this disorder as you do. It behooves you to read and study everything you can get hold of concerning this disorder. If you have not already done so, join the CFIDS Association, P.O. Box 220398, Charlotte, North Carolina 28222-0398, (704) 362-2343 and request a list of resources."

301

SECTION **VII**

The Yeast Connection Controversy

If you review medical history, you'll find countless examples of new ideas that helped sick people get well, and that were stumbled on "accidentally." Some of these discoveries were made by scientists working in their laboratories and others by practicing physicians. Still others were made by nonphysicians. *But regardless of who makes a discovery, or what the discovery is, if a full scientific explanation of the mechanism isn't forthcoming, it tends to be rejected by the establishment.*

This seems to be the situation with the yeast connection. Here's a brief summary of the story:

The Truss Observations

In the early 1960s, C. Orian Truss, M.D., a board-certified internist, first observed that the common yeast, *Candida albicans* could be related to fatigue, depression and many other systemic and nervous symptoms. During the next 15 years, Truss found that many of his patients with complex medical problems responded to a sugar free special diet and the oral antifungal medication *nystatin*.

Word of the Truss experiences spread to a handful of physicians following his presentation at a medical conference in Toronto in 1977. Subsequently, he published his observations in a 1978, 1980, 1981 and 1984 little known medical journal* from Canada and in a 1983 book, *The Missing Diagnosis*. However, because this journal was not peer-reviewed, the Truss reports were not listed in the *Index Medicus*. Accordingly, his observations were not available in the medical libraries and most physicians remained unaware of them.

Countless therapies that helped sick people get well were stumbled on "accidentally."

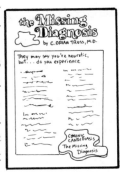

The Public Learns About the Yeast Connection

Then in the early 1980s, one of Truss' patients, Diane Thomas, wrote an article entitled "New Hope for Allergy Patients," which was published in *Atlanta Magazine* and subsequently in *Inn America* (a publication of the Holiday Inn Corp.). Further reports of the Truss observations were discussed in a health food magazine and on a popular interview program, the Freeman Report (CNN).

**Journal of Orthomolecular Psychiatry*, 7375 Kingsway, Burnaby, B.C., V3N 3B5. Present journal name, *Journal of Orthomolecular Medicine*.

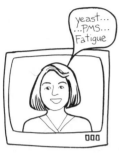

Subsequently, millions of Americans (and people all over the world) learned about the relationship of *Candida albicans* to fatigue, depression, PMS and other symptoms through reports in the press and media and through popular books, including *The Yeast Connection* and *The Yeast Syndrome.*

Concurrently, a scattering of reports appeared in the peer-reviewed literature which provided support for the relationship of *Candida albicans* to a variety of health problems. These ranged from immune and endocrine dysfunction to psoriasis and Crohn's Disease.

Skepticism and Controversy

In spite of these reports, the candida hypothesis was rejected by most physicians. For example, in a report on what they termed "the candidiasis hypersensitivity syndrome," the Practice Standards Committee of the American Academy of Allergy and Immunology (AAAI), stated,*

The concept is speculative and unproven. American Academy of Allergy and Immunology.

"This concept is speculative and unproven.

"The basic elements of the syndrome would apply to almost all sick patients at some time

"The complaints are essentially universal:
  a. The broad treatment program will produce remission in most illnesses regardless of cause.
  b. There's no published proof that *Candida albicans* is responsible for the syndrome.
  c. Elements of the proposed treatment program are potentially dangerous."

Following the AAAI statement, I wrote to the chairman of the AAAI committee and answered the committee's criticisms point by point. Yet, he did not reply and he gave no indication that the committee would like additional information.

So the controversy has continued. On one side, there are a few thousand professionals who have found that a special diet and antifungal therapy helps many of their patients. On the other side are a much larger number of physicians who continue to say in effect, "The yeast connection is a fad disorder."

Journal of Allergy and Clinical Immunology, 78:271-73, 1986.

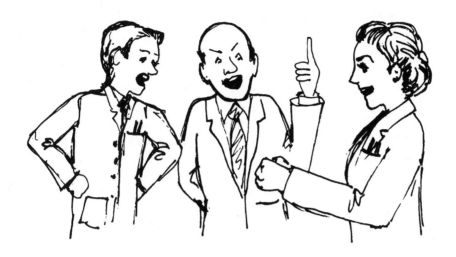

The Dismukes Report and the Bennett Editorial

In the December 20, 1990, issue of the *New England Journal of Medicine*, William E. Dismukes and associates of the University of Alabama published findings of a "randomized, double-blind trial of nystatin therapy for the candidiasis hypersensitivity syndrome." They evaluated a group of women with vaginitis who complained of fatigue, depression, PMS and other symptoms. In treating them, they only used oral and vaginal nystatin. They made no changes in diet and in their opinion, their results were "negative."

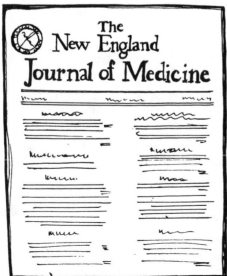

In an accompanying editorial, "Searching for the Yeast Connection," John E. Bennett, M.D., of the National Institute of Allergy and Infectious Diseases, Bethesda, Maryland said,

"Few illnesses have sparked as much hostility between the medical community and a segment of the lay public as the chronic candidiasis syndrome. Those who argue for the existence of this complex of symptoms . . . have leveled a serious charge against the medical community, claiming that it is not fulfilling one of its most important obligations to its patients. The charges simply put: You physicians are not listening to your patients. . . . Physicians pay more attention to the patient's normal laboratory test-results than to what the patients say. . . .

"Even more damaging is the profession's apparent refusal to study chronic candidiasis. How can science reject an idea that has not been tested when science is purportedly open to new ideas?"

In his continuing comments, Bennett said,

"The study by Dismukes et al. was carefully designed and the data thoughtfully analyzed. This will not end the controversy, however. The absence of a washout period between therapeutic regimens . . . will be criticized by those who design drug studies. Those who argue for the existence of the chronic candidiasis syndrome will complain that diet was not controlled and that it is an important aspect of treatment.

"In addition, candida allergy shots, injunctions to avoid moldy environments, and other therapeutic approaches are often included in treatment regimens. In fact, *none of the proponents of the syndrome have recommended the use of nystatin alone and they are not likely to consider the Dismukes study an adequate test of their hypothesis.* [emphasis added] . . .

" . . . The study by Dismukes is only a beginning. Additional scientifically sound studies will be needed to determine whether this syndrome does or does not exist and if it does, what the optimal treatment is for patients."

Responses in the *New England Journal of Medicine*

A number of professionals took exception to the Dismukes observations and wrote letters to the editor of the *New England Journal of Medicine* and to other publications. Some were pub-

A serious charge has been leveled against the medical community: You physicians are not listening to your patients.

The study by Dismukes is only a beginning. Additional scientifically sound studies will be needed. John E. Bennett, M.D.

lished and some were not. Here are excerpts of several letters published in the May 30, 1991, issue of *NEJM*.

"We see, in these data, strong support for the proposal that generalized symptoms caused by toxins or other mechanisms may accompany mucosal yeast infections."

C. Orian Truss, M.D., and associates,
Birmingham, AL

"I challenge the conclusion by Dismukes et al. that the candidiasis hypersensitivity syndrome 'is not a verifiable condition.' This negative conclusion is not substantiated by the results of their clinical study, which shows a strikingly positive effect of the all nystatin regimen in women with the presumed syndrome."

Marjorie Crandall, Ph.D.,
Torrance, CA

> *I challenge the conclusion of the Dismukes study. Marjorie Crandall, Ph.D.*

"As the author of the controversial and often maligned book *The Yeast Connection*, I would like to shine more light (and less heat) on the candida related complex. . . . Does (their study) mean that nystatin is of no value as part of a comprehensive program for patients with fatigue, premenstrual tension, gastrointestinal symptoms and depression?

"In my experience, and that of hundreds of other physicians and thousands of patients, the answer is a resounding 'No.' With few exceptions, the patient with a chronic health problem requires multimodal therapy. . . . And as noted by Bennett, 'None of the proponents have recommended the use of nystatin alone.'

"Additional scientifically sound studies are desperately needed. I hope that pharmaceutical companies or the National Institutes of Health will provide funds for carrying out such studies. . . . I would especially urge the investigators to look at the important role and intricacies of diet. A diet low in sugar (and other simple carbohydrates) was an essential part of the treatment program first outlined by Truss."

William G. Crook, M.D.,
Jackson, TN

> *The patient with a chronic health problem requires multi-modal therapy.*

Other Responses to the Dismukes Study

Here are excerpts from other letters I received which were not published in *NEJM* or which were published in other periodicals.

"It is hard to imagine why (the investigators) would go to all that trouble when only 14% of the women had positive vaginal cultures for the yeast and only 12% had positive rectal cultures on entry to this study."

Michael L. McCann, M.D.,
Parma, OH

> **"Any researcher who evaluates Truss' protocol, should use Truss' protocol." Dennis W. Remington, M.D.**

"I would like to report that I have now treated over 5000 patients using the Truss protocol. I have seen the dramatic multi-system improvement in the majority of my patients. Not one of Truss' critics referenced by Dismukes and Bennett has ever reported treating a single patient using Truss' complete protocol. I would like to recommend that any researcher who evaluates Truss' protocol, should use Truss' protocol."

Dennis W. Remington, M.D.,
Provo, UT

"It is very difficult to treat a yeast problem with a one-pronged approach. The startling aspect (of the Dismukes) paper is they ignored the diet. . . . This study is sort of analogous to designing a study on diabetes and insulin while letting the patients eat sugar."

Doris J. Rapp, M.D.,
Buffalo, NY

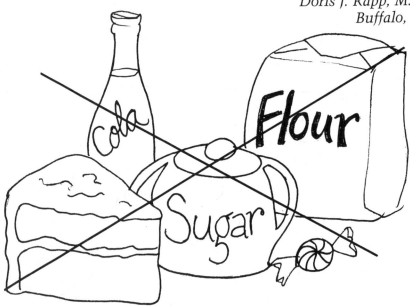

The overwhelming majority of candida-related illnesses are not hypersensitivity syndromes at all, but complex problems involving non-IgE related immune intolerance to the organism, probably coupled with direct toxicity.

" . . . Candida-related illness must always be treated, at least initially, with stringent dietary control, in addition to any anti-fungal therapy. In my experience, there's practically no hope of successful treatment of this problem without dietary restrictions."

W. A. Shrader, M.D.,
Kamula, HI

Keith W. Sehnert, M.D., St. Louis Park, Minnesota, sent me a copy of a three-page letter to Dr. Dismukes. In this letter he described his experiences based on his study and treatment of 1500 patients with the Candida-Related Complex (CRC). In his letter to Dr. Dismukes he outlined a comprehensive treatment program which included a low-sugar, yeast-free diet and lifestyle changes. In the closing paragraph, Dr. Sehnert said,

> "It's my fervent hope that you shall remain 'curious' about CRC and your research into this complex and common health problem will continue."

In his response to Dr. Sehnert, Dr. Dismukes said,

> "I appreciate your thoughtful letter of December 31, 1990. . . . I do understand the positive nature of your comments and accept them in that spirit. As we discussed in the paper, our study design was complex but did not incorporate all of the treatment approaches which have been advocated for CRC. Future studies should address these and other issues such as diagnostic criteria. Thanks for your input."

Since the Dismukes article and the Bennett editorial, I've knocked on many doors including the American Medical Association, the American Academy of Allergy and Immunology, and the National Institute of Allergy and Infectious Diseases. My goal has been to get studies started that everyone agrees are needed. I've also written to Pfizer, Janssen and other pharmaceutical companies that manufacture antifungal medications. Although there is nothing concrete to report as yet, I am encouraged.

The Candida Controversy Isn't Limited to the U.S.A.

You'll find a superb 34-page discussion of the candida controversy in the January 1991 issue of *Meeting-Place*. Here are excerpts from editor Jim Brook's introduction:

> "How is it not possible for medicine and science to solve a tantalis-

Candida-related illness must always be treated . . . with stringent dietary control.
W. A. Shrader, M.D.

I've written to pharmaceutical companies that manufacture antifungal medications. Nothing concrete to report, but I am encouraged.

311

ing mystery which has split doctors into two camps? Some doctors are skeptical that the fungus/yeast *Candida albicans* is a problem—except in some easily recognized situations.

"Others, the converts, have come to believe that *Candida albicans* is responsible for more undiagnosed illness than any other organism in the world; they treat for it even without clear evidence that there is any problem. They claim that 'response to therapy' is the best test at the present time."

In the material presented in *Meeting-Place* are comments by candida proponent, Dr. David Dowson of Southampton, England who said,

> *Treatments are so effective— often dramatic— that it is worrying that treatment for candida is not more readily available.*

"In the view of the prevalence of overgrowth of candida in the gut, particularly in M.E., I find it surprising that my orthodox colleagues largely reject such a diagnosis. The symptoms are so typical and treatments are so effective—often dramatic—that it is worrying that treatment for candida is not more readily available."

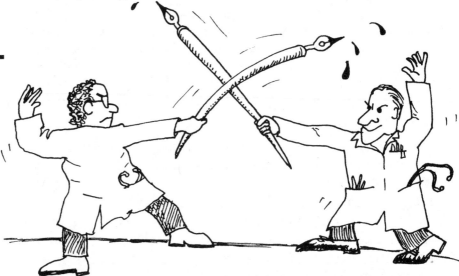

Dr. Charles Shepherd*, is an ex-M.E. sufferer and GP, and Vice-President of the M.E. Association. He is also author of *Living with M.E.,* and in presenting a different point of view said,

"One aspect of the M.E. debate that's guaranteed to create more hot air (and angry letters) is the yeast called candida. It's also an

*C. Shepherd, *Living With M.E.*, Mandarin Paperbacks, Michelin House, 81 Fulham Rd., London, SW3 6RB.

important reason why some doctors refuse to take M.E. seriously. They regard candida as yet another bogus illness. . . . My feeling is that the candida connection is probably another blind alley for desperate sufferers searching for a cure. By all means, weigh up the arguments carefully, but remember—the case for candida is nowhere as watertight as the advocates suggest."

How Should the Efficacy of a Therapy Be Determined?*

In answering this question, I'd like to quote from a statement by the Office of Technology Assessment, Congress of the United States. In a September 1978 publication entitled, "Assessing the Efficacy and Safety of Medical Technologies," appeared the following comments:

". . . Despite the increasing need to formally estimate the efficacy and safety of medical technologies, the majority of such evaluations are still based on informal approaches. White** estimated that 80% to 90% of all procedures . . . have been evaluated by informal methods.

"It has been estimated that only 10 to 20% of all procedures currently used in medical practice have been shown to be efficacious by controlled trials. . . . Personal experience is perhaps the oldest and most common informal method of judging the efficacy and safety of a medical technology. . . . Despite its limited statistical value, this technique does have some advantages compared to some of the more rigorous methods used in certain situations. . . . It is important to point out that many medical advancements have properly and successfully proceeded without rigorous statistical methodology of evaluation."

Personal experience is perhaps the oldest and most common informal method of judging the efficacy and safety of a medical technology.

And in an article in the *Journal of the American Medical Association*,*** James S. Goodwin, M.D. and Jean M. Goodwin, M.D. M.P.H., of the University of New Mexico talked about tomatoes and how no one ate them in North America during the 16th, 17th and 18th centuries. Here's why: People thought they were poisonous and 'it simply did not make sense to eat poisonous food.'

*See also the comments of Eugene Stollerman, M.D. in Section VI.
**K. L. White, International Comparison of Health Service Systems. Millbank Mem. Fund Q 46:117, 1968.
***J. Goodwin and J. Goodwin, "The Tomato Effect—Rejection Of Highly Efficacious Therapies." *JAMA* 251:2387-90, 1984.

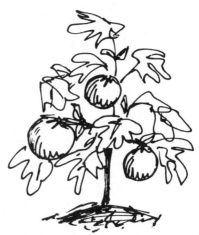

These doctors used the tomato story to explain the derivation of the term "tomato effect" and they defined it as follows:

The tomato effect in medicine occurs when a efficacious treatment for a certain disease is ignored or rejected.

"The tomato effect in medicine occurs when a efficacious treatment for a certain disease is ignored or rejected because it does not make sense in the light of accepted theories of disease mechanism and drug action."

In their continuing discussion, Drs. Goodwin and Goodwin said,

"Modern medicine is particularly vulnerable to the tomato effect. Pharmaceutical companies have . . . turned to theoretical over practical arguments for using their drugs. Therefore, we're asked to use a new arthritis drug because it stops monocytes from crawling through a filter . . . and an oral diabetes drug because it increases insulin receptors on monocytes.

Only three issues matter in picking a therapy. Does it help? How toxic is it? How much does it cost?

"What gets lost in such discussions are the only three issues that matter in picking a therapy. *Does it help? How toxic is it? How much does it cost?* In this atmosphere we are at risk for rejecting a safe, inexpensive, effective therapy in favor of an alternative treatment, perhaps less efficacious and more toxic."

So when a sugar-free special diet and safe, prescription and nonprescription substances, such as nystatin, Nizoral, Diflucan, caprylic acid, aged garlic extract and acidophilus are rejected, in favor of less effective treatment measures which are also more toxic, we see a clear example of "the tomato effect."

Other Topics of Interest

Intestinal Microbes and Systemic Immunity

According to Dr. Leo Galland, the intestinal tract is the largest organ of immune surveillance and response in the human body. He stated that we should not be surprised that events in the lumen or on the mucosal surfaces have systemic effects on immune function and disease resistance.

In a recent comprehensive discussion,* Dr. Galland stated that over 500 species of bacteria live in the digestive tract and in the average adult they weigh over two pounds. I was surprised to learn that these intestinal tract inhabitants synthesize at least seven essential nutrients, which supplement those that a person obtains from diet. Included are folic acid, biotin, pantothenic acid (vitamin B$_5$), riboflavin (vitamin B,) pyridoxine (vitamin B$_6$), cobalamin (vitamin B$_{12}$) and vitamin K. Apparently, the gut microflora do a lot of other good things for us: they help us get rid of carcinogens and they metabolize drugs and mercury and other toxic substances.

In discussing the important role of intestinal microbes, Dr. Galland commented,

> "The gut flora of healthy individuals is very stable.... Alteration in the level of normal flora by antibiotics has long been known to allow secondary infection by pathogenic bacteria and yeasts....** Ionescu, et al., (1986) studied fecal flora in children and adults with atopic eczema. Compared with healthy controls there was marked reduction in *Lactobacillus, Bifidobacterium* and *Enterococcus* species in the great majority of cases. This was associated with increased concentration of *Candida* species (and other organisms).... In neither of these studies is it possible to determine whether abnormal bowel flora caused allergy or whether food-allergic disease destabilized gut flora."

Microflora do many good things for us.

*Adapted and excerpted from *The Effect of Microbes on Systemic Immunity* by Leo Galland, M.D., from the book, *Post-viral Fatigue Syndrome*, edited by R. Jenkins and J. Mowbray, copyright 1991, John Wiley and Sons, Ltd.
**C.S. Keefer, *American Journal of Medicine*, 11, 665-66, 1951, Seelig, M., Bacteriological Reviews, 30, 442-59, 1966.

Giardia lamblia

During my many years of pediatric practice, I saw fewer than five patients with giardiasis. At least, if I saw such patients, I didn't recognize them. Although I had the hospital laboratory in my community carry out stool studies on patients with persistent diarrhea and other digestive symptoms, they were usually negative for *Giardia*.

Yet, a number of studies reported in the medical literature during the past two decades suggest that giardiasis occurs commonly and affects 5 to 10% of people world wide. Moreover, according to Galland, giardiasis is the commonest cause of parasitic disease in the United States with an overall prevalence at 7.4%.

Giardiasis is the commonest cause of parasitic disease in the United States with an ovarall prevalence at 7.4%.

Why isn't giardiasis diagnosed more frequently? According to Galland, it's due to the techniques used. And he said, "Single stool specimens have a sensitivity of zero to 50%."

However, Galland and associates have developed a different technique that they have found to be extremely adequate. Rectal mucus obtained at anoscopy is stained with a monoclonal antibody to giardia cysts and examined by "epifluorescence microscopy."*

In discussing his findings using this type of examination Galland said,

> "We recently conducted a two-year retrospective study of 218 patients who presented to our medical clinic with the chief complaint of chronic fatigue. G. *lamblia* infection was identified by rectal swab in 61 patients. . . . Sixty one percent of fatigued patients with *giardiasis* had been diagnosed elsewhere as suffering from chronic fatigue syndrome (CFS) or M.E., compared to only 19% of fatigued patients without giardiasis.

Cure of giardiasis resulted in clearing of fatigue in 70% of 218 patients.

> "Cure of giardiasis resulted in clearing of fatigue and related 'viral' symptoms (myalgia, sweats, flu-like feeling) in 70% of cases, some palliation of fatigue in 18%, and was of no benefit in 12%.

*L. Galland and H. Bueno, "Advances in laboratory diagnosis of intestinal parasites," *American Clinical Laboratory*, p. 18-19, 1989.

318

"This study shows that giardiasis can present with fatigue as the major manifestation accompanied by minor gastrointestinal complaints and sometimes by myalgia and other symptoms suggestive of M.E. It indicates that *G.lamblia* infection may be a common cause of CFS, at least in the U.S. It is noteworthy that tricyclic antidepressants, a standard treatment for CFS, suppress the growth of *Giardia* in vitro. (Weinbach, et al, 1985)

In analyzing this relationship, Galland pointed out that some of the symptoms in patients with giardiasis may be related to pre-existing atopic disease. It may also be related to the effects of giardia on nutritional status, including protein loss and deficiencies of carotene, folate, vitamin A and vitamin B_{12}. Also bacterial overgrowth in the small intestine in patients with giardiasis may contribute to malabsorption and nutritional deficiencies and may also promote the colonization of *Candida albicans*. In one report 30% of the patients with giardiasis showed *Candida albicans* in the jejunum whereas none of the controls showed such colonization.

Candida albicans

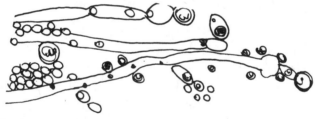

During the past decade Galland has studied and treated hundreds of patients with candida-related health problems. He served as a keynote speaker at the Candida Update Conference, Memphis, September 1988. In his presentation he summarized data on 91 patients with what he described as "impeccable evidence for the Candida Related Complex." Symptoms in these patients included fatigue (89%), food intolerance (86%), GI disturbances (81%), alcohol intolerance (71%), chronic vaginitis (61%), memory impairment (55%), depression (54%), chemical hypersensitivity (46%), premenstrual sydrome (44%), anxiety (39%), headache (29%), carbohydrate cravings (19%). Antibiotics were a precipitating factor in 82% of the patients.

Symptoms in patients with candidiasis included fatigue, food intolerance, chronic vaginitis, memory impairment and depression and headache.

In discussing candida-related problems in his chapter in the book *Post Viral Fatigue Syndrome*, Galland said,

319

"Serious infection with *Candida albicans* has increased dramatically over the past 40 years; this increase is largely iatrogenic [caused by physicians] and may be attributed to the widespread use of antibiotics and immunosuppressive drugs. (Seelig, 1966; Kirkpatrick, 1984, Host factors in defense against fungal infections, *American Journal of Medicine*, 77, 4D, 1-12.) *Candida albicans* is an opportunist *par excellence* and its ability to exploit pre-existing immune deficiency in a host animal is well known."

Candida albicans *exploits pre-existing immune deficiencies.*

Galland then reviews a lot of the literature which shows that *C. albicans* is a potential allergen. Included in these reports were those showing that hyposensitization to candida helped patients with asthma, eczema and urticaria. In the latter group, oral antifungal medication was combined with a special diet and immunotherapy. Other reports showed that oral nystatin helped people with gastrointestinal symptoms.

"These studies ... indicate that candida allergy is not a rare disease with limited symptoms ... but a relatively common disorder with protean manifestations."

He then discusses the relationship between candida allergy and vaginal infections. And after reviewing the observations of many researchers and summarizing some of their studies, he said,

"There are numerous and complex immunologic responses to *Candida* constituents, both antigenic and non-antigenic, which may follow colonization or infection; These cause release of inflammatory mediators and alterations in CMI (cell mediated immunity). Local infections may have systemic affects."

In concluding his review of the effect of intestinal microbes on systemic immunity, Galland stated,

Fungal infection may play an important role in many CFS patients. Leo Galland, M.D.

"Our results demonstrate that some patients with CFS have *Giardia lamblia* infection as a primary, and unexpected diagnosis. The excellent response to ketoconazole reported by Jessop suggests that fungal infection may play an important etiologic role in many CFS patients. Mowbray's group has found chronic enteroviral antigenemia in the majority of patients with post-viral fatigue syndrome.

"It is possible that bacterial dysbiosis, enteric protozoan or yeast infection, or intestinal allergy may alter normal immune responses of the gut, allowing persistence of viral replication. The probable importance of enteric factors in the pathogenesis of M.E. should guide diagnostic and treatment strategies."

CFS and Fibromyalgia (FM)

In his article "Fibromyalgia Syndrome, an emerging but controversial condition,"* Don L. Goldenberg, M.D., of the Boston University School of Medicine, 71E Concord St., Boston, MA 02118, described the clinical manifestations, laboratory findings and treatment results of 118 patients with fibromyalgia (FM). Here are excerpts from his article:

An estimated 3 to 6 million people in the U.S. show symptoms of fibromyalgia.

"Fibromyalgia is one of the most common diagnoses in ambulatory practice. Recent estimates of the incidence of fibromyalgia in the United States have ranged from 3 to 6 million. . . .

"The Gold Standard for diagnosis . . . has been the presence of a minimum number of tender points. . . . From four of 40 to 12 of 14 possible tender points.

"Common symptoms noted in our series and other recent reports have included neck and shoulder pain, morning stiffness, sleep disturbances and fatigue. Seventy to 90% of patients have been women and the mean age of diagnosis have varied from 34 to 55 years.

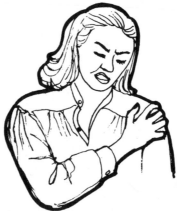

"The following basic concepts are important: 1. Fibromyalgia is a clinical syndrome . . . cannot be explained on current pathophysiologic grounds and lack specific or other diagnostic tests. 2. Fibromyalgia causes chronic pain and fatigue but is not degenerative or

*JAMA, 257, 2782-2787, May 22/29, 1987.

deforming, it has no excess mortality. 3. Fibromyalgia is a diagnosis that is best entertained over time; there is no definitive diagnostic test and no specific therapy and therefore no urgent reason to make the diagnosis.

"The diagnosis should be considered in any patient with chronic poorly defined, diffuse musculoskeletal pain. Most patients are women age 20 to 50. . . . Common symptoms have included neck and shoulder pain, morning stiffness, sleep disturbances and fatigue; hypersensitivity to cold or heat; frequent bouts of abdominal pain, constipation and diarrhea; frontal or occipital headaches; sensations of numbness or swelling in the hands and feet; and anxiety and depression. These disturbances have been reported in 60% to 90% of patients."

The diagnosis should be considered in any patient with chronic poorly defined, diffuse musculo-skeletal pain.

In discussing natural history and treatment, Goldenberg said,

"Fibromyalgia is a chronic condition. The average duration of symptoms at the time of diagnosis has been five years. . . . Most patients reported little change in their symptoms (while taking various medications) and 90% of patients were symptomatic after 3 years of followup. Most patients continued to have significant symptoms whatever medication is used."

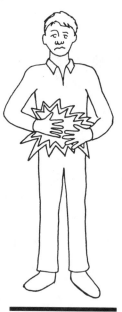

In his concluding remarks Goldenberg said,

"Since fibromyalgia shares many common features with other poorly described, chronic pain conditions, including low back pain, tension headaches and irritable bowel syndrome, each of these disorders should be evaluated in similar pathophysiologic fashion and compared with fibromyalgia. Investigators should continue to search for possible common neurochemical alterations in these conditions also thus far, no specific abnormalities have been noted."

In an editorial in the same issue of *JAMA* (pages 2802-2803), Robert M. Bennett, M.D., FRCP, Oregon Health Sciences University, Portland, said,

"There are lessons to be learned from the fibromyositis-fibromyalgia saga. Not the least is granting patients credibility when symptoms and signs do not conform to contemporary medical prejudices. Willful fabrication of symptoms and outright ma-

Patients should be granted credibility when symptoms and signs do not conform to contemporary medical prejudices.

lingering are distinctly uncommon. Yet, the straightjacket of current medical thought sometimes leads to such considerations."

Are FM and CFS the same disorder? You'll find one of the best discussions of this subject in the Spring/Summer 1990 issue of the *CFIDS Chronicle* on pages 16 and 21-24. Here's a brief summary:

On April 20-22, 1990, the FM Association of Central Ohio, held the first national conference for persons with FM. (Over 300 attended.) More than a dozen professionals spoke at the three-day conference, including Drs. Don L. Goldenberg, Robert M. Bennett, Ernest O. Vasquez, George Waylonis, and Harvey Moldofsky. Varying points of view were expressed and different treatments were recommended. The general consensus seemed to be that fibromyalgia and CFIDS were closely related—if not the same.

In discussing terminology, Kristin Thorson, Publisher, *Fibromyalgia Network*,* said,

FM could be another name for CFIDS or vice versa . . . depending on which diagnosis you happen to have.

"Dr. Don Goldenberg made the following comment during an interview in 1989: 'What you call it (FM or CFIDS) depends on the eyes of the beholder'. I'm convinced that Dr. Goldenberg is correct. FM could be another name for CFIDS . . . or vice versa . . . depending on which diagnosis you happen to have."

In commenting on the relationship of CFS to Fibromyalgia, Lt. Col. Kurt Kroenke,** M.C., USA, Department of Medicine, Uniformed Services, University of Health Sciences, 4301 Jones Bridge Rd., Bethesda, MD, 20814, said,

"Fibromyalgia is one of the most common rheumatalogic conditions seen in office practice, with an estimated prevalence of 3 to 6 million cases in the United States. Like Chronic Fatigue Syndrome, Fibromyalgia occurs primarily in young to middle aged women . . . Although myalgia is often predominating in cases of

---

*For additional information including a six-page brochure, "Fibromyalgia Syndrome (FMS)—a Patients Guide" write, 7001 School House Lane, Bakersfield, CA 93309 (805/833-8387) or FM Association at Central Ohio, Riverside Methodist Hospital, Suite 8, 3545 Olentangy River Rd., Columbus, OH 43214 (614/262-2000)
**K. Kroenke, *Post Graduate Medicine*, Vol. 89/No. 2, February 1, 1991, pp. 44-55.

Fibromyalgia, and fatigue is the dominant symptom of Chronic Fatigue Syndrome, the overlap between the two disorders is none the less striking."

When I think about CFIDS, FM and related disorders I'm reminded of the varied streptococcal manifestations in children I saw during my medical school, internship and residency days and in my early years of practice.

I can remember examining and treating four brothers between the ages of six and twelve. The 12-year-old seemed perfectly well, although his throat culture was positive; the 10-year-old had a mild sore throat. The 8-year-old developed a high fever, enlarged cervical lymph glands and a severe headache, and the 6-year-old developed similar symptoms, plus a fine red rash. All four brothers were infected by the same "strep" germ.

When I think about CFIDS, FM and related disorders I'm reminded of the varied streptococcal manifestations in children.

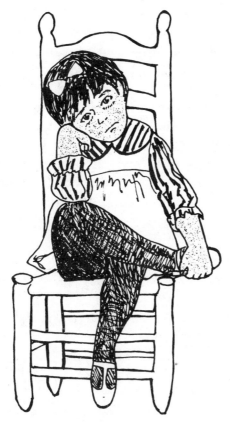

Taking things one step further. Following a community epidemic of streptococcal infections, three weeks after an acute sore throat, an occasional child would develop hot swollen, tender, red joints. Moreover the swelling would jump from one joint to another. The right elbow and left knee might swell the first day; the left shoulder and both ankles would swell the next and wrists on the third day. Then the cycle would repeat itself. We called the disease *"rheumatic fever."*

Following a strep infection, some children developed rheumatic fever; others developed neurological symptoms; still others developed kidney inflammation.

Other children with rheumatic fever showed only mild joint pains but developed inflammation of the heart. Sometimes such children would become dangerously—even critically—ill. Other children in the community who experienced the same streptococcal infection would develop still other symptoms.

These included grimacing and purposeless movements of the arms and legs. We labeled children with this type of affliction, *Sydenham's chorea.* Other children following streptococcal infection would develop blood in the urine, severe headaches, puffiness of the face and legs and elevated blood pressure. The diagnostic label for this streptococcal-related disorder is *acute glomerulonephritis.*

All of these disorders were clearly related to or caused by streptococcal infections. Yet, other factors were important in the development of the diseases which occurred in different persons. Here are a few of them. *Rheumatic fever* appeared to be largely an urban disease and it developed more often in people who were crowded together. It also seemed more apt to attack undernourished children. Finally, in some families there appeared to be a genetic factor.

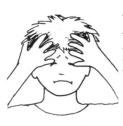

And so it is with CFS, CFIDS, M.E., FM and related disorders. *People with these disorders, seem to develop them because their immune systems are disturbed.* When their immune systems are weakened, viruses are activated, candida yeasts multiply, food and chemical allergies become aggravated and nutritional deficiencies develop. *Each person is unique.* Some individuals will be bothered more by fatigue, headache and depression; others will experience more muscle aching; still others will be bothered especially by cognitive dysfunction and/or other symptoms.

People with CFS and FM develop these disorders because their immune systems are disturbed.

Viral Studies

During the last several years, researchers in North America and overseas have been searching for viruses in persons with CFS. Exciting progress has been made and the results of many of their studies were presented on November 17-18, 1990, at the CFIDS Association Research Conference in Charlotte, North Carolina. Here are the titles of a few of these presentations:

- "Clinical and Epidemiological Features of CFIDS," Paul R. Cheney, M.D., Ph.D.
- "Levels of Lymphokines, Soluble Receptors and IL-2 Inhibitors in Sera from CFIDS Patients," Irina Rozovsky, Ph.D.
- "Detection of Viral Sequences Using Gene Amplification," W. John Martin, M.D., Ph.D.
- "Retroviral Sequences in Children with CFIDS," David S. Bell, M.D.
- "Association of an HTLV-II-Like Virus with CFIDS," Elaine DeFreitas, Ph.D. and Brendan Hilliard, Ph.D.
- "Retroviruses in Human Disease," Hilary Koprowski, M.D.
- "The Role of HHV6 in CFS," Anthony L. Komaroff, M.D.

In a letter introducing the Spring 1991 issue of The *CFIDS Chronicle*, K. Kimberly Kenney, Director of Operations and Managing Editor said,

"This is the *Chronicle* that everyone has been waiting for . . . This *Chronicle* documents the best of the best. Those most closely involved with CFIDS research and the diagnosis and treatment of this illness are brought to life in these next one hundred plus pages. This issue is more than our conference *Chronicle*. It is a reference manual for those who are truly interested in learning about a disease process whose (as yet) unknown causative agent has been likened to the stealth bomber because of its ability to attack and then elude detection by the most modern and sensitive medical technology available."

I attended the Charlotte conference and took many pages of notes. I also read and reread the comprehensive report of the conference presentations in the Spring 1991 issue of the *CFIDS Chronicle*. I must confess however, that much of what I heard and read was—to put it simply—over my head. So I'll make no attempt to summarize the viral studies other than to quote the comments of researcher Elaine DeFreitas, Ph.D., of the Wistar Institute in Philadelphia.

In closing her presentation, Dr. DeFreitas said,

> "In summary I'd like to tell you what we think we know and what we think we don't know. Unfortunately, the second list is going to be longer than the first. What we *know* is we are seeing an association with certain sequences with HTLV-II with CFIDS patients and to a *lesser* extent in exposure controls . . . but not non-exposed controls. We know that this gene is functional; that it is making messenger RNA.

> "The things we don't know are as follows:

> - If this agent we're detecting or this gene we're detecting is part of a *complete* live virus;
> - If the virus is infectious and is moving in and out of cells;
> - What *cell* this virus is in—we know it's in blood because we exclusively studied blood, but we don't know what cell of the blood it's in;
> - If this agent is bona fide HTLV-II or, as some of the data suggests, it's different from HTLV-II, possibly a new strain of HTLV-II, or a more distantly related virus that warrants a new name;
> - If this virus is live and infectious, how is this virus transmitted? . . .

> "Finally we don't know if this agent *causes* the disease. The epidemiological data suggests that there may be horizontal transmission, casual transmission—we do not know if retroviruses can even be spread this way in humans. It may be that people have this agent or this gene, and then what triggers the disease is a *second* virus which is casually transmitted. . . . So it may be a two-hit event that must take place in order for people to become ill. We hope that isolating, sequencing and identifying this virus . . . being able to call it by a *name* . . . will give us some clues as to its biologi-

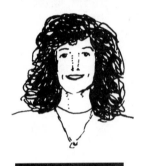

The Spring 1991 issue of the CFIDS Chronicle *is a reference manual for those interested in this disease.*

Dr. DeFreitas described, "what we think we know and what we think we don't know."

We're seeing an association with certain sequences with HTLV-II with CFIDS patients.

cal behavior and what it could be doing in the cells and, ultimately, what it may be doing to patients."

More on Viruses

In an article in the Monday, September 16, 1991, issue of the *Wall Street Journal*, "Virus May Have Role in Causing Chronic Fatigue," staff reporter Ron Winslow, discussed the observations of a University of Southern California researcher, John Martin. Here are excerpts from the Winslow report:

U.S. Researcher Says He's Identified Virus Possibly Linked to Chronic Fatigue Illness

By Ron Winslow
Staff Reporter

NEW YORK — A University of Southern California researcher says he has identified a virus that may cause or play another important role in a mysterious ailment

meeting is whether researchers who appear to be considering different viruses as a possible cause of the syndrome may actually be looking at the same

"It's too early to a cause of

and therapies, and the These are

"John Martin, chief of molecular pathology at USC Medical Center, Los Angeles, says he found the virus in the cerebral spinal fluid of about 10 patients with severe neurological abnormalities that mimic problems associated with brain ailments such as multiple sclerosis. . . . The virus, from a family known as spumaviruses, hadn't been previously linked to human disease."

In his continuing report, Winslow said that controversy surrounds Martin's observations and three prominent medical journals have declined to publish his current data. And chronic fatigue researcher Dr. Paul Cheney of Charlotte, North Carolina, is quoted as saying that,

"It's too early to say a spumavirus is a cause of Chronic Fatigue Syndrome, but it's a very appealing candidate as a cause."

In his continuing report, Winslow said,

"But other scientists say that even if Dr. Martin's findings are replicated, it isn't clear that his seriously ill patients suffer from the syndrome as opposed to an atypical neurologic disease. . . . Many scientists investigating the syndrome say they are now convinced that it reflects the immune system's response to an invading infectious agent, possibly a virus. They suspect that the agent engages the immune system and keeps it from shutting down with the re-

Many scientists investigating the syndrome say it reflects the immune system's response to an invading infectious agent, possibly a virus.

329

sulting biological activity consuming the body's energy at the molecular and cellular level."

Chronic Fatigue Syndrome and Immune Activation

In a recent report in *The Lancet,* researchers told of their findings in studying 147 individuals with CFS. Sophisticated immunological studies were carried out on these patients. Similar studies were carried out on 80 healthy individuals, 22 contacts of CFS patients and 43 patients with other diseases. Here are brief excerpts from this report:

"A viral cause of CFS has been suspected because several viral infections are characterised by a chronic post-infection fatigue and because the onset of CFS often resembles an acute viral illness. However, in other viral infections, in contrast to CFS, the symptoms do not generally persist after several weeks. Initial studies showed that CFS was associated with high concentrations of antibodies to Epstein-Barr Virus (EBV).

No conclusive evidence of a common causative agent in CFS has been presented . . . The findings suggest that immune activation is associated with many cases of CFS.

"However, subsequent studies suggested that high antibody titers to EBV were not found in all CFS patients, and that polyclonal activation of B cells was a common finding with antibodies to several viruses, especially herpes viruses. . . . Lately, serological and polymerase chain reaction methods have pointed to an association of human T-lymphotropic virus-like agent with the syndrome. Nevertheless, no conclusive evidence of a common causative agent in CFS has been presented . . .

"To see whether we could resolve some of this conflicting data, we evaluated certain viral and immunological indices in a clinically well-defined cohort of patients with CFS and compared them with control populations. A reduced CD8 suppressor cell population and increased activation markers (CD38, HLA-DR) on CD8 cells were found. The differences were significant ($p = 0.01$) in patients with major symptoms of the disease. Similar immunological indices were not observed in the control group of healthy individuals, contacts of CFS patients and the patients with other diseases. . . .

"No correlation of these findings in CFS patients with any known viruses could be detected by serology. The findings suggest that immune activation is associated with many cases of CFS."[*]

[*]A.L. Landay, C. Jessop, E.T. Lennette and J.A. Levy, "Chronic Fatigue Syndrome: Clinical Condition Associated with Immune Activation," *The Lancet,* 1991; 338:707-12. (September 21st.)

Mercury/Amalgam Fillings and CFS

If your CFS is yeast-connected, you'll nearly always improve if and when you . . .

If your CFS is yeast-connected, you'll nearly always improve if and when you change your diet and take anti-yeast mediations.

- change your diet. This means cutting out (or sharply limiting) sugar and junk food, eating more vegetables and identifying (and avoiding) the foods that cause sensitivity reactions.
- take prescription medications, including nystatin, Nizoral or Diflucan. And/or take nonprescription substances, including caprylic acid products, citrus seed extract, *Lactobacillus acidophilus*, bifidobacteria (and other probiotics), garlic and/or other substances that discourage yeast proliferation in the gut.

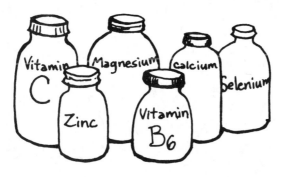

- take nutritional supplements, including vitamins and minerals (especially zinc and magnesium and the essential fatty acids).

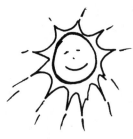

- clean up your environment, especially your home and your workplace. This means avoiding tobacco smoke, perfumes, insecticides, kitchen gas stoves, laundry chemicals and other indoor pollutants.
- get adequate amounts of fresh air and sun or skylight.
- walk and take limited amounts of other exercise as your health improves.
- obtain psychological support.

If you have CFS and are at a standstill, it could be because you are absorbing toxins from mercury/silver amalgam fillings.

But, if you have CFS and you are doing all these things and are at a standstill, it could be because you are absorbing toxins from the mercury/silver amalgam fillings in your mouth.

The hazards of silver-mercury fillings have been talked about by a handful of dentists during the past decade. According to those who oppose the use of these fillings, they can cause toxic reactions and play a part in making people sick. Symptoms attributed to these fillings include fatigue, headache, central nervous system dysfunction, muscle and joint pains and disturbances in other parts of the body.

An opposite point of view is expressed by the American Dental Association, which represents at least 75% of the nation's dentists. This organization continues to support the use of amalgam as a safe, effective method of tooth restoration. Recently this controversy was brought into the public "mainstream" on CBS's "60 Minutes," December 15, 1990.

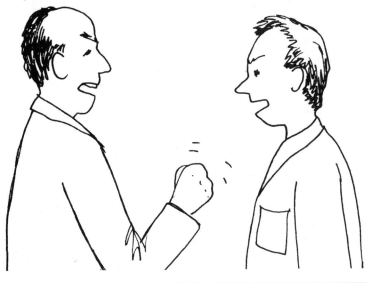

On this program, Dr. Murray J. Vimy of the University of Calgary Medical School and and Alfred Zamm, M.D., of Kingston, New York, presented information on the potential and actual toxic effects of mercury-amalgam fillings. Vimy had placed silver fillings in the mouths of pregnant sheep. Three days later, mercury was found in the blood of mothers and fetuses and in the amniotic fluid. Two weeks later, it was found in other tissue samples.

Along with their comments and presentation of scientific data were testimonials from patients whose fatigue and other chronic health problems were "turned around" following the removal of mercury amalgam fillings.

In February 1991, Dr. Zamm sent me a copy of a 21-page, carefully referenced monograph entitled "Anticandida Albicans Therapy: "Is There Ever An End To It?, Dental Mercury Removal: An Effective Adjunct." And in a subsequent conversation with me Dr. Zamm said,

> "Mercury from dental amalgam induces symptoms in a sensitive group of the population that has been observed to be sentisitive to xenobiotic* substances. This sensitive group serves as a marker of the potential danger of dental mercury to the rest of the population who are also at risk but may not yet exhibit symptoms. I've found that in many severely ill patients, including those with chronic fatigue, candidiasis and allergies that removal of silver/mercury dental fillings is an effective way of improving their health."

In April 1991, I attended a seminar sponsored by the Environmental Dental Association, (9974 Scripps Ranch Blvd., Suite #36, San Diego, CA 92131). During this seminar, Joyal Taylor, D.D.S., President of EDA, gave a demonstration that impressed me.

Volunteers from the audience were tested with a special probe which measured the release of mercury vapor following chewing. One of the volunteers had no fillings in her mouth and the second had a number of fillings. (The machine for testing mercury vapors is used in submarines by the U.S. Navy, as well as the Envi-

Silver fillings were placed in the mouths of pregnant sheep. Three days later mercury was found in sheep fetuses.

Some patients with chronic fatigue, allergies and yeast-related problems are helped by the removal of silver mercury dental fillings.

---

*Xenobiotic substances are those which are foreign to the natural state of an organism. Examples of such foreign substances include petrochemical vapors, chlorinated hydrocarbons, sulfites and metals which are not metabolically useful.

If you suffer from chronic health disorders which haven't improved, a silver/mercury illness relationship should be considered.

ronmental Protection Agency, EPA.) The woman with dental fillings showed a high level of mercury, while the other woman showed none.

During the meeting, several people in the audience told of their improvement in fatigue, muscle aches and other symptoms following the replacement of their dental amalgam fillings.

Should you have your dental fillings removed? In *The Yeast Connection* (third edition), in responding to this question, I said, "I don't know. Yet, if you suffer from chronic health disorders which haven't improved in spite of all your efforts and those of your physicians, I feel a silver/mercury illness relationship should be considered."

Based on the observations of Drs. Joyal Taylor, Murray Vimy, Alfred Zamm and others, I would suggest that the possibility of dental mercury toxicity be investigated by a dentist familiar with this problem. The names of mercury-free dentists in your area can be obtained by writing to the Foundation for Toxic Free Dentistry, P.O. Box 608010, Orlando, Florida 32860. Include a long SASE with first-class postage.

Further information about the toxic effects of mercury/amalgam dental fillings can be obtained from:

Alfred V. Zamm, M.D., III Maiden Lane, Kingston, N.Y. 12401. Enclose a long, SASE with first-class postage.

The Environmental Dental Association (EDA) at (800) 388-8124. Call for a free packet of information.

Books that provide information on mercury/amalgam dental fillings include:

The Complete Guide to Mercury Toxicity from Dental Fillings, Joyal Taylor, D.D.S., EDA Publishing, 9974 Scripps Ranch Blvd., Suite #36, San Diego, CA 92131. $14.95 plus $3.00 shipping.

Are Your Dental Fillings Poisoning You?, Guy S. Fasciana, D.M.D., Keats Publishing Co., 27 Pine St., New Canaan, CT 06840.

The Toxic Time Bomb, Sam Ziff, D.D.S., 4401 Real Court, Orlando, FL 32808.

Almost every day I learn something about CFS, yeast-connected health disorders and food allergies that I didn't know before. In fact, books on these subjects (like those on Russia) might well be published in loose-leaf form. In this section you'll find information on a variety of topics which are related to CFS.

Chronic Fatigue Syndrome: A Working Case Definition

During the years 1985, 1986 and 1987 many physicians felt that people with chronic fatigue, muscle aches, memory loss and many other symptoms were suffering from a chronic Epstein-Barr virus infection. The term applied to these patients at that time was Chronic Epstein-Barr Virus Syndrome.

Laboratory studies, however, failed to confirm this relationship. In March 1988, Dr. Gary Holmes from the Division of Viral Diseases, Centers for Disease Control (CDC), Atlanta, and a group of other scientists and clinicians developed a consensus of the salient characteristics of this disorder and devised a definition for it. Here's a brief summary of their report:*

"The Chronic Epstein-Barr Virus Syndrome is a poorly defined symptom complex characterized primarily by chronic or recurring debilitating fatigue and various combinations of other symptoms. . . . We propose a new name for the chronic Epstein-Barr virus syndrome—the chronic fatigue syndrome—that more accurately describes this symptom complex as a syndrome of unknown cause characterized primarily by chronic fatigue.

We propose a new name for the Chronic Epstein-Barr virus syndrome—the Chronic Fatigue Syndrome.

"We also present a working definition for the chronic fatigue syndrome designed to improve the comparability and reproducibility of clinical research and epidemiologic studies and to provide a rational basis for evaluating patients who have chronic fatigue of undetermined cause. . . .

"Because this syndrome has no diagnostic test, the definition at the present is based on signs and symptoms only. This definition is intentionally restrictive to maximize the chances that research studies will detect significant associations if such associations truly exist. It identifies persons whose illnesses are most compati-

*G.P. Holmes, et al., "Chronic Fatigue Syndrome: A Working Case Definition," *Annals of Internal Medicine,* 108:387-89, 1988.

A reprint of the two and a half page article is available from Division of Viral Diseases, Center for Infectious Diseases, Centers for Disease Control, Atlanta, Georgia 30333.

ble with a possibly unique clinical entity; persons who may have less severe forms of the syndrome or who have less characteristic clinical features may be excluded by the new definition."

Here's an abbreviated summary of the criteria listed in the CDC report:

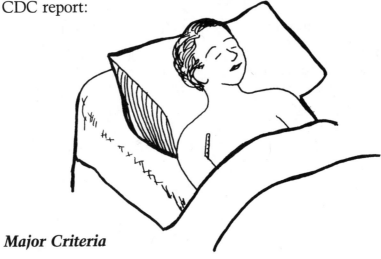

Major Criteria

New onset of debilitating fatigue severe enough to impair average daily activity below 50% for at least 6 months.

1. New onset of persistent or relapsing, debilitating fatigue or easy fatigability in a person who has no previous history of similar symptoms, that does not resolve with bedrest, and that is severe enough to reduce or impair average daily activity below 50% of the patient's premorbid activity level for a period of at least 6 months.
2. Other clinical conditions that may produce similar symptoms must be excluded by thorough evaluation, based on history, physical examination and appropriate laboratory findings.

Minor Criteria

In addition to fulfilling both major criteria, the CDC stated that patients should report 6 or more symptoms (listed below), plus 2 or more characteristic physical signs; or 8 or more of the 11 symptom criteria.

Symptom Criteria: To fulfill a symptom criterion, a symptom must have begun at the time of onset of increased fatigability, and must have persisted or recurred over a period of at least 6 months. Symptoms include:

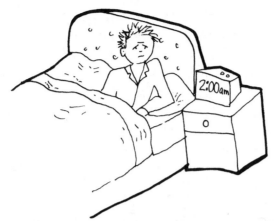

Mild fever; sore throat; painful lymph nodes; unexplained general muscle weakness; muscle discomfort or myalgia; prolonged general fatigue after mild exercise; generalized headaches; migratory joint pains; neuropsychologic complaints including excessive irritability, confusion, difficulty in thinking, inability to concentrate, depression; sleep disturbance; development of the main symptom complex over a period of a few hours to a few days.

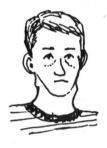

Physical Criteria: These criteria must be documented by a physician on at least two occasions, at least 1 month apart. Symptoms include:

Low grade fever; inflammation of the mucous membrane; palpable or tender lymph nodes.

Comments on the Definition of CFS

The CDC report played a significant role in bringing CFS into the medical mainstream. It accomplished this by providing clear clinical guidelines for making a diagnosis in people with severe forms of this illness. In so doing, it helped counteract criticisms from professional and nonprofessionals who sometimes said, "People with this disorder aren't really sick" or "Depression is the cause of their problems."

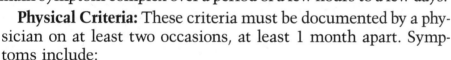

The CDC report played a significant role in bringing CFS into the medical mainstream.

Yet, the authors of the CDC report pointed out that "periodic reconsideration of conditions such as those listed under Major Criteria, Part 2, should be standard practice in the long-term follow-up of these patients."

During the past four years other physicians interested in CFS, including Dr. Carol Jessop, have found that many of their patients

339

do not have an acute onset and enlarged glands. And at her presentations at the CFS conferences in San Francisco and North Carolina, Dr. Jessop pointed out that the past medical history of CFS patients may represent the key to understanding this illness.

In her reports at the San Francisco CFS Conference in April, 1989 and at the Charlotte CFS Conference in November, 1990 she stated that 80% of her CFS patients gave a history of recurrent antibiotic treatment (as a child, adolescent or adult). Almost half of them had experienced recurrent hives. She also noted that the great majority had "serious sugar addictions or alcohol abuse many years prior to the onset of CFS and many gave a history of irritable bowel syndrome, vaginal yeast infections, headaches, PMS and anxiety attacks."

Eighty percent of Dr. Jessop's CFS patients gave a history of recurrent antibiotic treatment.

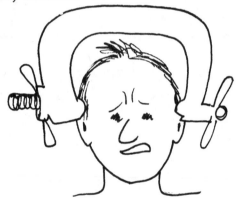

Comments on CFS From the National Institutes of Health

In an October 1990 publication, *Chronic Fatigue Syndrome—A Pamphlet for Physicians,* * appeared the following comments:

Most investigators studying CFS believe that the syndrome has many possible causes . . .

"Most investigators studying CFS believe that the syndrome has many possible causes. . . . Preliminary research also shows a variety of immunologic disturbances in some patients. . . . Several different latent viruses also appear to be reactivated in some CFS patients, although reactivation has not been shown in all patients and it is not clear that any of these viruses are causally related to CFS or its symptoms.

" . . . Most cases of CFS are sporadic: the patient does not have a

---

*For a copy of this pamphlet and other information on CFS contact the N.I.H., Office of Communications, National Institute of Allergy and Infectious Disease Division, Bldg. 31, Room 7A32, 9000 Rockville Pike, Bethesda, MD 20892. (301) 496-5717.

close contact who has developed a similar illness. Frequently, however, close contacts, including family members, become ill with CFS at about the same time.

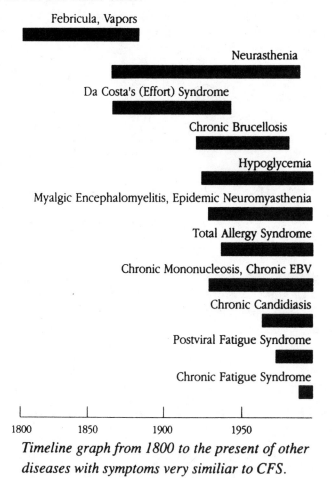

Febricula, Vapors

Neurasthenia

Da Costa's (Effort) Syndrome

Chronic Brucellosis

Hypoglycemia

Myalgic Encephalomyelitis, Epidemic Neuromyasthenia

Total Allergy Syndrome

Chronic Mononucleosis, Chronic EBV

Chronic Candidiasis

Postviral Fatigue Syndrome

Chronic Fatigue Syndrome

1800   1850   1900   1950

Timeline graph from 1800 to the present of other diseases with symptoms very similiar to CFS.

CFS does not appear to be a new disorder.

"Although interest in this illness has grown tremendously since the mid-1980's, CFS does not appear to be a new disorder. . . . Furthermore, case reports describing similar illnesses date back several centuries. These sporadic cases of fatigue syndromes have often been linked to a bacterial, viral or protozoal infections. . . . But fatigue syndromes also appear outside the setting of an infectious illness . . . Many patients have a history of allergies years before the onset of CFS and occasionally allergic symptoms worsen after these patients become ill. Allergies are so prevalent in CFS patients that it is important to differentiate those symptoms that are allergy related and thus amenable to treatment."

In discussing etiologic theories, the pamphlet stated,

> *Allergies are prevalent in CFS patients . . . the symptoms that are allergy related are amenable to treatment.*

"Several theories have been postulated as to the etiology of CFS. Most investigators currently believe that no single etiologic agent will prove to be the cause of all cases. . . . Preliminary evidence suggests that several latent viruses may be actively replicating more often in CFS patients than in healthy [control] subjects. . . . If subsequent studies confirm that several viruses are active more often in people with CFS than in healthy individuals, it will then be needed to determine if this activity is a primary or secondary event . . . Most investigators believe reactivation of these viruses is probably secondary to some immunologic disturbance."

Here's an excerpt of the discussion of patient management:

> *Both the physician and the patient need to be open to reasonable treatment alternatives.*

"The patients need both symptomatic treatment and emotional support. . . . It is vitally important for the physician to be the patient's advocate. In the absence of any proven treatments, empiric therapy should be tried.

"In brief, no strict recipe for treating CFS exists and sometimes several different treatment approaches may have to be tried before the patient reports benefit. *Both the physician and the patient need to be open to reasonable treatment alternatives and appreciate the difficulty in assessing their benefit in CFS.*"

Comments by Marc Iverson, President of the CFIDS Association, Inc.

In his Annual Report published in the Fall 1991 issue of *The CFIDS Chronicle* Iverson described the current status of CFIDS research and advocacy and summarized the operating policies and financial results of this organization. He also said that his report is a "blatant attempt to enlist your continuing support! We seek your help because we're entirely dependent on you."

In describing the organizational structure and guiding principles of the CFIDS Association he said,

"There are many factors that distinguish The CFIDS Association from hundreds of the other organizations working exclusively on behalf of PWCs (persons with CFIDS). This association is the largest such organization by any meaningful measure. . . . [It] is an independent non-profit corporation which has earned a "definitive" ruling from the IRS granting 501 (C) (3) tax exempt status.

"The association is governed by a large all-volunteer Board of Directors . . . [and] managed by the Executive Committee of its Board of Directors and an Executive Director, Kim Kenney who is an experienced health professional. . . . We directly fund CFIDS research, [and] allocate every dollar earmarked for research or advocacy to the targeted application . . . with no overhead or administrative 'fees' taken out; [we] publish the largest, most comprehensive CFIDS journal, *The CFIDS Chronicle* (and its supplement, the *Physicians' Forum*). . . . The major thrust (mission) of The CFIDS Association is educational."

> *The CFIDS Association, Inc. is the largest organization working to help persons with this illness.*

In his continuing discussion, Iverson pointed out that the efforts of the association have attracted the attention of international media including *Newsweek, Wall Street Journal, USA Today, Reader's Digest,* and *New York Times.* In discussing CFIDS research he said,

"Far too many of us, myself included, are "battered patients" who have been victimized by conventional medical institutions, their practitioners and their rigid and arrogant doctrines. (If a condition does not fit accepted patterns and is not understood, then it is deemed to be nonexistent or of psychiatric origin.) And in the interest of PWCs and the public, this association aggressively resists a 'medical establishment' which continues to trivialize and 'psychologize' CFIDS."

In discussing milestones and financial results for 1990 and 1991, Iverson said,

"Financially, The CFIDS Association is a conduit. We have no endowment; intangible assets are limited to office furniture, inventories of educational materials, computers and related equipment. By design we spend the revenue we receive . . . investing it in research, advocacy and dissemination of information.

"1990 was an extraordinary year for our association. Our total revenue increased by 50% over 1989. . . . 1991 is proceeding according to plan . . . an extremely aggressive one. We have already raised over a half million dollars and funded $238,000 in research and $21,000 in advocacy. In addition, we've employed our first Ex-

> *We spend the revenue we receive. . . . investigating it in research, advocacy and dissemination of information.*

ecutive Director, introduced a new journal (*The CFIDS Chronicle Physicians' Forum*) and implemented both our toll-free and information [telephone] lines."

In discussing "What You Can Do", Marc Iverson said,

"The question I'm most often asked by PWCs and those who love them is 'What can I do to advance the cause?' The short answer is donate money, become a fund raiser yourself. Help us 'spread the word' and reach out to others with CFIDS.

"Donate what you can. Help us build the knowledge we need to beat CFIDS. There is no cause that is more important. There are many creative ways to raise money for CFIDS causes. So far the most effective method has been to simply and directly ask family and friends to contribute. Tell them what CFIDS has done to you and how much you want to get well."

> *Donate money . . . become a fund raiser . . . help us "spread the word."*

Iverson suggested other ways to help, including writing or visiting your representative in the U.S. Congress and contacting the media. He also thanked the many, many people who have contributed to the success of this preeminent organization which is working to help people with this still misunderstood illness.

After reading his letter I picked up the phone and called five people including relatives of PWCs and related disorders. In 48 hours I received checks made out to the CFIDS Association, Inc., ranging from $25 to $200 with a total of $500. So if you want to support this organization, *the most effective method to raise money is to ask for it.**

Hormonal Disorders in CFS

According to an Associated Press report from Washington, December 3, 1991,

"Researchers have found a hormonal disorder that may play a role in the symptoms of Chronic Fatigue Syndrome. . . . Federal scientists report that blood studies of a group of patients with CFS showed that they had lower levels of cortisol, a hormone that acts to control the immune system and is secreted in response to stress.

> *A group of CFS patients had lower levels of the hormone cortisol.*

*P.O. Box 220398, Charlotte, North Carolina 28222-0398. Fax #704-365-9755 or 1-800-442-3437.

"Further tests, said Phillip W. Gold of the National Institute of Mental Health, showed that the patients also had a low level of corticotropin releasing hormone, a brain chemical that plays a key role in the production of cortisol . . .

"Gold said a shortage of cortisol is known to cause lethargy and fatigue and corticotropin releasing hormone is a key hormone in the body's 'fight or flight' reaction, the automatic response to fear of a sense of danger. The imbalance of the chemicals could leave patients in a permanent state of lethargy. . . .

"The study provides a biological explanation for the symptoms observed in sufferers and 'takes it away from the impression that these patients are malingering'. . . .

"Chronic Fatigue Syndrome usually has been treated as a result of some infection, with a virus considered the most likely candidate. The hormone study does not show what initiates the imbalance, but it helps explain symptoms that might have started from infection or malfunction."

CFS, Hormonal Disorders and the Yeast Connection

In his book, *The Missing Diagnosis*, in discussing candida-related health problems in women, C. Orian Truss, M.D.* commented,

"Once the yeast problem has become chronic in women, hormone function is almost always abnormal. . . . Premenstrual tension and diminishing libido often herald the beginning of interference with the tissue response of the ovarian hormone. . . .

"Hormone administration not only fails to correct the problem, but may indeed aggravate it. The endocrine system is complex and administration of one hormone affects the function and production of the other endocrine glands. . . . The many manifestations of poor female hormone function will disappear when interfering factors—in this case, yeast—are removed."

Further observations on the possible relationship of candida yeasts to hormonal dysfunction were made by Steven S. Witkin, Ph.D.,** Cornell University Medical College who said:

The Missing Diagnosis, pages 29-31.
**"Defective Immune Responses in Patients With Recurrent Candidiasis", *Infections in Medicine*, May/June 1985, pages 129-132.

"Recent studies suggest that the (vaginal yeast) infection itself may cause immunosuppression resulting in recurrences in certain patients. In addition to creating an increased susceptibility to candida reinfection, the immunological alterations may also be related to subsequent endocrinopathies . . ."

Vaginal yeast infections were found to be related to hormonal dysfunction.

Jay S. Schinfeld, M.D., Temple University also noted the relationship between vaginal candidiasis and hormone dysfunction—including PMS, loss of libido and infertility.* (See Section III).

The observations of Truss, Witkin and Schinfeld show that hormonal problems may be yeast-connected. Accordingly, persons with CFS who are troubled by such problems may benefit from a comprehensive treatment program which includes a sugar-free special diet and antifungal medication.

Lyme Disease

During the past several years a strange and often puzzling disease has received national attention. It first appeared in the town of Lyme, Connecticut, and has received the name Lyme Disease (LD). It is an infectious disease caused by the spirochete *Borrellia burgdorferi*, a slow-growing, fastidious microorganism which is difficult to culture. It is transmitted by ticks which typically attach to the white-tailed deer and deposit eggs from which larvae are hatched 6 to 8 weeks later. Then in a few months, these larvae feed on white-footed mice.

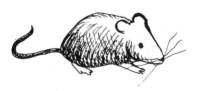

---

*Thyroid dysfunction may also be present even though routine blood studies (T-3, T-4 and TSH) may be normal. (See The Yeast Connection, 3rd edition, pages 244, 337-338.)

Humans are an accidental host for this tick and may come in contact with it in wooded areas where deer or mice are abundant. The disease occurs in several stages. Initially there is a flu-like illness which is often associated with a red expanding rash which may appear days to weeks after the tick bite. Weeks to months later, neurologic or cardiac symptoms develop. Months to years later arthritis and other symptoms may develop.

The diagnosis is difficult to make because the organism is hard to culture. Accordingly, serologic and immunologic methods, including the ELISA test, are the mainstays of diagnosis. Yet, consistent results using these tests may be difficult to reproduce between different laboratories and sometimes within the same laboratory. Antibiotics, including tetracycline, ampicillin and erythromycin have been found effective in treating patients with LD—especially when given during the acute stage. Yet, in spite of such treatment,many patients with this illness continue to experience health problems.

> *The diagnosis is difficult to make because the organism is hard to culture.*

In answering the question "Are prolonged courses of antibiotics useful when treating LD," two University of Pennsylvania researchers said,

"At this time there is no evidence to suggest that many months of antibiotic treatment are better than the current standard therapy. They may actually be harmful. . . . Some manifestations of LD are the result of persistent infections, whereas *other symptoms are a consequence of immunologic changes secondary to the infection.* Most disease manifestations are not specific to this illness. . . . The disease is overdiagnosed and overtreated."*

> *Prolonged antibiotic treatment of Lyme disease may be harmful.*

CFS and Lyme Disease

In a report in the October 29, 1991 issue of *The Medical Post,* Lyme Disease was noted to be a cause of CFS according to presentations at the annual meeting of the American Neurological Association in Atlanta.

In a study carried out in Stony Brook, New York, Drs. P.K. Coyle and Lauren Krupp linked the spirochete *B. burgdorferi* to Chronic Fatigue Syndrome. Twelve of 20 CFS patients from a group living in an area endemic for the spirochetes showed anti-B.

*B.E. Ostrov, and Balu-Athreya, "Lyme Disease, Difficulties in Management and Treatment", *Pediatric Clinics of North America*, 38:535-53, June 1991.

burgdorferi antibodies by enzyme-linked immunoabsorbent assay (ELISA). In commenting on their observations, Dr. Coyle concluded that "*B. burgdorferi* may act as a trigger in susceptible hosts to precipitate CFS."

Lyme Disease, CFS and the yeast connection

Recently a 36-year old chronically ill Wisconsin woman wrote me a several page letter describing multiple health problems. In 1987 she developed a rash, fatigue, cardiac palpatations and neurologic symptoms. She saw a number of different physicians during the ensuing years. Her complaints included chronic diarrhea and sinus infections for which she received many courses of antibiotic drugs. Due to her persistent symptoms other tests were run, including a test for Lyme Disease. This was reported as "positive" in April, 1990. Further antibiotics were prescribed.

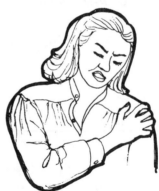

Symptoms of fatigue, food sensitivities, muscle aches and tender trigger points also appeared. A diagnosis of fibromyalgia was suggested by another physician. Then in the fall of 1991, still another physician prescribed nystatin and a sugar-free special diet. Within a few days she began to improve even though a moderate number of symptoms persisted.

Although I've never treated a patient with Lyme disease, it seems logical to assume that the long-term broad spectrum antibiotics given to persons with LD promote yeast overgrowth. And in such persons with persistent symptoms (including those with CFS), a comprehensive treatment program which includes anticandida therapy and a sugar-free special diet may help them regain their health.

Sugar Promotes Yeast Growth

In 1984, Horowitz[*] and Horowitz et al. carried out a study that showed that women with recurrent candida vulvovaginitis showed a higher dietary sugar intake and higher urinary sugar than women with non-candida vaginitis.

Then in 1984, Reed[**] and associates found a correlation between carbohydrate intake and calories and a history of recurrent vulvovaginitis.

Still, another study by Gilmore[***] and associates showed that growing *Candida albicans* in a higher glucose medium augmented the appearance of a receptor which enhanced resistance to phagocytosis.

All these studies mean that if you're bothered by vaginal yeast infections or yeast overgrowth in the gut, you must avoid sugar.

If you're bothered by yeast infections, stay away from sugar.

Several years ago one of my adult patients, Karen, who had conquered most of her yeast-related health problems, commented, "Dr. Crook, I was doing fine and had had no vaginal symptoms for many months. Then, just before Christmas, I baked some chocolate sugar cookies for my four children. I ate four of them. Within a few hours, my vaginal symptoms returned and it took me three weeks to get back to normal."

And Doris Rapp, M.D. commented: "Some women need only to eat a bar of candy and they develop an immediate vaginal discharge."[****]

Recently completed research studies[*****] carried out in mice with suppressed immune systems provide support for the relationship of sugar to yeast proliferation. Here's a summary of the 1991 study:

Thirty six mice, colonized with gastrointestinal candidiasis as infants, were randomized into three groups. One group was allowed plain water; a second was given water containing dextrose, while the third group was given water with xylitol.

---

[*]B.J. Horowitz, et al., *J. Reproduct. Med.*, 29:441-43 (1984).

[**]B. Reed, et al., *J. Family Practice*, 29:509-15 (1989).

[***]B.J. Gilmore, et al., An ic3b Receptor On *Candida albicans:* Structure, Function and Correlates For Pathogenicity, *J. Infect. Dis.*, 157:38-46 (1988).

[****]*Healthline*, Vol. 3, No. 2, page 3. Published by the International Health Foundation, Box 3494, Jackson, TN 38303.

[*****]S.L. Vargas, and W.T. Hughes, Department of Infectious Diseases, St. Jude Research Hospital, 332 N. Lauderdale, Memphis, TN 38101-03184.

Gastrointestinal growth and invasion of candida was approximately 200 times greater in the mice receiving dextrose.

Cyclophosphamide had been used to suppress the immune system. Stool colony counts were serially determined.

The mice were then sacrificed and cultures of the stomach wall were carried out. *The results showed that gastrointestinal growth and invasion of candida was approximately 200 times greater in the mice receiving dextrose than in the control or xylitol group.*

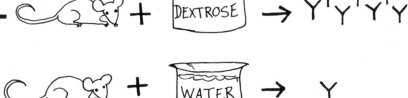

In their conclusion these investigators stated, *"Results suggest that dietary dextrose may increase* Candida albicans *GI growth and invasion."*

More on Prozac

In her presentation at the November 1990 CFIDS Association Research Conference, Nancy Klimas, M.D., discussed the immunological markers in CFS and the use of Prozac in CFS. In her discussion, she reviewed the various components of the immune system, including macrophages, T-helper cells, T-cytotoxic cells, B cells and natural killer (NK) cells. And she said,

> "Natural killer cells are your primitive immune system. Natural killer cells are always charged up and going. They're looking for stuff all the time and they're not specific. . . . Natural killer cells attack anything that's not part of you. . . . The NK cell is a very critical cell in chronic fatigue syndrome because it clearly is negatively impacted. . . .
>
> "The most compelling finding was that natural killer cell toxicity in chronic fatigue syndrome was as low as we've ever seen in any disease. . . . These cells seem to feel the way that CFS patients do . . . they're exhausted."

Dr. Klimas then discussed neuropsychiatric complications and stated that the more depressed people were, the worse their immune function was. She also discussed studies using Prozac and she found that depression in many CFS patients who took this drug improved. She also made this surprising observation: *People with CFS who had little or no depression had better clinical improvement while taking Prozac than those with high depression scores.*

Although Dr. Klimas found that Prozac was not a panacea for all patients and caused side effects in some, she found that the patients who improved showed a normalization of their NK cell cytotoxicity.

CFS patients who improved while taking Prozac showed a normalization of their NK cell cytotoxicity.

Candida albicans laboratory studies in CFS

In commenting on the yeast connection to CFS, Edward E. Winger, M.D.* said,

> "Crayton, Winger and Rippon have provided evidence that individuals with symptoms of depression, irritability, muscle and joint complaints, headaches, depression and other somatic complaints are associated with serologic findings of *Candida albicans*. Serum antibody levels, in a group of symptomatic individuals, of the IgG and IgA classes directed against *Candida albicans* were elevated above those in a group of control at a very high level of significance.
>
> "This study provides the first evidence, under controlled-blind experimental conditions, of the relationship between *Candida albicans* and the chronic fatigue syndrome. With the demonstration of abnormalities in Candida serology, it is now appropriate to add the Candida-related complex to the differential diagnosis of the chronic fatigue syndrome.

This study . . . under controlled-blind experimental conditions provided evidence of the relationship between Candida albicans and CFS.

In the Spring 1991 issue of The *Journal of Advancement in Medicine*,** David S. Bauman, Ph.D., and Howard E. Hagglund, M.D., reported their findings on studying 43 women who were classified as "Polysystem Chronic Complainers." These women had 10 or more symptoms, including poor memory, fatigue, mood swings, head pressure, muscles aches, digestive symptoms, inability to concentrate (they were given 67 complaints to choose

---

*Immunopathologist, Director Immunodiagnostic Laboratory, Inc., 488 McCormick St., San Leandro, CA 94577.
**Reprints of this article can be obtained by writing to the Cerodex Laboratories, Inc., P.O. Box 1151, Norman, OK 73070-1151.

from). They were compared with 53 volunteers who had four or fewer complaints.

In taking a history of these patients, 29 out of 43 who gave a history of prolonged antibiotics were chronic complainers as compared to only 5 out of 33 of the controls.

The test subjects had increased levels of antibodies to two antigens (extract from *Candida albicans*) significantly more often than did control subjects as measured in an enzyme immunoassay with the antigens. In a second part of the study, those with high questionnaire scores were treated with nystatin. Ninety-two percent of these patients with high enzyme immunoassay scores showed symptomatic improvement while only 5% of those with lower scores showed improvement. In commenting on their findings, these observers said, "The findings of this study suggest that *C. albicans* may be the etiologic agent in a group of polysystem complainers, but in no way does the study explain the process by which the complaints are produced."

Polysymptomatic patients showed significant elevations in antibodies to Candida albicans.

Tests for Food Sensitivities

The ALCAT Test: This new cellular test for food sensitivity was reported by British investigators in 20 patients (16 female, 4 male) who had a longer than three year history of irritable bowel syndrome, often associated with joint pains, headache and fatigue.* They'd all been fully investigated by endoscopy and barium enema and no major pathology was demonstrated.

The ALCAT test measures changes in cell size/volume following incubation with food extracts using a computer.

The basis of the ALCAT test** is the accurate measurement in changes in cell size/volume following incubation with food extracts using the modified Coulter ZF linked to a computer. (The manufacturers of the ALCAT test have since designed their own specialized instrument.)

Foods that caused positive reactions on the test were eliminated from the diet for two weeks. At that time, ⅔ of the patients described improvement. In an 18 months followup, 50% of the patients were symptom free.

In a previous report, "Gastrointestinal Complaints Related to

---

*P. J. Fell, S. Soulsby and J. Brostoff, *Journal of Nutritional Medicine* (1991) 2, 143-49.
**American Medical Testing Laboratories, One Oakwood Blvd., Suite 130, Hollywood, FL 33020.

Diet," (*International Pediatrics*, 5:21-29, 1990), Douglas H. Sandberg, M.D., stated,

"Certain gastrointestinal disorders are now accepted as related to sensitivities to food components. Published reports have indicated additional diseases in which dietary elements may play a role in pathogenesis. Diagnosis and treatment of food sensitivity-related illness has been a cumbersome and imperfect process. Use of a combination new blood test, the antigen Leukocyte cellular antibody test, and titration skin testing is suggested as a more efficient and effective approach to these disorders."*

A Patch Test for Delayed-type Food Allergy:** In a recent report, James C. Breneman, M.D., Professor of Immunology, Western Michigan University, Kalamazoo, Michigan, Michael Sweeney, Ph.D., and Andre Robert, Ph.D., described a diagnostic patch test for food allergens. Here's an excerpt from their report in the June 1991 issue of *Immunology & Allergy Practice:*

"For two decades, immediate (IgE) food allergy has been adequately diagnosed by using history, aqueous ID antigens and RAST. Delayed type food allergy (DTFA) has also been shown to be of immune origin; however, lack of an inexpensive, practical diagnostic test has delayed progress in the study of this type of allergy.

"Twelve years of experience with DMSO (Dimethysulfoxide) mixed with specific food antigens as patch tests provides convincing evidence that it is a safe, reliable screening test for immune responses to ingestants.

". . . Results of this study may not be specific for every ingestant intolerance situation; however, they did apply to every patient we tested. . . . Our thesis is based on a limited number of biopsies, therefore, further investigation for substantiation needs to be carried out. The safety of the patch test, however, is certainly established in that over 42,000 tests have been applied with no detectable systemic symptoms, not even in severely anaphylaxis-prone individuals."

> *"Certain gastrointestinal disorders are now accepted as related to sensitivities to food components."*
> *Douglas H. Sandberg, M.D.*

> *Over 42,000 food allergy-patch tests have been applied without detectable systemic symptoms.*

*Department of Pediatrics, Director, Division of Gastrointerology and Nutrition, Allergic and Environmental Disease Unit, University of Miami, Children's Hospital Center, Miami, Florida.
**This test is not yet commercially available. Further information can be obtained by writing to James C. Breneman, M.D., P.O. Box 177, 9880 E. Michigan Ave., Galesburg, MI 49053-0177.

Rubella Virus Vaccine Therapy for Patients with CFS

During the 1980s Allan D. Lieberman, M.D.,* collected data on 512 chronically fatigued patients. He especially evaluated these patients for evidence of an Epstein-Barr virus infection (EBV). One out of seven patients showed EBV titers of 1:80 or greater. Then in 1988, he reported on the observations of Allen,** who had studied 200 patients presenting with symptoms of the alleged Chronic Epstein-Barr Virus infection. He found abnormally high levels of antibody to the rubella virus which correlated with the patient's clinical condition. "The sicker they were the more evidence of rubella virus activity there was."

Based on these observations, Lieberman went back and did rubella titers on 114 patients whose diagnoses were compatible with the Chronic Fatigue Syndrome. When he compared his data with those of Allen, he found that they coincided in that 60% or more of the patients with the Chronic Fatigue Syndrome appeared to be affected by the rubella virus.

Sixty percent or more of the patients with chronic fatigue were affected by the rubella virus.

These patients were then given viral neutralization therapy using killed Rubella viral vaccine in dilutions of 1:5 to 1:125. This vaccine was administered by sublingual drops given two to four times daily. In most patients, the dilution was 1:125.

Lieberman stated,

> "We found that for a select group of patients, rubella virus neutralization was dramatically effective in reversing their chronic fatigue syndromes. . . . Treatment with the wrong neutralizing dose resulted in some patients exacerbating many of their signs and symptoms and becoming quite ill."

> "In the end there is one observation which is remarkably consistent with this population of patients: they are highly sensitive and/or allergic to the whole spectrum of the environment, but especially to foods and chemicals. It is these sensitivities which provide the myriad of signs and symptoms that we see in our ecologically ill patients . . . Viruses can alter the immune response and set up the pathophysiology for the development of IgE and non-IgE mediated altered reactivity or allergy."

*A. D. Lieberman, "The Role of Rubella Virus in the Chronic Fatigue Syndrome," *Clinical Ecology*, Volume VII, No. 3, P. 51-54, 1990.
**A. Allen, "Is RA27/3 a Cause of Chronic Fatigue?", *Med. Hypothesis* 1988; 27:217-20.

Comments about CFS by Physicians

Sidney MacDonald Baker, M.D.[*], Skillman, New Jersey: Dr. Baker, a former member of the Clinical Faculty at Yale University and former Head of the Gesell Institute of Human Development has long been interested in the multiple factors which contribute to illness. He was also co-sponsor of conferences on the yeast/human interaction in Birmingham in 1983 and in San Francisco in 1985. Much of my book, *The Yeast Connection*, includes concepts I learned from Dr. Baker. In commenting on CFS he said,

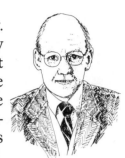

> "In modern medicine there is some confusion between *naming* and *understanding* certain chronic illnesses. It is comforting for CFS patients to know that they belong to a group of individuals with similar symptoms. It is misleading, however, to call CFS an 'entity' and to believe that all CFS patients have 'the same thing'.

> "Chronic fatigue is a global signal that something is wrong. I approach the problem with simple biological common sense such as one would apply to any living thing, whether it be a person or a potato plant: maybe there is something that doesn't agree with the individual, and/or maybe there is something she lacks or has a special need for."

Robert Cathcart, M.D., Los Altos, California: For over two decades, Dr. Cathcart has been interested in the causes of illness, including the role played by vitamin deficiencies, food and chemical sensitivities. He has been especially interested in the effectiveness of large doses of vitamin C in strengthening the immune system. In discussing CFS he said,

> "Chronic fatigue can be initiated by many causes, including viruses, yeast, toxic chemicals, stress, malnutrition, allergies, chronic bacterial infections, etc. Over the past few years, the cause of extreme sudden-onset fatigue has been ascribed to various viruses, such as EBV, HHV6 and now a retrovirus.
> "Of the patients I see with off and on, slow-onset fatigue, yeast (candida) is either the prime cause or one of multiple causes. A high percentage of the sudden-onset, viral fatigue cases developed

---

[*]Dr. Baker is the Director of Medical Computer Science, Princeton Biocenter, 862 Rt. 518, Skillman, New Jersey 08558.

355

All CFS patients either have or are in danger of developing the yeast syndrome. Robert Cathcart, M.D.

yeast problems as part of the problem after several months. Unless a patient is bedridden with fatigue, I estimate that the yeast cases are 5 to 10 times more frequent than the viral cases. All chronic fatigue patients either have or are in great danger of developing the yeast syndrome."

Robert A. Hallowitz, M.D.,[*] Gaithersburg, Maryland: For a number of years this physician has been interested in immune dysfunction, food sensitivities, stress management and the Chronic Fatigue Syndrome. Since 1985 he has been a health and wellness advisor for U.S. Senator Claiborne Pell and he was one of the sponsors and speakers at the Rhode Island CFS Conference in October 1988. In his presentation he discussed a comprehensive approach to the management of persons with the chronic fatigue syndrome, including the use of antiyeast medications and a special diet. Since that time, his interest in CFS has continued. In a recent report to me he said,

"The immune system of the person with CFS resembles a tired, cranky, irritable child. The child is inert and grouchy and rarely prone to do anything productive. He'll pick a fight with anyone and once the fighting starts it's hard to stop.

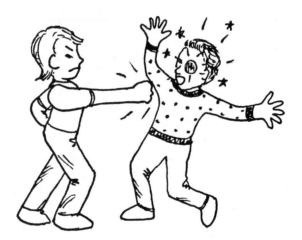

[*]Dr. Hallowitz is the medical director of Applied Immune Technologies (AIT). His company provides remote consultation services to persons with CFS and the health providers who care for them. For more information, write to AIT, 19211 Montgomery Village Ave., B-24, Gaithersburg, MD 20879.

"Here are some of the immune system battles of the person with CFIDS: Candida yeasts, food sensitivities, airborne allergens, microbes of various kinds, one's own tissues (like the thyroid) and viruses. A host of viruses that reside in the body may generate a battleground within the immune system. They attack the immune system and then the immune system overacts, attacks itself and loses its ability to keep the viruses asleep.

"A person with Chronic Fatigue Syndrome needs to find out which battles are being fought and do what can be done to minimize or stop those battles.

"In my practice, by sorting out and prioritizing these issues, I've been able to help most of my patients stabilize and strengthen their immune systems. In so doing, the 'irritable, cranky child' regains its strength. And the person with CFS is on the road to getting well."

A host of viruses that reside in the body may generate a battleground within the immune system.

Ronald Hoffman, M.D., New York, New York: In her 1991 book, *What Really Killed Gilda Radner?,* Neenyah Ostrom tells of her 2½ years of investigating the Chronic Fatigue Syndrome and related disorders. She reviewed dozens of reports in the medical and lay literature and talked to many people, including Ronald Hoffman, M.D., a physician interested in the many factors that play a part in causing CFS. These include viruses, parasites, candida yeasts and food allergies.

Ms. Ostrom asked Dr. Hoffman to describe the immune profile of the person with chronic viral fatigue syndrome. Here are excerpts from Dr. Hoffman's response:

I diagnose by symptoms . . . After all I'm treating the patient, not the lab test.

"First of all let me say that you can have a pretty normal immune profile and still have chronic viral fatigue syndrome. I also diagnose by symptoms. . . . After all I'm treating the patient, not the lab test."

Dr. Hoffman also stated that he had found elevated titers to viruses, particularly HHV and sometimes to CMV and the early antigen fraction of Epstein-Barr Virus. In his continuing comments, he said,

"You also may find a lack of natural killer cells. The real precise test to do would be to test not only for a number of these cells present, but to also test their activity. . . . People with sophisticated laboratories can do these tests. But I'm in the trenches here and I can't say to my patients, 'Well, let's do $2500 worth of tests and *then*

357

we'll start talking about making you better. Real patients . . . often don't have the money for such testing. They just want to feel better."

Dr. Hoffman also told of his experiences in treating a woman whose illness was triggered by an insecticide spray and about many other people who were troubled by "tons of food allergies." In treating them, Dr. Hoffman uses a combination of traditional, pharmaceutical and holistic therapies. These include vitamin A, vitamin C, zinc, selenium, vitamin B_6 and other nutritional supplements, anti-candida therapy and measures to boost the immune system.

You'll find a detailed report of Ms. Ostrom's interview with Dr. Hoffman on pages 106-17 of her book. Dr. Hoffman also discusses Chronic Fatigue Syndrome in his newsletter, *Hoffman Center News*, 40 East 30th St., New York, NY 10016 (212-779-1744).

Dan Kinderlehrer, M.D., Newbury, Massachusetts: For a number of years, Dr. Kinderlehrer has been interested in nutrition. In a way, you might say he "inherited" his interest from his mother, Jane, who for many years served as an editor of *Prevention Magazine*. Here are brief excerpts from a recent conversation with him.

"I've seen many patients with the Chronic Fatigue Syndrome during the past several years. Patients with this syndrome seem to develop it because of immune dysfunction. Some give a history of recurrent viral and/or other infections, as well as recurrent allergies.

"Some of my patients developed well documented infectious mononucleosis or other viral infections such as CMV. Following this infection, a few of them had symptoms for years. Then following an elimination diet, plus treatment for candida, their symptoms are totally resolved.

"I've also seen patients in whom CFS developed in other ways. Such patients started off with multiple allergies and then began to develop recurrent viral infections. Regardless of the sequence, most patients with CFS are bothered by multiple allergies,— including food sensitivities. And I have seen patients go into total remission simply by controlling their food allergies . . . in which case the diagnosis of CFS was inaccurate. Chemical sensitivities have also been prominent."

Most patients with CFS are bothered by multiple allergies . . . including food sensitivities.

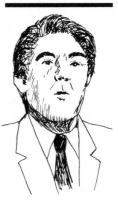

Anthony Komaroff, M.D.,* Boston, Massachusetts: In the Spring of 1987 I wrote to Dr. Komaroff about the Candida-Related Complex. I sent him reprints and other information including reports of patients I had treated. Here are excerpts from a letter I received from him on June 3, 1987:

"It is impressive how similar the symptoms are in patients with the diagnosis of chronic candidiasis and patients given the diagnosis of chronic mononucleosis. Conceivably they all have the same disease and the same cause. . . .

"There are some features of the 'chronic mononucleosis' condition that suggest to me the probability that the condition is caused by an infectious agent, probably a virus. I wonder if these clinical findings apply to the patients you've seen with chronic candidiasis. . . .

During the past five years Komaroff has been a leading chronic fatigue syndrome investigator. And in a December 31, 1991 letter I received from him he said,

"At this time we have evidence that HHV-6 is actively replicating in the white blood cells of patients with chronic fatigue syndrome

*Director, Division of General Medicine and Primary Care, Department of Medicine, Brigham and Women's Hospital, Harvard Medical School, 75 Francis St., Boston, MA 02115.

359

more frequently than in healthy adults of the same age and sex. We believe this reflects a secondary reactivation of a long-standing chronic infection, since most human beings become infected permanently with this virus in childhood. At this time, we cannot tell whether reactivation of this virus contributes to the suffering that patients experience."

Richard M. Podell, M.D., New Providence, New Jersey: In 1987 this board certified internist published a remarkable book, *Doctor Why Am I So Tired?* I call this book "remarkable" because the author comprehensively, yet succinctly, discusses many causes of fatigue which are *not* related to chronic viral infections. Topics covered include caffeine, sugar, hypoglycemia, vitamins, minerals, prescription drugs and stress. In commenting on the yeast connection to fatigue he said,

"About 50% of patients with the typical history of repeated antibiotics and multiple symptoms improve substantially on candida treatment." Richard M. Podell, M.D.

"The candida yeast theory stems from the work of C. Orian Truss, a Birmingham, Alabama allergist. Several persons told me that Truss' treatment had helped them . . . so I decided to offer it to selected patients after carefully explaining my skepticism. Most of the original patients improved. Four years later, my experience is that about 50% of patients with the typical history (repeated antibiotics, multiple symptoms) who adopt the candida treatment program improve substantially.

"I believe it is legitimate to try the candida treatment even though its effectiveness has not been proved. If properly supervised, the candida program should be extremely safe. A low-sugar, low-yeast diet is boring, but nutritionally adequate. Nystatin used at manufacturer's recommended doses is less likely to cause serious harm than almost any other drug. . . ."

Sherry Rogers, M.D., Syracuse, New York: In a presentation at the Candida Update Conference, Memphis, Tennessee, September 1988, Dr. Rogers stated she had successfully treated hundreds of polysymptomatic patients (including many with CFS) using a sugar-free special diet and antifungal medication. Although most patients improved, many continued to experience problems until the "total" load was reduced.

Like other physicians interested in CFS and in the Candida Related Complex, Dr. Rogers has observed that magnesium deficiency occurs commonly in these patients. She has also found that deficiencies of zinc, potassium, chromium and other minerals may also be present. And for those with persistent problems, she recommends that still other causes of the patient's illness need to be investigated. These include hidden hormone deficiencies, hidden chemical sensitivities and toxicities and stress.

George E. Shambaugh, Jr., M.D., Hinsdale, Illinois: For many years food and chemical sensitivities, zinc deficiency and other nutritional problems have interested this 89-year-old physician. Dr. Shambaugh, Professor and Chairman of the Department of Otolaryngology, Emeritus, Northwestern University, is the recipient of many honors in the United States and abroad. He is one of my heroes for many reasons. Here are a few of them:

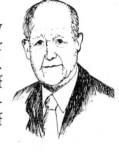

He continues in active practice, carries out research and writes a newsletter. And he has just signed a 2-year lease on his office. In a recent letter to me he said,

"Chronic Fatigue Syndrome is now recognized by the medical profession as a frequent cause of many chronic medical complaints. Yeast overgrowth in the intestinal tract (and sometimes in the vagina, mouth and throat) is a major cause of this syndrome and accounts for the majority of the cases seen in our country.

"The medical profession, as a whole, does not agree because there's no laboratory test that proves whether or not one has the candida problem. . . . In my practice, the majority of patients with CFS respond to the anti-candida regimen."

Chronic Fatigue Syndrome is now recognized as a frequent cause of many chronic medical complaints.

Intravenous Immunoglobulin (IVIG)—Conflicting Results

In the March 1991 *Annals of Internal Medicine,* Dr. P. K. Peterson, Department of Medicine, Hennepin County Medical Center, 701 Park Ave., Minneapolis, MN 55401 (and associates) reported their studies using intravenous gamma globulin in 30 patients who had been recruited from the local chronic fatigue research program. Seventy-three percent of these patients were women and 43% of them were unable to work.

The mean age of the patients was 40.8 years and the mean duration of illness was 3.8 years. Twenty-eight patients completed the trial. Intravenous IgG (1 gram per kilogram body weight) was infused over several hours every month for six treatments. *These*

361

investigators concluded that no benefit could be demonstrated from intravenous IgG in these patients with CFS.

An editorial in the February 9, 1991, issue of *The Lancet* (pages 331-332) reviewed this study and compared it with a similar study which showed positive results. Here are excerpts from *The Lancet* editorial.

Australian studies were positive while American studies showed no benefits from IVIG.

"Two trials have lately addressed the value of intravenous immunoglobulin (IVIG) treatment for patients with the Chronic Fatigue Syndrome (CFS). An Australia group reported a favorable outcome whereas a U. S. team found no beneficial effect. . . .

"The Australian workers studied 49 patients who had had an acute viral-like illness and gave a history of symptoms lasting at least 6 months. . . . Symptoms were assessed by a physician and a psychiatrist and psychological performance indicators and measures of cell mediated immunity were followed. Symptomatic improvement was found by the physician in 43% of patients receiving IVIG compared with 12% of those receiving placebo.

"IVIG responders also showed significant improvements in psychological and immunological variables. Psychiatrists-rated responses did not differ significantly between the groups. Although benefits were found in IVIG responders, overall improvements in physical, psychological and immunological measures could not be shown.

"The U. S. trial was in 30 patients randomized to monthly IVIG for 6 months. (43% and 64% of patients had low concentration of IgG 1 and IgG 3, respectively.) IVIG restored IgG 1 values to normal but symptoms, physical and social status and mental health did not improve.

"Patients were allowed to continue all other treatments prescribed by their primary carers . . . Headaches were reported more often in the U.S. IVIG treated patients; phlebitis developed in 55% and constitutional symptoms in 82% of IVIG recipients from Australia.

Conflicting results—and high frequency of side effects militate against recommending IVIG for patients with CFS.

"*The conflicting results, lack of long-term follow up, and high frequency of side effects all militate against recommending IVIG for patients with CFS* [emphasis added]. However, these trials have confirmed both disorder immunoregulation in some patients and the importance of affective symptoms in others. While a biological explanation continues to be sought, a problem oriented approach to each patient seems most appropriate."

Food Sensitivities and Brain Dysfunction

In the foreword of the book *Allergy and the Nervous System*,* edited by Frederic Speer, M.D., Walter C. Alvarez, M.D. (a former member of the staff of Mayo Clinic) told about a 20-year old boy he saw in consultation with fatigue, inability to concentrate and other symptoms which caused him to drop out of college. Because of his interest in the relationship of food sensitivities to nervous symptoms, Dr. Alvarez advised the parents to put the boy on a diet that eliminated a number of his favorite foods.

A 20-year-old boy with fatigue and inability to concentrate had to drop out of college

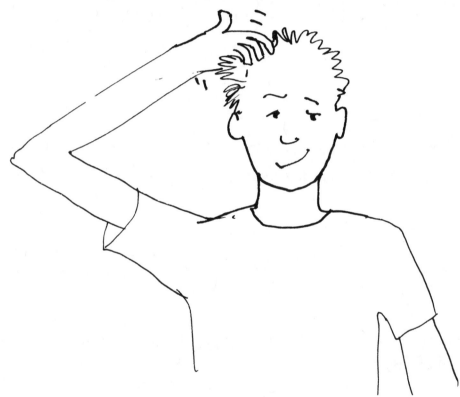

After a few days, the boy's symptoms disappeared and he "became bright." Following a few tests and further dietary experimentation, a marked sensitivity to eggs was detected. This young man's physical and mental health problems had begun when his mother started giving him an omelet each morning made with five eggs.

When he stopped eating an omelet each morning his symptoms disappeared and he became bright.

*F. Speer, *Allergy and the Nervous System*, Springfield, Ill., Charles C. Thomas, 1970.

I've already talked about the many patients I've seen with fatigue, irritability, headache, muscle aches and nasal congestion who improved—often dramatically when they avoided one or more common foods. In addition to these patients I saw an occasional patient with even more severe brain dysfunction. Here's the story of such a patient:

Neal experienced multiple problems during the early years of life. These included rhinitis, irritability, wheezing and digestive problems. He didn't walk until he was 18 months old and his speech was delayed. Because of multiple problems he was seen at a university child development center. Here's a summary of their report:

> Neal's current level of intellectual functioning is within the borderline of an approximate dull-normal range. His greatest difficulties aside from speech production, appear to inattention and visual motor skills. These difficulties suggest an organic impairment. Diagnosis: Mental retardation (mild).

At the age of 4, Neal was placed on the "Cave Man" Diet. His response was immediate and dramatic. Following food challenges his mother noted that milk, chocolate, chicken and several other foods provoked symptoms. When these foods were eliminated Neal's nasal congestion and other symptoms disappeared.

Neal gradually regained tolerance to trouble-making foods over the next several years. And except for minor allergic rhinitis his health remained good. Moreover, in the spring of 1990 he received his Masters Degree from the University of Tennessee.

Neal's attention defects and apparent mental retardation disappeared when he avoided food trouble-makers.

MEETING-PLACE—A Journal for Professionals and Nonprofessionals

During a visit to New Zealand in March 1988, I met Jim Brook and Toni Jeffreys. Since that time, I've corresponded with them and I've read their superb journal *Meeting-Place*. Here's a description of this journal in their words:

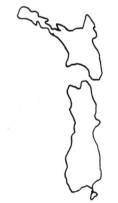

> *"MEETING-PLACE is a journal produced (from time to time) for members of ANZMES (NZ) Inc., their health advisers and for people wanting health information not readily available from other sources.*
>
> *"By bringing together:*

- people who are otherwise separated by distance and illness;
- patients and their professional advisers;
- the scientific and the speculative;

it is hoped to contribute to the support network for sufferers from M.E. Syndrome/CFS/CFIDS and similar chronic ill health, and, as well, to bring about improvements in awareness, diagnosis, treatment and care.

"While every effort has been made by the editors to present all the information in a balanced way, any advice, either explicit or implied, is not intended to replace qualified medical advice, which should always be sought. All claims that particular treatment options are helpful must be seen in the light of the fact that illness will spontaneously remit in many cases.

"MEETING PLACE is produced and edited by Jim Brook, published by ANZMES (N.Z.), Inc., and printed by Corporate Press, Glenfield, Auckland. All contributions and enquiries to: C/ ANZMES (N.Z.), Inc., P.O. Box 35-429, Browns Bay, Auckland 10, New Zealand. SUBSCRIPTION/MEMBERSHIP: New Zealand NZ$30, OVERSEAS AIRMAIL: AUST$35; $US35; CAN$40, UK£24. OVERSEAS SURFACE, AUST$32; US$28, CAN$32, UK£16. (Other countries please enquire.) Payment in personal cheques in own currency. Overseas members must belong to their local ME/CF(ID)S Group. These rates will be current for 1992 and 1993 but please inquire in 1994 and later for possible changes in above prices."

This New Zealand journal is loaded with helpful information for people with CFS/M.E.

I am impressed by the quality and diversity of information found in this superb publication. It should be of great help to persons with CFS and professionals who care for them. Included in this journal are reprints of entire articles and/or book chapters by physicians with impeccable academic credentials, along with all sorts of practical, tremendously helpful information. Here are examples:

The 60-page March 1990 issue contains a beautifully printed 18-page copy of a discussion entitled "The Chronic Fatigue Syndrome: An immunological mystery disease" which was published in *The Body at War,** by Dr. John Dwyer.

---

*Professor Dwyer is ex-chief of the section of clinical immunology at the Yale University School of Medicine, and now head of the same school of medicine at the University of New South Wales in Sydney. The book was published by Allan and Unwin, Sydney, in 1988 and was reproduced by kind permission of the publisher and after the payment of a copyright fee.

In the same issue appeared a copy of an article by Michael B.A. Oldstone, "Viral Alteration of Cell Function," which was reprinted from the August 1989 *Scientific American**

Included also are two brief but complete reports from major British medical journals on the effectiveness of homeopathic therapy. The first of these, "Effect of homeopathic treatment on fibrositis (primary fibromyalgia)" by Peter Fisher and colleagues from the Department of Rheumatology and Clinical Pharmacology, St. Barthlomew's Hospital, London, EC1A 7BE, was reprinted from the *British Medical Journal* (5, August 1989).

The second of these reports, "Homeopathy, a Placebo Response?—Controlled Trial of Homeopathic Potency, with Pollen and Hay Fever as Models," came from David Taylor Riley and associates from the University of Glasgow.

> *This journal contains a diverse group of scientific articles and patient reports.*

A third article, "The Immune System and Pesticides" by Leon John Olsen was reprinted from the *Journal of Pesticide Reform.*** Included also are excerpts from the Fall 1989 issue of the Nightingale Research Foundation, 383 Danforth Ave., Ottawa, Canada K2A 0E1, which reviews the viral causes of M.E. in a comprehensive manner.

I liked the section "This and That" and I was delighted with the informality and open-mindedness of the authors. The topics discussed included giardiasis, hydrogen peroxide, the Vega test, evening primrose oil, vitamin C, water purifiers, book reviews, including a review of Toni Jeffreys' delightful books, *The Last of the Green-Toed Fruit-Bats* and *The Mile-High Staircase.*

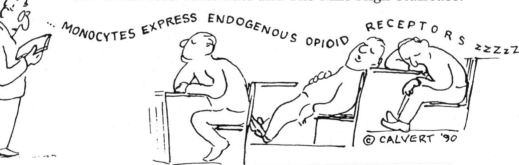

*Michael B. Oldstone, M.D., a member of the Departments Immunological and Neuropharmacology at Scripps Clinic and Research Foundation in La Jolla, CA, where he heads a laboratory of viral immunology.

**Leon John Olsen is a toxicologist and research scientist with the Wisconsin Department of Health and Social Services.

Trying to describe this magnificent publication is difficult. Yet, I'll put my thoughts into these few words: *Authentic, scientific, open-minded, readable, comprehensive, informal* and done with a light touch. In addition, it's delightfully illustrated by Oliver Calvert. If you're a professional or nonprofessional with CFS/CFIDS/M.E./FM, food allergies, environmental sensitivities, candida-related health problems and/or other chronic disorders, you'd do well to subscribe to this publication and order as many back copies as you can afford.

CACTUS—A Coalition of CFIDS Organizations and Leaders

As I've discussed elsewhere in this book persons with CFS have often experienced difficulty in getting family members, physicians (and other professionals) and government leaders to listen. Too often, their complaints have been ignored. At other times, they've led to such diagnoses as "hypochondriasis," "depression" or "psychoneurosis."

Persons with CFS have often experienced difficulty in getting family members, physicians and government leaders to listen.

Happily, during the past several years, things have been improving. And scientific presentations by researchers and clinicians at conferences in California, England, North Carolina and elsewhere have brought CFS into the medical mainstream.

Leading the battle for credibility is an organization with the acronym CACTUS (CFIDS Action Campaign for the United States). This organization "is a national coalition of CFIDS organizations and leaders formed to wage a campaign of advocacy and activism by and for people with CFIDS (PWCs*)." The CACTUS coalition includes national, regional and local organizations and support groups.

CACTUS is a coalition of CFIDS leaders formed to wage a campaign of advocacy and activism.

Here are some of the organizing principles of CACTUS:

- CFIDS is a serious disease of immune dysfunction;
- It is a newly emerging epidemic in many parts of the world;
- It is transmissible;
- The federal government has been slow to address CFIDS;
- The word "fatigue" in the name trivializes the disorder;
- PWCs should be primary decision- and policy-makers in the CFIDS movement.

*PWCs is an abbreviation for Persons with CFIDS.

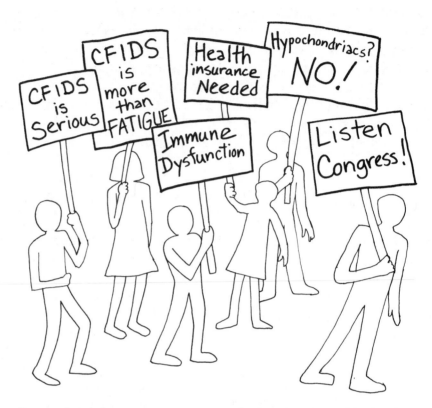

The goals of this organization include advocating funds for programs and services for PWCs; providing timely information; raising funds for research; training PWCs in leadership skills and activist strategies; diversifying the leadership of the CFIDS movement; protecting and promoting the civil rights of PWCs; collaborating with other activist, health and disability rights organizations.

Here's a partial list of current CACTUS projects:

- Meeting with members of Congress and developing support on Capitol Hill;
- Developing timely communication among CFIDS groups;
- Working to improve insurance availability and adequate reimbursement for CFIDS related medical expenses;
- Developing a support group manual;
- Working for a name change for this disease
- Publishing *CAN*, The CACTUS Action News, and
- Fund raising.

A special note: The day before this book was scheduled to be sent to the printer, I learned that because of a lack of funding CACTUS had become inactive.

If you're interested in CFIDS advocacy and other goals expressed by CACTUS leaders, write to the CFIDS Association, P.O. Box 220398, Charlotte, NC 28222-0398 (see also pages 343-344).

POSTSCRIPT

In July 1982 the relationship of *Candida albicans* to a diverse group of health problems was the subject of a small conference in Dallas. In discussing the candida/human interaction, one of the conference participants, the late Phyllis Saifer of Berkeley, California commented, "I have more questions than answers."

As I look at Chronic Fatigue Syndrome (CFS) in early 1992 a similar comment seems appropriate, especially when I think about the many complex factors which lead to the development of this illness. Yet, in spite of many unanswered questions (based on research studies and clinical observations of both physicians and non-physicians) I'm certain that. . . .

- *CFS is an illness characterized by disturbances in your immune system.* When your immune system is "out of kilter," you get sick. Because other systems of your body are closely related to your immune system, you feel "sick all over." You're usually bothered by symptoms in your nervous system, your endocrine system and your musculoskeletal system. And, like every person with this illness, your respiratory and digestive systems and other parts of your body are also affected.

- *CFS is an illness which can develop from many different causes.* These include acute viral infections and infections by other microorganisms, including bacteria, spirochetes and parasites. It can also develop in people who have received repeated or prolonged courses of broad spectrum antibiotic drugs, leading to overgrowth of the common yeast, *Candida albicans.* Nutritional deficiencies, chemical toxins and other factors may also play a role in aggravating CFS.

- *CFS often develops following an acute viral infection in a previously healthy person.* Or it can come on insidiously over a period of weeks, months or years.

- *This illness is much more than "fatigue."* And even though I use the name Chronic Fatigue Syndrome in this book, I agree with those who say that including "fatigue" in the name of this illness may "trivialize" it and cause some observers—including physicians—to ignore it or to blame it on psychological causes.

- *CFS is not "simply a state of mind."* Nor is it a "somatization disorder." Admittedly, depression—even suicidal depression—may develop in persons with CFS. Yet, observations by Dr. Carol Jessop show that depression, when present in the person with CFS, almost always develops as a consequence of organic changes in the immune, endocrine, nervous and other systems of the body.

Most people with CFS can be helped by a simple but comprehensive treatment program. Parts of this program include:

> **Most people with CFS can be helped by a simple but comprehensive treatment program.**

- A diversified nutritious diet which features vegetables and other complex carbohydrates and avoids sugar and foods loaded with fats and additives of various types.

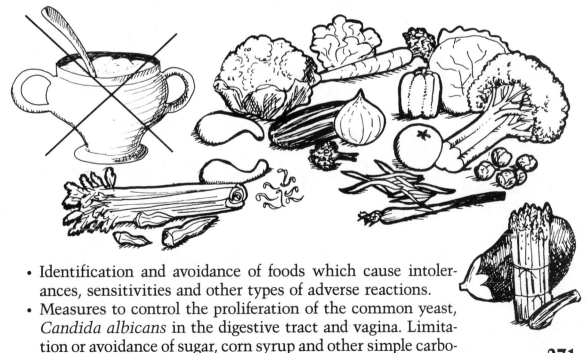

- Identification and avoidance of foods which cause intolerances, sensitivities and other types of adverse reactions.
- Measures to control the proliferation of the common yeast, *Candida albicans* in the digestive tract and vagina. Limitation or avoidance of sugar, corn syrup and other simple carbo-

371

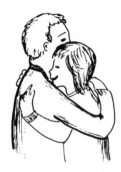

hydrates and prescription and nonprescription agents are essential parts of anti-candida therapy.

• Environmental control measures—especially in the home and work place.

• Lifestyle changes, fresh air and rest with gradually increasing exercise.

• Psychological support including love, praise, laughter (even when you feel like crying) and a PMA (Positive Mental Attitude).

• Nutritional supplements—including a comprehensive, multi-vitamin-mineral preparation along with essential fatty acids (EFAs) and magnesium.

Other treatment measures may also help, including medications prescribed or administered by your physician for sleep disturbances, muscle pain, depression and/or other symptoms. Yet, if you personally "take charge" and follow the treatment program outlined above, your health will gradually—even rapidly—improve. Then, like the overloaded camel who sheds some of his burdens, you'll soon be off and running!

BIBLIOGRAPHY

Books

*Bahna, S.L. and D.C. Heiner. *Allergies to Milk*. Springfield, Ill.: Charles C. Thomas, 1980.

Barnard, N.D. *The Power of Your Plate*. Summertown, Tenn.: Book Publishing Company, 1990.

Beasley, J. and J. Swift. *The Kellogg Report—The impact of nutrition, environment and lifestyle on the health of all Americans*. Amityville, N.Y.: Institute of Health Policy and Practice, Bard College, 1990.

Beasley, J. *The Betrayal of Health*. New York: Times Books, 1991.

Berne, Katrina H. *CFIDS Lite*. Mesa, Ariz.: BHB Communications, 1989.

Bliznakov, E.G. *The Miracle Nutrient: Coenzyme Q$_{10}$*. New York: Bantam, 1987.

Bolles, E.B. *Learning to Live with Chronic Fatigue Syndrome*. New York: Dell Publishing, 1990.

*Breneman, J.C. *Handbook of Food Allergy*. New York: Marcell Dekker, Inc., 1987.

Brooks, Barbara and Nancy Smith. *CFIDS: An Owner's Manual*, 2nd ed. Self-published, 1990. Available from BBNS, P.O. Box 6456, Silver Springs, MD 20916-6456.

*Brostoff J. and S.J. Challacombe, eds. *Food Allergy and Intolerance*. Eastbourne, East Sussex, Eng.: Balliere Tindall, 1987.

Brostoff, J. and L. Gammlin. *The Complete Guide to Food Allergy and Intolerance. London:* Bloomsbury, 1989.

Chaitow, L. Candida albicans: *Could Yeast Be Your Problem?* Wellingborough, Eng.: Thorsons, 1985.

Cheraskin, E. *Health and Happiness*. Wichita: Bio Communications Press, 1989.

Cheraskin, E., W.M. Ringsdorff and A. Brecher. *Psychodietetics*. New York: Bantam Books, 1976.

Conant, S. *Living with Chronic Fatigue*. Dallas: Taylor Publishing Co., 1990.

373

Crook, W.G. *Detecting Your Hidden Allergies.* Jackson, Tenn.: Professional Books, 1988.

Crook, W.G. *The Yeast Connection,* 3rd ed. Jackson, Tenn.: Professional Books, 1986.

Crook, W.G. and M.H. Jones. *The Yeast Connection Cookbook: A Guide to Good Nutrition and Better Health.* Jackson, Tenn.: Professional Books, 1989.

Cousins, N. *Anatomy of an Illness.* New York: Norton, 1979.

Cousins, N. *The Healing Heart.* New York: Norton, 1985.

Dadd, D.L. *Non-toxic Natural and Earth Wise.* Los Angeles: J. P. Tarcher, Inc., 1990.

Davies, S. and A. Stewart. *Nutritional Medicine.* London: Pan, 1987.

Dawes, B. and D. Downing. *Why M.E.?* London: Grafton Books, 1989.

DeSchepper, Luc. *Candida: The Symptoms, the Causes, the Cure.* Self-published. Available from the author at 2901 Wilshire Blvd., Suite 435, Santa Monica, CA 90403.

Erasmus, U. *The Complete Guide to Fats and Oils in Health and Nutrition.* Vancouver: Alive Books, 1987.

Faelten, S. and editors of *Prevention Magazine. Allergy Self-Help Book.* Emmaus, Pa.: Rodale Press, 1983.

Fasciana, G.S. *Are Your Dental Fillings Poisoning You?* New Canaan, Conn.: Keats Publishing Co., 1986.

Feiden, K. *Hope and Help for Chronic Fatigue Syndrome.* New York: Prentice Hall, 1990.

Fisher, G.C. *Chronic Fatigue Syndrome: A Victim's Guide to Understanding, Treating and Coping with This Debilitating Illness.* New York: Warner Books, 1989.

Galland, L. with D.D. Buchman. *Superimmunity for Kids.* New York: Copestone, 1988.

Gardner, D.C. and G. J. Beatty. *Never Be Tired Again: The famous 7-day high-energy program and diet explained in full.* New York: Macmillan Publishing Co., 1988.

*Gerrard, J.W., ed. *Food Allergy: New Perspectives.* Springfield, Ill.: Charles C. Thomas, 1980.

Goldbeck, N. and D. Goldbeck. *The Goldbecks' Guide to Good Food.* New York: New American Library, 1987.

Goldstein, J.A. *Chronic Fatigue Syndrome: The Struggle for Health.* Beverly Hills, Calif.: CFIDS Institute, 1990.

Goldstein, J.A. *Could Your Doctor Be Wrong?* New York: Pharos Books, 1991.

Griffin, G.G. and W. Castelli. *Good Fat, Bad Fat—How to Lower Your Cholesterol and Beat the Odds of a Heart Attack.* Tucson: Fisher Books, 1989.

Gunn, D.M. *Out of the Maze—A Holistic Approach to the M.E. Syndrome.* Self-published, 1988. Available from the Bay of Plenty Multiple Sclerosis Society, Inc., and Bay of Plenty Myalgic Encephalomyelitis Support Group, Inc., 13 Tynan St., Te Puke, New Zealand, 3071.

Jacobs, G. Candida albicans—*Yeast and Your Health.* London: Macdonald Optima, 1990.

Jacobson, M.F., L.Y. Lefferts, and A.W. Garland. *Safe Food— Eating in a Risky World.* Los Angeles: Living Planet Press, 1991.

Jeffreys, T. *The Last of the Green-Toed Fruit-Bats.* Auckland: Waiake Wordsmiths, 1989. Available from ANZMES, P.O. Box 35-429, Browns Bay, Auckland 10, New Zealand.

Jeffreys, T. *The Mile-High Staircase.* Auckland: Hodder and Stoughton, 1982. Available from ANZMES, P.O. Box 35-429, Browns Bay, Auckland 10, New Zealand.

Jones, M. *The Allergy Self-Help Cookbook.* Emmaus, Pa.: Rodale Press, 1984.

Kasl, C.E. *Many Roads, One Journey:* Moving beyond the 12 steps. New York: Harper Collins, 1992.

Langer, S.E. and Scheer, J.F. *Solved: The Riddle of Illness,* Keats Publishing Co., New Canaan, CT 1984.

Langer, S.E. *Solved: The Riddle of Weight Loss.* Rochester, VT: Healing Arts Press, 1988.

Lee, W.H. *Coenzyme Q_{10}—Is it our new fountain of youth?* New Canaan, Conn.: Keats Publishing Co., 1987. (booklet)

Levin, A.S. and M. Zellerbach. *Type 1/Type 2 Allergy Relief Program.* Los Angeles: Jeremy Tarcher, Inc., 1983. Distributed by Houghton Mifflin Company, Boston, Mass.

Lieberman, S. and N. Bruning. *The Real Vitamin and Mineral Book.* Garden City Park, N.Y.: Avery Publishing Group, Inc., 1990.

McDougall, J.A. *McDougall's Medicine—A Challanging Second Opinion*. Piscataway, N.J.: New Century Publishers, 1985.

McDougall, J.A. *McDougall's Medicine—12 Days to Dynamic Health.* New York: Plume-Penguin, 1991.

*Miller, J.B. *Food Allergy: Provocative Testing and Injection Therapy.* Springfield, Ill.: Charles C.Thomas, 1972.

Miller, J.B. *Relief at Last.* Springfield, Ill.: Charles C. Thomas, 1987.

Null, G. *Healing Your Body Naturally—Alternative treatments to illness.* Four Walls Eight Windows Publishing, P.O. Box 548, Village Station, New York, NY 10014. 1992.

*Odds, F.C. *Candida and Candidosis.* 2nd ed. Baltimore: Baltimore University Park Press, 1988.

Ornish, D. *Dr. Dean Ornish's Program for Reversing Heart Disease.* New York: Random House, 1990.

Oski, F. *Don't Drink Your Milk.* Castle Hill, Australia: Beta Books, 1983.

Passwater, R. *EPA—Marine Lipids.* New Canaan, Conn.: Keats Publishing Co., 1985.

Podell, R.N. *Doctor Why Am I So Tired?* New York: Fawcett-Ballantine, 1987.

Rapp, D.J. *Allergies and Your Family.* New York: Publishers Press, 1990.

Rapp, D.J. *Is This Your Child?* New York: William Morrow, 1991.

Remington, D.W. and B.W. Higa. *Back to Health: Yeast Control.* Provo, Utah: Vitality Health, 1986.

Rogers, S.A. *The E.I. Syndrome.* Syracuse, N.Y.: Prestige Publishers, 1990.

Rogers, S.A. *Tired or Toxic.* Syracuse, N.Y.: Prestige Publishers, 1990.

Rona, Z.P. *The Joy of Health—A Doctor's Guide to Nutrition and Alternative Medicine.* Hownslow Press, 124 Parkview Ave., Willowdale, Ontario, Canada M2N 3Y5.

Rosenbaum, M. and M. Susser. *Solving the Puzzle of Chronic Fatigue Syndrome.* Tacoma, Wash.: Life Science Press, 1992.

Rousseau, D.W., W.J. Rae and J. Enwright. *Your Home, Your Health and Well-Being.* Hartley and Marx Publishers, 3663 W. Broadway, Vancouver, BC, V6R 2B8, Canada, 1988.

Rudin, D.O. and C. Felix. *The Omega III Phenomena*. New York: Rowson and Associates, 1987.

Shepherd, C. *Living with M.E.* London: Cedar, 1989.

Siegel, B.S. *Love, Medicine and Miracles*. New York: Harper and Rowe, 1986.

Siegel, B.S. *Peace, Love and Healing*. New York: Harper and Rowe, 1989.

Solomon, N. *Sick and Tired of Being Sick and Tired*. Paris, N.Y.: Wynwood, 1989.

*Speer, F., ed. *The Allergic Child*. New York: Hoeber, 1963.

*Speer, F. *Allergy of the Nervous System*. Springfield, Ill.: Charles C. Thomas, 1970.

Stoff, J. and C. Pellegrino. *Chronic Fatigue Syndrome: The Hidden Epidemic*. New York: Random House, 1988.

Taylor, J. *The Complete Guide to Mercury Toxicity from Dental Fillings*. San Diego: EDA Publishing, 1989.

Trowbridge, J.P. and M. Walker. *The Yeast Syndrome*. New York: Bantam Books, 1987.

Truss, C.O. *The Missing Diagnosis*. Self-published, 1983. Available from the author at P.O. Box 26508, Birmingham, AL 35226.

Weiner, M.A. *Maximum Immunity*. Boston: Houghton Mifflin, 1986.

Weissman, J.D. *Choose to Live*. New York: Grove Press, 1988.

Wilkinson, S. *Chronic Fatigue Syndrome: A Natural Healing Guide*. New York: Sterling Publishing Co., 1988.

Wunderlich, R.C., Jr. *Fatigue Revisited.* Self-published, 1990. Available from the author at 666 Sixth St. South, Suite 206, St. Petersburg, FL 33701.

Wunderlich, R.C., Jr. *Sugar and Your Health*. St. Petersburg, Fla.: John E. Reeds, Inc., Good Health Productions, 1982.

Wunderlich, R.C., Jr. and D. Kalita. Candida albicans *and the Human Condition*. New Canaan, Conn.: Keats Publishing Co., 1984.

*Of particular interest to physicians.

Articles

Alexander, J.G. "Allergy in the Gastrointestinal Tract." *Lancet* ii (1975), 1264.

Crook, W.G. "Adverse Reactions to Food Can Cause Hyperkinesis." *American Journal of Diseases in Children* 132 (1978), 819 (letters).

Crook, W.G. "The Allergic Tension-Fatigue Syndrome." In *The Allergic Child*, edited by F. Speer. New York: Hoeber, 1963.

Crook, W.G. "The Allergic Tension-Fatigue Syndrome." *Pediatric Annals* (October 1974).

Crook, W.G. "Candida Colonization and Allergic Phenomena." *Hospital Practice* 19 (1984), 20 (letters).

Crook, W.G. "Candidiasis and Depression." *Hospital Practice* 20 (1985), 12 (letters).

Crook, W.G. "The Coming Revolution in Medicine." *Journal of the Tennessee Medical Association* 73 (March 1983), 3.

Crook, W.G. "Depression Associated With *Candida Albicans* Infections." *Journal of the American Medical Association* 251 (1984), 2928 (letters).

Crook, W.G. "Food Allergy—the Great Masquerader." *Pediatric Clinics of North America* 22 (1975), 227.

Crook, W.G. "Is Remote Disease Associated with Candida Infection a Tomato?" *Journal of the American Medical Association* 254 (1985), 2891 (letters).

Crook, W.G. "Plight of Imprisoned Youth." The Pharos 46 (1983), 39 (letters).

Crook, W.G. "PMS and Yeasts: An Etiologic Connection?" *Hospital Practice* 18 (1983), 21.

Crook, W.G., W.W. Harrison, S.E. Crawford and B.S. Emerson. "Systemic Manifestations Due to Allergy. Report of Fifty Patients and a Review of the Literature on the Subject." *Pediatrics* 27 (1961), 790-99.

Davison, H.M. "Cerebral Allergy." *Southern Medical Journal* 42 (1947), 712.

Deamer, W.C. "Pediatric Allergy. Some Impressions Gained over a 37-Year Period." *Pediatrics* 48 (1971), 930.

Dees, S.C. "Neurologic Allergy in Childhood." *Pediatric Clinics of North America* 1 (1954), 1017.

Egger, J., C.M. Carter, J. Wilson, J. Soothill et al. "Is Migraine Food Allergy? A Double-Blind Trial of Oligoantigenic Diet Treatment." *Lancet* ii (1983), 865.

Egger, J., et al. "Oligoantigenic Diet Treatment of Children with Epilepsy and Migraine." *Journal of Pediatrics* (January 1989), 51-58.

Holti, G. "Candida Allergy." In *Symposium of Candida Infections*, edited by H. I. Winner and R. Hurley, 74-81. Edinburgh and London, E. & S. Livingstone, 1966.

Hosen, H. "Focal Fungal Infections Treated by Immunological Therapy with Emphasis on Vaginal Moniliasis." *Texas Medicine* 67 (1971), 58.

Hunter, J.O. "Food Allergy—or Enterometabolic Disorder?" *The Lancet* 338 (1991), 495-96.

Iwata, K. "Fungal Toxins and Their Role in the Etiopathology of Fungal Infections." In *Recent Advances in Medical and Veterinary Mycology*. Tokyo: University of Tokyo Press, 1977.

Iwata, K. "A Review on the Literature on Drunken Symptoms Due to Yeast in the Gastrointestinal Tract." In *Yeasts and Yeast-like Microorganisms in Medical Science, Internal Specialized Symposium on Yeasts*, edited by K. Iwata, 184-90. Tokyo: University of Tokyo Press, 1976.

Iwata, K. and K. Uchida. "Cellular Immunity in Experimental Fungus Infections in Mice." *Medical Mycology* (January 1977).

Iwata, K. and Y. Yamamoto. "Glycoprotein Toxins Produced by *Candida albicans*." Proceedings of the Fourth International Conference on the Mycoses, June 1977. *PAHO Scientific Publication No. 356*.

James, J. and R.P. Warrin. "An Assessment of the Role of *Candida albicans* and Food Yeast in Chronic Urticaria." *British Journal of Dermatology* 84 (1971), 227-37.

Kniker, W.T. "Deciding the Future for the Practice of Allergy and Immunology." *Annals of Allergy* 55 (1985), 106-13.

Kudelko, N.M. "Allergy in Chronic Monilial Vaginitis." *Annals of Allergy* 29 (1971) 266.

Liebeskind, A. "*Candida albicans* as an Allergenic Factor." *Annals of Allergy* 20 (1961) 394-96.

Miles, M.R., L. Olsen, and A. Rogers. "Recurrent Vaginal

Candidiasis—Importance of an Intestinal Reservoir." *Journal of the American Medical Association* 238 (1977), 1836-37.

Miller, J.B. "The Management of Food Allergy." In *Food Allergy: New Perspectives*, edited by J.W. Gerrard, 274-82. Springfield, Ill.: Charles C. Thomas, 1980.

Palacios, H.J. "Desensitization for Monilial Hypersensitivity." *Virginia Medical Journal* (June 1977), 393-94.

Palacios, H.J. "Hypersensitivity as a Cause of Dermatologic and Vaginal Moniliasis Resistant to Topical Therapy." *Annals of Allergy* 37 (1976), 110-13.

Randolph, T.G. "Allergies as a Causative Factor of Fatigue, Irritability and Behavior Problems in Children." *Journal of Pediatrics* 32 (1948), 266.

Rosedale, N. and M.B. Browne. "Hyposensitization in the Management of Recurring Vaginal Candidiasis." *Annals of Allergy* 43 (1979), 250-53.

Rosenberg, E.W., and associates, and S. Baker and associates. Letters to *Archives of Dermatology* (April 1984.)

Rosenberg, E.W., P.W. Belew, R.B. Skinner, Jr. and N. Crutcher. Letters to *New England Journal of Medicine* 308 (1983), 101.

Rowe, A.H. "Allergic Toxemia and Migraine Due to Food Allergy." *California and Western Medicine* 33 (1930), 785.

Rowe, A.H. "Clinical Allergy and the Nervous System." *Journal of Nervous and Mental Disease* 99 (1944), 834.

Speer, F. "The Allergic Tension-Fatigue Syndrome in Children." *International Archives of Allergy* 12 (1958), 207.

Truss, C.O. "Metabolic Abnormalities in Patients with Chronic Candidiasis." *Journal of Orthomolecular Psychology* 13 (1984), 66-93.

Truss, C.O. "Restoration of Immunologic Competence to *C. albicans.*" *Journal of Orthomolecular Psychology* 9 (1980), 287-301.

Truss, C.O. "The Role of *Candida albicans* in Human Illness." *Journal of Orthomolecular Psychology* 10 (1981), 228-38.

Truss, C.O. "Tissue Injury Induced by *C. Albicans:* Mental and Neurologic Manifestations." *Journal of Orthomolecular Psychology* 7 (1978), 17-37.

Walker, W.A. "Role of the Mucosal Barrier in Antigen Handling by the Gut." In *Food Allergy and Intolerance*, edited by J. Brostoff and S.J. Challacombe, 209-22. Eastbourne, East Sussex, Eng.: Balliere Tindall, 1987.

Witkin, S.S. "Defective Immune Responses in Patients with Recurrent Candidiasis." *Infections in Medicine* (May/June 1985), 129-32.

Zwerling, M.H., K.N. Owens, and N.H. Ruth. "Think Yeast—the Expanding Spectrum of Candidiasis." *Journal of the South Carolina Medical Association* 80 (1984), 454-56.

Index

Other Booklets and Books
William G. Crook, M.D.

Additional copies of this booklet, as well as other helpful booklets and books by Dr. Crook, are available from your health food store, bookstore or pharmacy. Or you can order them by phone or by mail. (See below.)

- -

ITEM	QTY.	PRICE	TOTAL
BOOKS:			
The Yeast Connection		12.95	
Tracking Down Hidden Food Allergy		7.95	
The Yeast Connection Cookbook		13.95	
Help for the Hyperactive Child		14.95	
Solving the Puzzle of Your Hard-to-Raise Child		19.95	
Chronic Fatigue Syndrome and The Yeast Connection		14.95	
Detecting Your Hidden Allergies		10.95	
BOOKLETS:			
Yeasts		2.95	
Allergy		2.95	
Hypoglycemia		2.95	
Hyperactivity/ADD		2.95	
Chronic Fatigue Syndrome		2.95	
Add $3.50 shipping and handling (single) Add $5.00 shipping and handling (multiple)		S/H	
		TOTAL	

SHIP TO:

(   )
_____
Name   Phone

_____
Street Address

_____
City   State   Zip

To order these publications, call 1-800-227-2627 or 1-205-879-6551. (Visa or Mastercard accepted.)

Or you can mail your check or money order along with this form to:
Wellness Health & Pharmaceuticals, 2800 S. 18th St., Birmingham, AL 35209.

If you order 5 or more copies of a single title, you will be given a 30% discount on that title.

Prices subject to change without notice.